Pharmacology

for the

Tech

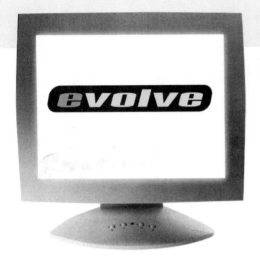
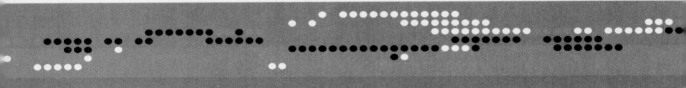

Pharmacology for the Surgical Technologist

SECOND EDITION

Katherine C. Snyder, CST, BS
Surgical Technology Program Director
Laramie County Community College
Cheyenne, Wyoming

Chris Keegan, CST, MS
Professor and Chair
Surgical Technology and Surgical First Assisting Programs
Vincennes University
Vincennes, Indiana

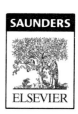

SAUNDERS

ELSEVIER

SAUNDERS
ELSEVIER

11830 Westline Industrial Drive
St. Louis, Missouri 63146

PHARMACOLOGY FOR THE SURGICAL
TECHNOLOGIST, REVISED SECOND EDITION   ISBN: 978-1-4160-5431-3

Notice

Knowledge and best practice in this field are constantly changing. As new research and
experience broaden our knowledge, changes in practice, treatment, and drug therapy may
become necessary or appropriate. Readers are advised to check the most current
information provided (i) on procedures featured or (ii) by the manufacturer of each product
to be administered, to verify the recommended dose or formula, the method and duration
of administration, and contraindications. It is the responsibility of the practitioner, relying
on his or her own experience and knowledge of the patient, to make diagnoses, to
determine dosages and the best treatment for each individual patient, and to take all
appropriate safety precautions. To the fullest extent of the law, neither the publisher nor
the authors assume any liability for any injury and/or damage to persons or property
arising out or related to any use of the material contained in this book.

The Publisher

ISBN: 978-1-4160-5431-3

Acquisitions Editor: Michael Ledbetter
Developmental Editor: Katherine Judge
Publishing Services Manager: Julie Eddy
Project Manager: Kelly E.M. Steinmann
Designer: Julia Dummitt

Printed in the United States of America

Last digit is the print number: 9 8 7 6 5 4 3 2

This textbook is dedicated to the students and the instructors of surgical technology and surgical first assisting—and to the patients we serve.

Kathy and Chris

REVIEWERS

Jeff Bidwell, CST/CSA
Madisonville Community College
Madisonville, Kentucky

Pam Buff, CST
Platt College
Tulsa, Oklahoma

Joseph F. Burkard, DNSc, CRNA
Naval School of Health Sciences
Naval Medical Center
San Diego, California

Kathleen A. Case, MSN, RN
Corinthian Colleges, Inc.
Santa Ana, California

Melissa W. Coughlin, MS, CRNA, ACLS, PALS certification
Erie County Medical Center
School of Nurse Anesthesia
State University of New York at Buffalo
Buffalo, New York

Mauro da Fonte, MD
Gateway Community College
Phoenix, Arizona

Stacey May, CST
South Plains College
Lubbock, Texas

Ann Marie McGuiness, CST, MSEd, CNOR
Shawnee Mission Medical Center
Shawnee Mission, Kansas

Renee Nemitz, CST, RN
Western Iowa Tech Community College
Sioux City, Iowa

Simon Nixon, BA, MSc, PGDIP (SRM), ODP
Association of Operating Department Practitioners Council
Lewis, United Kingdom

Julie Orloff, CPC, RMA, CMA, CPT
Career Education Corporation
Miami, Florida

Rebecca Pieknik, CST, BS
William Beaumont Hospital
Royal Oak, Michigan

Janet Sesser, RMA, CMA, BS Ed Admin
High-Tech Institute
Phoenix, Arizona

Clifford W. Smith, MSN, RN, ONC, CRNFA, CRNP
Mount Aloysius College
Cresson, Pennsylvania

Nancy H. Wright, RN, BS, CNOR
Virginia College
Birmingham, Alabama

Samuel Yanofsky, MD, MSEd
Children's Hospital Los Angeles
University of Southern California
Keck School of Medicine
Los Angeles, California

PREFACE

More than 10 years ago, a committee of instructors met to work on revisions to the *Core Curriculum for Surgical Technology*. During the meeting, the topic of textbooks surfaced—in particular pharmacology textbooks. It generally was agreed that no adequate pharmacology textbook for surgical technologists existed. As the discussion progressed and we complained about the situation, a question was posed: "Well, are you going to be part of the problem or part of the solution?" This second edition of the textbook is our continuing response to that question. It offers a distinct combination of subject matter. The text is organized into three units, each focusing on information specific to the surgical environment. Students will review basic math skills; learn a framework of pharmacologic principles to apply the information in surgical situations; learn commonly used medications by category, with frequent descriptions of actual surgical applications; and learn basic anesthesia concepts, not previously presented at this level, to function more effectively as a surgical team member.

Special learning tools used in this text include the following:
- Tables of medications covered in the chapters
- Key Terms, which are then boldfaced in the chapters
- Learning Objectives, stated at the beginning of each chapter
- Insight boxes that offer additional information on the subject
- Illustrations, including surgical photographs, designed to familiarize the student with the surgical environment
- Tables that condense information to facilitate learning
- Chapter Key Concept summaries that emphasize critical content
- Advanced Practices emphasizing the role of the surgical first assistant

These features have been developed to assist the student in learning this new and often unfamiliar material. Key terms are listed at the beginning of each chapter for quick reference, and students are encouraged to consult a medical dictionary as needed for routine medical terminology used throughout the text. Learning objectives are used to guide the students through the material, emphasizing important concepts. Chapter review questions and additional learning activities contained in the accompanying

Study Guide are designed to help students think about concepts from a broader perspective and to apply content at a more personal level, particularly their local clinical facilities.

The authors would appreciate comments and suggestions from practitioners, instructors, and students using this text. Please contact us through Elsevier, c/o Michael Ledbetter, 11830 Westline Industrial Drive, St. Louis, MO 63146.

ACKNOWLEDGMENTS

We would like to acknowledge and sincerely thank the following people for their valuable input and assistance in the development and completion of this second edition of our textbook. Thanks to the staff at Elsevier for continuing to share our vision and for helping us make this textbook's second edition a reality. We are especially grateful to Michael Ledbetter and Katherine Judge for their patience and guidance throughout the entire project. Thanks to our students for good-naturedly using various drafts of this text and for their helpful input. Our gratitude goes to Dorothy Corrigan, CST, for helping us realize the need for our text and challenging us to "be the solution."

Our special thanks goes to Renee Nemitz, CST, RN; Jeffrey Ware, CST/CFA; and Clifford W. Smith, MSN, RN, ONC, CRNFA, CRNP, for their contributions of the Advanced Practices sections.

Our sincere gratitude goes to June Gross, CRNA; Karyn Domenici, RPh; Claire Fitzgerald O'Shea, RN, MS; and the operating room crew at Brigham and Women's Hospital for their generous contributions to this project.

CONTENTS

Unit One

Introduction to Pharmacology

As a surgical technologist, you will mix and measure medications and deliver them to and from the sterile field. This means you will be dealing with *pharmacology*—the science of drugs. In Unit One, we look at general pharmacologic information, including how medications are measured, what kinds of medications are used, what laws pertain to them, how they are labeled, and how they are administered to the surgical patient. Chapter 1 gives a look at the medications themselves—their sources, names, classifications, routes by which they are administered, and their forms. This chapter provides a framework of pharmacologic terms, concepts, and principles—a framework that helps you understand current information about medications and prepares you to assimilate new information effectively. In Chapter 2, we focus on laws, regulations, and medication labels. You will see the importance of laws to regulate medications and the information found on medication labels, what types of laws exist, and which government agencies enforce the laws. You will also learn what acts govern your scope of practice in regard to medications. In Chapter 3, we address precision because it is critical to delivering exactly the right quantity and strength of any medication. Thus, we review mathematics that you need to do the job. We include a refresher on basic computation techniques and a review of the measurement systems used in medicine. Patient safety depends on accuracy, and the surgical technologist is the last line of defense against medication errors at the sterile field. Then in Chapter 4, we concentrate on methods you will use when handling medications, including aseptic technique, proper medication identification, and clear labeling of all medications on the sterile field.

BASIC PHARMACOLOGY

Medications Covered in Chapter 1

Generic Name	Brand or Trade Name	Category
atropine	Atropisol	Anticholinergic
digitalis	Digoxin	Cardiac agent
morphine	Duramorph	Analgesic
thyroglobulin	Proloid	Hormone
thrombin	Thrombogen	Topical hemostatic
silver sulfadiazine	Silvadene	Dermatologic agent
aurothioglucose	Solganal	Antiarthritic agent
meperidine	Demerol	Analgesic
amoxicillin	Amoxil, Biomax	Antibiotic
human insulin	Humulin	Hormone
human growth hormone	Nutropin	Hormone
human thyroid-stimulating hormone	Thyrogen	Hormone
alteplase	Activase	Thrombolytic
ranitidine	Zantac	Gastric agent
heparin	Calciparin	Anticoagulant
lidocaine	Xylocaine	Anesthetic
bacitracin, neomycin, polymixin B	Neosporin	Antibiotic

(continued on following page)

Medications Covered in Chapter 1   *(continued)*

Generic Name	Brand or Trade Name	Category
dantrolene	Dantrium	Muscle relaxant
neomycin, polymixin B, hydrocortisone	Cortisporin	Combination antibiotic and anti-inflammatory agent
betamethasone	Celestone	Anti-inflammatory agent
propofol	Diprivan	Sedative/hypnotic anesthetic agent
desflurane	Suprane	Anesthetic agent
sodium citrate	Bicitra	Antacid
tetracaine	Pontocaine	Anesthetic
phenylephrine	Neosynephrine	Vasoconstrictor
methylene blue	Urolene Blue	Diagnostic agent (dye)
ketorolac	Toradol	Nonsteroidal anti-inflammatory
bupivicaine	Marcaine	Anesthetic
epinephrine	Adrenalin	Hormone
warfarin	Coumadin	Anticoagulant
succinylcholine	Anectine	Muscle relaxant
mannitol	Osmitrol	Diuretic

OBJECTIVES

After completing this chapter, you should be able to:

1. Define terms and abbreviations related to pharmacology.
2. List sources of drugs and give an example of each.
3. List four drug classification categories and identify several subcategories in each.
4. Discuss medication orders used in surgery.
5. List the parts of a medication order.
6. Describe the drug distribution systems used in hospitals.
7. List types of drug forms.
8. Discuss the medication administration routes used in surgery.
9. Describe the four processes of pharmacokinetics.
10. Discuss aspects of pharmacodynamics.

KEY TERMS

absorption	emulsion	pharmacokinetics
adverse effect	enteral	plasma protein binding
agonist	excretion	reconstituted
antagonist	hypersensitivity	side effects
bioavailability	idiosyncratic effect	solubility
biotechnology	indication	solution
biotransformation	local effect	suspension
bolus	metabolism	synergist
contraindication	onset	systemic effect
distribution	parenteral	topical
duration	pharmacodynamics	

The science of pharmacology is a diverse study of the interaction between chemicals and biological systems. In the broadest sense, it includes toxicology, food science, agriculture, and medicine. When chemicals are used to treat diseases, we call them drugs or medications. Medical pharmacology is a rapidly expanding field of study because new drugs are being developed nearly every day. An understanding of basic principles in pharmacology can help the surgical technologist deal with such constant developments. Students should seek to build a framework of principles so they can incorporate new information more easily. When a new drug is introduced into surgical practice, the surgical technologist should be able to understand information about the drug by applying the principles of pharmacology. This chapter presents an introduction to the foundations of pharmacology that can be applied throughout a professional career in surgical technology.

DRUG SOURCES

Drugs in use today come from three main sources: natural sources, chemical synthesis, and **biotechnology.** Natural sources include plants, animals, and minerals.

At one time, plants were nearly the only source of medicines available. Today, however, only a few prescription drugs are still derived directly from plant sources (Fig. 1–1). Examples of current drugs made from plants include atropine from the roots of the belladonna plant (deadly nightshade), digitalis from the leaves of the purple foxglove, and morphine from the seeds of the opium poppy. The trend toward alternative medicines has initiated a

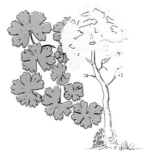

Figure **1–1.**   Plants are sources of some drugs in use today.

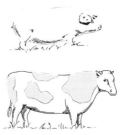

Figure **1–2.**   Animals are sources of some drugs in use today.

closer look at plants as sources of important and helpful chemicals in the natural state.

Animals (Fig. 1–2) provide a source for some drugs, particularly hormones. Cattle and hog endocrine glands were the best available source of hormones prior to the advent of biotechnology. We describe drugs derived from hogs as *porcine* and those from cattle as *bovine*. Thus, thyroglobulin (Proloid)—a purified extract of hog thyroid gland—is porcine in origin, whereas thrombin (Thrombogen)—a topical hemostatic—is bovine in origin. The early form of insulin is both bovine and porcine because it was obtained from the pancreas of cattle and hogs.

Minerals (Fig. 1–3), such as calcium, magnesium, and silver salts in several forms, are used in some pharmacologic agents. For example, Tums and Mylanta are antacids that contain calcium (Tums) and magnesium (Mylanta) hydroxides. Silvadene cream is an antimicrobial agent used in dressings for burn patients that contains silver salts. Even gold is used, as in Solganal, an antiarthritic agent.

The second major source of drugs is chemical synthesis in the laboratory (Fig. 1–4). There are two ways for drugs to be *synthe-*

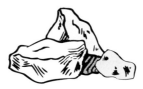

Figure **1–3.**   Minerals are sources of some drugs in use today.

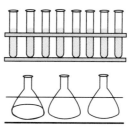

Figure **1–4.**   Synthetic and semisynthetic drugs are produced in a chemical laboratory.

sized, that is, put together. *Synthetic drugs* are drugs that are synthesized from laboratory chemicals. *Semisynthetic drugs* are drugs that start with a natural substance that is extracted, purified, and altered by chemical processes. The vast majority of modern drugs are either synthetic or semisynthetic. Meperidine (Demerol) is an example of a synthetic drug; it is made from chemicals, yet its pain-relieving effects are similar to those of opium. Many penicillins—such as amoxicillin—are semisynthetic drugs. The penicillin group of drugs was originally derived from a natural mold *(Penicillium),* the active substance of which is extracted and purified in the chemical laboratory. Another example of semisynthetic drugs is the aminoglycoside group of antibiotics, the active substance of which is obtained from the bacterial species *Streptomyces.*

An increasing source of drugs has been provided by the science of biotechnology. The term *biotechnology* is used to refer to the concepts of genetic engineering and recombinant DNA technology. Biotechnology is a process that allows scientists to produce proteins from bacteria—proteins that were previously available only from animals. Molecular biologists use bacteria as tiny factories to produce the proteins they need to make drugs. They do this by altering the DNA of bacteria such as *Escherichia coli (E. coli).* How? By physically inserting a gene into the DNA of a single *E. coli* cell— a gene that *codes for* (tells the cell to make) a certain protein (Fig. 1–5). When the bacterial cell has this gene incorporated into its

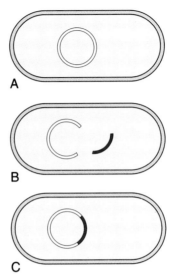

Figure **1–5.** **Biotechnology: (A)** *Escherichia coli* DNA. **(B)** Desired gene is inserted into bacterial DNA. **(C)** Bacterial DNA with recombinant gene.

DNA, it becomes a miniature copying machine, producing daughter cells that have daughter cells that have daughter cells—each with the new gene and each producing the desired protein. As this reproduction process occurs very rapidly, large volumes of the desired protein can be obtained quickly. The specific protein is extracted and purified in the laboratory and prepared for administration into a patient. Molecular biologists also use cultures of mammalian cell lines, such as genetically altered Chinese hamster ovary cells to produce various therapeutic proteins.

Among the drugs produced by biotechnology are human insulin (Humulin), human growth hormone (Nutropin), human thyroid-stimulating hormone (Thyrogen) and the thrombolytic agent alteplase (Activase). Such genetically engineered proteins do not cause the adverse side effects—for example, immune or allergic reactions—often seen in the long-term use of drugs from animal sources. Drugs such as these are always administered by injection; they cannot be taken orally because they are proteins, which are digested when consumed.

DRUG CLASSIFICATIONS

Drug classifications are used to group similar drugs, or drugs that are used for similar purposes. We can classify drugs by what they

Table 1–1   Drug Classification Categories and Subcategories

Therapeutic Action	Physiologic Action	Body System	Chemical Type
Analgesic	alpha-Adrenergic blocker	Cardiovascular agent	Barbiturate
Anticoagulant	Cholinergic	Dermatologic agent	Benzodiazepine
Antiemetic	Diuretic	Ophthalmic preparation	Hormone
Antihistamine	Hemostatic	Urinary tract agent	Narcotic
Antihypertensive	Histamine receptor antagonist		Oxytocic
Anti-inflammatory	Muscle relaxant antagonist		Steroid
Antineoplastic	Narcotic antagonist		
Antipyretic	Tranquilizer		
Antispasmotic	Vasoconstrictor		
Sedative			
Thrombolytic			

do, what they affect, and what they are; thus, common classification categories include the following:

- *Therapeutic action:* what they do for a patient; for example, analgesics relieve pain.
- *Physiologic action:* what they do in the body; for example, histamine receptor antagonists block histamine production.
- *Affected body system:* what they affect; for example, cardiovascular agents affect the heart and circulatory system.
- *Chemical type:* what they are; for example, barbiturates are a class of chemical compounds derived from barbituric acid.

Drugs can be cross-referenced in multiple categories. For example, ranitidine (Zantac) is categorized therapeutically as an antacid, physiologically as a histamine receptor antagonist, and by body system as a gastric agent. Each classification category has several subcategories, as shown in Table 1–1. Drugs having multiple therapeutic effects are classified in more than one subcategory. For example, aspirin relieves pain, fever, and inflammation, so it is classified as an analgesic, an antipyretic, and an anti-inflammatory agent—three different therapeutic subcategories. Therapeutic-action subcategories of drugs frequently used from the sterile back table include antibiotics, anticoagulants, anti-inflammatory agents, and local anesthetics.

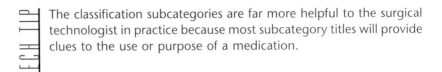

The classification subcategories are far more helpful to the surgical technologist in practice because most subcategory titles will provide clues to the use or purpose of a medication.

In addition, the subcategories of the classification "body system" may be helpful in clarifying appropriate surgical uses. For example, if a medication is subcategorized as an ophthalmic agent, it may be specially formulated for use in the eye only. An "otic" medication is specially formulated for use in the ear.

Drugs are also classified by how they may be obtained. The distinction between prescription and nonprescription or over-the-counter (OTC) drugs is a legal classification. In addition, some prescription medications are subcategorized as controlled substances. Legal classifications are discussed in detail in Chapter 2.

MEDICATION ORDERS

PRESCRIPTIONS

When treatment requires a specific drug, a licensed physician or designee such as a physician's assistant (PA) or nurse practitioner (NP) writes a prescription for the drug. State governments have the power to regulate which medical professionals write prescriptions, so there are variations in practice from state to state. Figure 1–6 shows a typical prescription form. As shown, prescriptions must include the date, name of the patient, name of the drug, dosage, route of administration, and frequency or time of administration. It must also bear the prescriber's signature. Notice that the printed form contains the name, address, telephone number, and DEA number of the prescriber. The Drug Enforcement Agency (DEA) requires that this number be listed on any prescription for a controlled substance (see Chapter 2). A written prescription usually designates the drug by trade name but may indicate that a generic substitution is permissible. When writing prescriptions, physicians (or their designees) use abbreviations and symbols (Table 1–2) for dosages, frequency, and administration routes. Pharmacists interpret these symbols and give the drugs to the patient, along with instructions for proper use. Many pharmacies use computer database systems that provide specific, detailed printouts to the patient of such important drug information as side effects, precautions, normal usage, and storage. Prescriptions

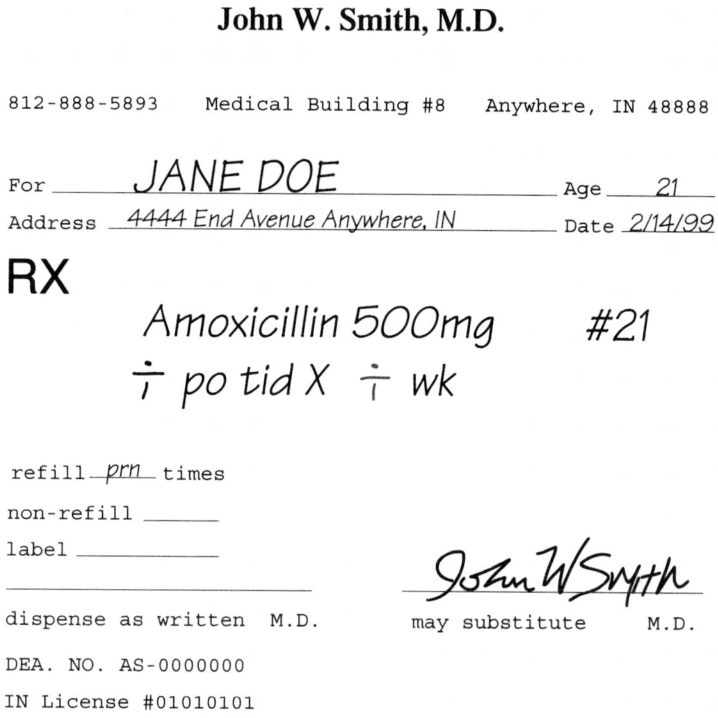

John W. Smith, M.D.

812-888-5893   Medical Building #8   Anywhere, IN 48888

For ___*JANE DOE*_____ Age ___*21*___

Address ___*4444 End Avenue Anywhere, IN*_____ Date *2/14/99*

RX

Amoxicillin 500mg   #21
ī̄ po tid X ī̄ wk

refill _*prn*_ times

non-refill _____

label _____

_____

dispense as written M.D.

John W Smyth

may substitute   M.D.

DEA. NO. AS-0000000

IN License #01010101

Figure **1–6.**   A typical prescription form.

such as shown are not generally used during a patient's hospitalization, so have little or no use during surgery.

HOSPITAL MEDICATION ORDERS

In the hospital setting, any medications to be administered to the patient must be ordered by a licensed physician or designee and written on a physician's order sheet. In surgery, the medication order may be one of several types:

Standing Orders

A standing order, or *protocol,* is used for common situations requiring a standard treatment. For example, a standing order may be in place for the preoperative holding area stating that all surgical patients are to receive 15 mL of sodium citrate (Bicitra) by mouth 30 minutes before surgery. In the operating room, surgeon's

Table **1-2**	Abbreviations for Anatomical and Administration Directions
os	mouth
aa	of each
ad	to, up to
ad lib	as desired
amt	amount
c̄	with
et	and
KVO, TKO	keep vein open, to keep open
npo, NPO	nothing by mouth (os)
per	by means of, by
qs	quantity sufficient
Rx	take
s̄	without
ss	one half
sig	label
sos	once if necessary
STAT	immediately

preference cards contain standing orders for specific surgical procedures. For example, Dr. Vigil's preference card for abdominal aortic aneurysm (AAA) repair may include a standing order for 5000 units of heparin in 1000 mL of NaCl for topical irrigation. A standing order of this type informs the operating room team that the indicated medication should be ready on the sterile back table as a standard part of the setup for that procedure.

Verbal Orders

Verbal orders are commonplace in surgery, as a surgeon may request a particular drug to be administered either from the sterile field or by the anesthesia provider. For example, during a AAA repair Dr. Vigil may give a verbal order to the anesthesia provider to administer 5000 units of heparin intravenously three minutes prior to cross-clamping the aorta. Verbal orders in surgery are usually for a one-time single administration of a medication.

STAT Orders

Often given verbally, STAT orders indicate that a drug is to be administered immediately and one time only. The most common use of STAT orders in surgery is during cardiac arrest resuscitation or other emergent situation.

PRN Orders

PRN stands for *pro re nata,* which means that the drug may be given as needed. For example, during septoplasty performed under local anesthesia, meperidine (Demerol) may be administered PRN to reduce patient discomfort.

In surgery, medications routinely needed during a procedure are listed on the surgeon's preference card. As shown in Figure 1–7, the preference card should list all pertinent information, such as drug strength and quantity. Surgical medication orders on preference cards usually contain the drug name, strength, and dosage. Unlike medication orders given in nursing care units, the surgeon administers all medications at the sterile field, so route of administration and frequency are not usually stated on surgeon's preference cards.

Many abbreviations are used to represent drug forms, dosages, routes, and timing of administration. Dosages are stated in a particular unit of measure, usually in the metric system, and abbreviated, such as 300 mg, 10 mL, or 1000 units. The dosage of a medication is the medication strength (usually expressed as a percent) multiplied by the volume administered. For example, lidocaine (Xylocaine) may be injected for local anesthesia and therefore is listed on the preference card as "lidocaine plain 1%— 30 mL." This indicates that a 30-mL vial of a 1% solution of lidocaine without epinephrine should be delivered to the sterile back table and prepared for use. It may not be necessary to use the entire 30 mL during the procedure, so the surgical technologist in the scrub role reports the final amount (volume) used to the circulator who records the dose.

For regular hospital medication orders, the route of administration is usually abbreviated; for example, if a drug is to be given intravenously, it is designated as IV. The frequency or time of administration is also clearly stated and is often abbreviated; for example, if the drug is to be taken four times a day, it is designated QID. Table 1–3 lists common abbreviations used to represent frequency of drug administration. Again, most surgeons' preference cards do not list the route or frequency because the surgeon is administering all medications given at the surgical site.

REGIONAL MEDICAL CENTER
SURGEON PREFERENCE CARD AND REQUISITION

Patient name: Jane Doe
Procedure date: 01/31/99
Scheduled time: 0730
Surgeon: Meier, C.
Procedure: Cataract extraction with IOL, O.D.

Item code	Item description	Req.	Quantity Picked	Chgd
	STERILE SUPPLIES			
001957	Steridrape 1060 3M	1	_____	_____
005006	Skin scrub tray	1	_____	_____
000574	Glove sterile 7	1	_____	_____
005890	Custom pack - eye	1	_____	_____
	INSTRUMENTS			
002040	Capsule polisher	1	_____	_____
001993	Irrigating cystitome	1	_____	_____
011005	Phaco tubing	1	_____	_____
009505	Cataract set - Meier	1	_____	_____
011013	Phaco handpiece	1	_____	_____
	MEDICATIONS			
002365	BSS 15 mL	2	_____	_____
012032	Bio-Cor Shield	1	_____	_____
002367	BSS Plus 500 mL	1	_____	_____
218965	Dexamethasone 4 mg	1	_____	_____
218966	Celestone 3 mg	1	_____	_____
	Hold if uses shield			
012164	Ancef 50 mg	1	_____	_____
	Hold if uses shield		_____	_____
444364	Carbastat 1 amp	1	_____	_____
417665	Maxitrol ointment	1	_____	_____
010433	Opthetic gtts	1	_____	_____
359003	Lidocaine 2% 50 mL			
	w/epi 1:200,000	1	_____	_____
359004	Bupivicaine 0.5%	1	_____	_____
010492	Epinephrine 1:1000 1 cc	1	_____	_____
437283	Wydase 150 units	1	_____	_____
455849	Healon .85 mL	1	_____	_____
455850	Healon .4 mL	1	_____	_____
	Hold			
238934	Tobradex gtts	1	_____	_____
567392	Vancomycin 10 mg	1	_____	_____

SURGEON SPECIAL REQUESTS
*Add 0.3 cc epinephrine, 2 mg dexamethasone, and 10 mg of Vancomycin to 500 cc bottle of BSS plus.
*Add remaining dexamethasone (2 mg) to celestone for injection at end of case (hold if using shield).
*Mix 1 gm Ancef with 10 cc NaCl⁻ give 0.5 cc of solution for injection at end of case (hold if using shield).
*Do not add Wydase to anesthetic agent until just prior to use.
*Combine 2% lidocaine w/epi (5 cc), bupivicaine 0.5% (5 cc), and Wydase 150 units for injection.

Figure **1–7.** A computerized surgeon's preference card lists medications required for the procedure.

Table **1–3**	Abbreviations for Frequency of Medication Administration
bid	twice a day
h, hr	hour
prn, PRN	as necessary *(pro re nata)*
q	every
qh	every hour
q2h	every 2 hours
qid	four times a day
tid	three times a day
stat	immediately

⚠ CAUTION

Some abbreviations have been the source of confusion and possible medication errors. The Joint Commission on Accreditation of Healthcare Organizations requires accredited facilities to publish a "do not use" list for potentially dangerous abbreviations, acronyms, and symbols (see Table 2–3). Before using what you may think are standard abbreviations, consult this list at your facility.

DRUG DISTRIBUTION SYSTEMS

Dispensing prescription drugs is the responsibility of a licensed pharmacist. That is, pharmacists must *release* drugs, either directly to patients or to the physician or surgeon who orders them. In hospitals, drugs are often released for secure storage in various patient care areas so they can be distributed as necessary.

☞ **Note:** In all medical facilities, *controlled substances* (such as morphine) must be stored in a double-locked cupboard, drawer, or box once they have been released from the pharmacy. Each shift, a designated person is usually in charge of the key to the controlled substances box or cupboard. At the beginning and end of each shift, two people count the drugs to verify proper documentation of use.

Distribution systems for drugs used in surgery vary among institutions. In large hospitals, a satellite pharmacy (Fig. 1–8) within the surgical suite may dispense drugs as needed for each procedure. Other, often smaller, facilities may maintain a medication room or cabinet where they store frequently used drugs, such as antibiotics and local anesthetics. In addition, many hospitals use a system of

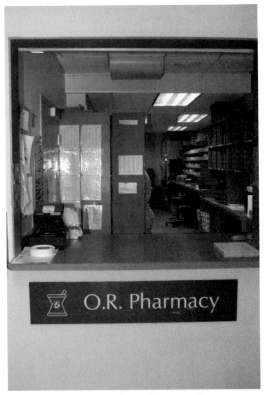

Figure **1–8.** A satellite pharmacy in surgery.

mobile drug carts, which must be exchanged for restocking after the drugs are used. For example, emergency-response drug carts, known as *crash carts,* are used for cardiac arrest and other emergency situations. Such carts may be restocked on an exchange basis to assure the immediate availability of all necessary drugs. One of the recent innovations in medication distribution has been the use of computer-automated dispensing systems. These systems have been developed to minimize medication administration errors. A barcode-scanning system allows an approved user access to particular medications for a particular patient.

DRUG FORMS OR PREPARATIONS

Drugs are available in several different forms or preparations. Drugs may be in solid, semisolid, liquid, or gas form (Fig. 1–9). The form of drug administered affects both the onset of drug actions and the intensity of the body's response to the drug.

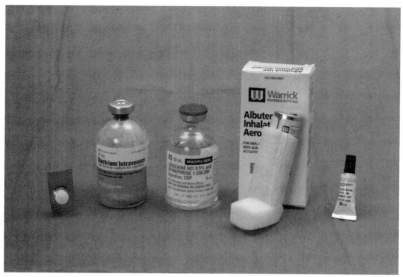

Figure **1–9.** Drugs are available in several forms or preparations.

Table **1–4** Abbreviations for Drug Forms or Preparations	
cap	capsule
gtts	drops
soln	solution
susp	suspension
tab	tablet
ung	ointment

Liquids, for instance, tend to act more quickly than solids, and gases or vapors tend to act even faster. Drug form also dictates route of administration. For example, the antibiotic Neosporin comes in ointment (semisolid) form, which must be applied topically only. Some drugs are available in more than one form. For example, lidocaine (Xylocaine) is available in jelly for topical application and in solutions of various strengths for injection. The names of drug forms are often abbreviated in drug orders. Table 1–4 lists several common abbreviations for drug forms.

SOLIDS

Many drugs come prepared in solid form. These drugs may be in capsule (cap) or tablet (tab) form and are administered orally.

Capsules are gelatin cases containing a drug in powder or granule form; tablets are a compressed form of the drug, usually combined with inert ingredients. Capsules and tablets are rarely used in surgery, because oral administration is required. In most cases surgical patients must be kept NPO (from the Latin *nil per ora*, nothing by mouth), or they may be under a general anesthesia and unable to swallow.

SEMISOLIDS

Some drugs come in powder form, which is considered semisolid form. These powdered drugs come in glass vials. Such powders must be mixed with a liquid (**reconstituted**) to form a solution so they can be administered by injection. For example, several antibiotics administered in surgery are powders that must be reconstituted with sterile water or a sodium chloride solution (saline) to make an injectable solution. Other drugs, such as dantrolene (Dantrium)—an infrequently used yet important skeletal muscle relaxant—also come in powder form and must be reconstituted before use (see Chapter 16). Therefore such medications come from the pharmacy in semisolid form but are administered in liquid form.

Other semisolid preparations include creams, foams, gels, ointments, and suppositories. Examples of semisolid drugs used in surgery include a number of antibiotics for topical irrigation, lidocaine (Xylocaine) jelly for topical anesthesia, Silvadene cream for burns, estrogen cream for vaginal packing, and Neosporin ointment for wound dressing.

LIQUIDS

Several types of liquid drug preparations are available. Many liquid medications are available in solution. A **solution** is a mixture of drug particles fully dissolved in a liquid medium (e.g., water, alcohol, or saline). Many solutions are used in surgery, including normal saline (0.9% NaCl) irrigation, antibiotic irrigation solutions, and heparin irrigation solution.

Drugs may also be in **suspension**. A suspension is a form in which solid particles float (are suspended) in a liquid. Suspensions should be shaken prior to administration to evenly distribute particles throughout the liquid. Suspensions used in surgery include Cortisporin otic, used in ear surgery, and Celestone, an anti-inflammatory used in ophthalmology.

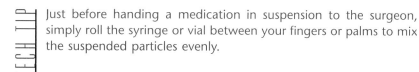
Just before handing a medication in suspension to the surgeon, simply roll the syringe or vial between your fingers or palms to mix the suspended particles evenly.

Another type of liquid medication form is an **emulsion,** in which the medication is contained in a mixture of water and oil bound together with an emulsifier. The most common emulsion used in surgery is propofol (Diprivan), an intravenous sedative-hypnotic agent used for anesthesia (see Chapter 15).

Drugs in liquid form may also be administered orally, as *elixirs* (sweetened solutions of alcohol) or *syrups* (sweetened aqueous solutions). But elixirs and syrups are rarely, if ever, used in surgery because of the NPO status for surgical patients.

GASES

The only common medications available in gas form are inhalation anesthetic agents. These agents include nitrous oxide and volatile liquids such as desflurane (Suprane) (see Chapter 15). The volatile liquid agents are vaporized through an apparatus on the anesthesia machine into gas form for administration.

DRUG ADMINISTRATION ROUTES

Medications are formulated for administration by a specific route. In addition to drug form, the route by which a drug is given can affect onset time and body response. Drugs may be administered by many different routes, only a few of which are used commonly in surgery. Medication orders state route of administration, usually in abbreviated form (Table 1–5). The three major categories of medication administration routes are **enteral, topical,** and **parenteral.** The enteral route indicates that the medication is taken into the gastrointestinal tract, either

Table **1–5** Abbreviations for Drug Administration Routes	
IM	intramuscular
IV	intravenous
PO, po	per os, orally
subQ	subcutaneously

orally or as a rectal suppository. Topical medications are applied to the skin surface or a mucous membrane-lined cavity. The term *parenteral* indicates any route other than the digestive tract, the most common of which are subcutaneous, intramuscular, and intravenous.

> Use medical terminology word-building techniques to help you understand the terms *enteral* and *parenteral.* The root word or combining form "enter/o-" means intestines, and the adjective ending "-al" means pertaining to. The combining form "/o" is not used when the suffix begins with a vowel, so the word *enteral* means pertaining to the intestines or intestinal tract. The prefix "para-" indicates beside or beyond (the "a" is dropped when the root word begins with a vowel) so the term *parenteral* means outside, or *not in,* the intestinal tract.

The oral route (PO, from the Latin *per ora,* "by mouth") is the simplest and most common way to administer many drugs. Tablets or capsules are swallowed and readily absorbed through the lining (mucosa) of the gastrointestinal tract. Certain drugs may irritate the gastrointestinal mucosa and should therefore be given with food. Other drugs may be inactivated by increased amounts of digestive enzymes and so are best taken between meals. When drugs are administered orally, onset of action is usually slower and duration of effect is usually longer than with other routes. Some drugs, however, are completely inactivated by the digestive process and therefore must not be given orally. Insulin, a hormone, and heparin, an anticoagulant, are not effective when administered orally.

The oral route is rarely used in surgery because the patient must be kept NPO before surgery and because many patients are under general anesthesia during surgery and so are unable to swallow. One exception is oral administration of sodium citrate (Bicitra), which may be given preoperatively to neutralize gastric acid (see Chapter 13).

Some medications are available in topical preparations, which are intended for application to the skin or a mucous membrane-lined cavity. The majority of topical agents work at the site of application; this is called a **local effect.** Some topical medications exert a **systemic effect,** that is, throughout the entire body. Examples of topical medications with local effect include steroid creams for rashes and antibiotic ointment for cuts. Hormone replacement, birth control, and motion sickness are applications for systemic topical agents. Topical medications are absorbed slowly through the skin, but are absorbed rapidly when applied to blood supply-rich mucous membranes.

☞ **Note:** Some medications, though taken orally, are actually topical in that the tablet (pill) is held in the mouth, either in the cheek (buccal) or under the tongue (sublingual), and allowed to dissolve. The medication is absorbed through the mucous membrane of the mouth and does not pass directly into the gastrointestinal tract.

Several topical medications are used in surgery. Antibiotic ointments, such as Neosporin, may be used on the surgical incision as part of the postoperative wound dressing. Estrogen cream may be applied to vaginal packing used as a pressure dressing after a vaginal hysterectomy.

Topical antibiotic irrigation is common in surgery, in which case an antibiotic solution is poured or squirted into the surgical site (Fig. 1–10). In many vascular procedures, a solution of heparin (an anticoagulant; see Chapter 9) is used as a topical irrigation to prevent the formation of blood clots in operative vessels during surgery.

☞ **Note:** Vascular procedures may also involve using intravenous heparin for systemic effect. But when used as a topical irrigation, heparin exerts a more significant local effect, because the opera-

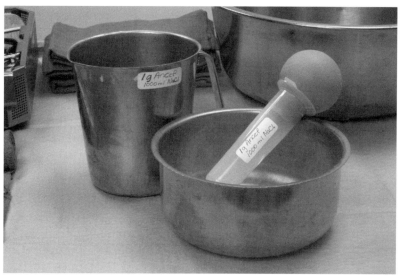

Figure **1–10.** Antibiotic irrigation used during surgery is an example of a topical application of a medication.

tive vessel is usually clamped off, preventing systemic absorption of the agent.

Instillation of a medication into a mucous membrane–lined cavity, such as the eye, nose, or urethra, may also be considered a topical route or application. A number of medications are instilled into body cavities intraoperatively, situations unique to surgery. For example, tetracaine (Pontocaine) drops may be instilled into the eye for local anesthesia for cataract extraction, phenylephrine (Neosynephrine) may be instilled into the nasal cavity for vasoconstriction during sinusoscopy, or lidocaine (Xylocaine) jelly may be instilled into the urethra as topical anesthesia for cystoscopy. During diagnostic gynecologic laparoscopy, a methylene blue solution may be instilled via a cervical cannula into the uterus. This procedure is known as a tubal dye study or chromotubation and is used to assess tubal patency in patients with infertility. The methylene blue solution fills the uterus and exits through the uterine tubes into the pelvic cavity when the tubes are patent (open). The laparoscope is used to observe the blue solution exiting the tubal fimbria. If the tubes are blocked by scarring, the solution cannot enter the pelvic cavity. Another example of medication instillation occurs during operative cholangiography. Although not as frequently performed currently due to the availability of endoscopic retrograde cholangiopancreatography (ERCP), intraoperative cholangiography involves the instillation of a radiographic contrast media into the common bile duct to detect gallstones under x-ray. If present, common bile duct stones will be evident on x-ray as shadows in the radiopaque contrast media. For additional information on diagnostic agents, see Chapter 6.

Inhalation is a means of medication administration that can be considered topical. Some asthmatic drugs are administered through a nebulizer—a device that converts liquid drugs into an inhalable mist. The drug is absorbed in the bronchi of the lungs, providing local relief of bronchoconstriction. In surgery, anesthetic gases and vapors are administered via inhalation, but these drugs exert systemic rather than local effects.

Most medications used in surgery are administered parenterally. The most common parenteral routes are subcutaneous, intramuscular, and intravenous. Subcutaneous injections are given beneath the skin into the subcutaneous tissue layer. Common sites for subcutaneous injections are the upper lateral aspect of the arm, the anterior thigh, and the abdomen. Depending on blood supply, absorption from subcutaneous tissue is fairly rapid. Only a few drugs are administered subcutaneously in surgery; for example, heparin may be injected subcutaneously preoperatively in some cases to help prevent pulmonary embolism.

A few drugs used in surgery are administered intramuscularly (IM). Intramuscular injections are usually given into a large muscle mass, such as the deltoid, gluteal, or vastus lateralis. Intramuscular absorption is usually rapid due to the large absorbing surface and good blood supply. An example of a drug given IM in surgery is ketorolac (Toradol), a nonsteroidal anti-inflammatory drug (NSAID) used for postoperative pain relief.

Probably the most common example of the parenteral route used at the surgical site is the administration (injection) of a local anesthetic agent for intraoperative pain control. Local anesthesia during a surgical procedure may be accomplished with lidocaine (Xylocaine) injected into multiple tissue layers as needed. Quite frequently, a longer-acting local anesthetic (such as bupivicaine) is used to inject the surgical site for postoperative pain control. For a more detailed discussion of local anesthetics, see Chapter 14.

Most medications administered parenterally during surgery are given intravenously (IV), that is, within a vein, as shown in Figure 1–11. A small catheter is inserted into a vein and connected to tubing called an infusion set. The infusion set is attached to a bag of intravenous fluid for administration. Drugs may then be injected as needed into sites along the tubing. Drugs may be given

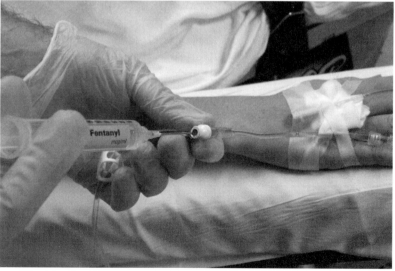

Figure **1–11.**   A drug may be administered by intravenous injection.

all at once, as a **bolus**, or by slow infusion. Absorption is immediate for medications administered intravenously because the agent goes directly into the bloodstream.

Other parenteral routes are used less frequently. *Intradermal* injections are given between layers of skin, as seen in tuberculin skin testing and allergy testing. A local anesthetic may be injected intradermally prior to placing an intravenous catheter, thereby reducing discomfort at the insertion site. *Intra-articular* injections (into the joint space) of anti-inflammatory agents or local anesthetics may be given after arthroscopy. *Intrathecal* injections of anesthetics or contrast media are administered into the spinal subarachnoid space. During cardiac arrest resuscitation, a drug such as epinephrine may be injected directly into the heart; this is called an *intracardiac* injection.

PHARMACOKINETICS

The study of **pharmacokinetics** focuses on how the body processes drugs, and the science of **pharmacodynamics** examines how the body responds to the action of the drug. The science of pharmacokinetics studies a medication from administration through four basic physiologic processes—absorption, distribution, metabolism, and excretion (Table 1–6). The patient's general health has a significant effect on how the body processes drugs. For example, if the patient's blood supply, liver function, or kidney function is compromised, the ability to process medications is also compromised.

ABSORPTION

To be effective, a drug must first be absorbed into the body. A drug is absorbed from the site of administration into the bloodstream and enters systemic circulation. Speed of **absorption** varies by

Table **1–6**   The Four Processes of Pharmacokinetics

Process	Body System
Absorption	Body system varies by administration route (e.g., integumentary, gastrointestinal, respiratory)
Distribution	Circulatory system
Metabolism	Liver
Excretion	Kidney

administration route and by blood supply to the area. **Solubility** of the drug (its ability to be dissolved) also affects absorption. If a drug is in solid or semisolid form, it must dissolve before it can be absorbed. Drugs in suspensions absorb faster than solid drugs, and solutions absorb faster than suspensions. For example, a solution instilled in the conjunctiva will absorb more quickly than an ointment applied to the conjunctiva.

Oral absorption varies depending on the drug's chemical structure as well as the pH (acidity) and motility of the gastrointestinal tract. If the digestive tract is highly motile, as in patients with diarrhea, ingested drugs may not be adequately absorbed. Conversely, if the patient is constipated drugs may be fully absorbed, sometimes to toxic levels. Intramuscular absorption is rapid if water-based drug solutions are injected and is slower if the solution is an oil-based emulsion. The amount and vascularization of muscle mass also affects the rate of absorption of medications given IM. Intravenous absorption is immediate because drugs are injected directly into the bloodstream. The absorption rate of drugs given subcutaneously depends on blood supply to the area of injection.

☞ **Note:** Rapid drug absorption can be undesirable in surgery when local anesthetics are used. The anesthetic agent must stay in the desired area instead of being carried away by the systemic circulation. Thus, a *vasoconstrictor,* usually epinephrine, may be added to the anesthetic agent to narrow the small blood vessels in the local area and delay absorption.

Absorption of drugs given by inhalation, especially inhalation anesthetics, is rapid, because of the huge numbers of capillaries in the alveoli of the lungs. Some drugs administered by inhalation (such as steroids for asthma) are specifically formulated for local effect, and so do not absorb rapidly. Mucosal tissues provide excellent absorption for some drugs because of the number of capillaries just under the mucosal surface. Common mucosal administration sites include the respiratory tract, oral cavity, and the conjunctiva.

Although most drugs are not absorbed easily through skin, some are specifically formulated to overcome the skin barrier. Such drugs are administered transdermally from patches. Scopolamine patches, for instance, are used to treat motion sickness; they release the drug slowly so it may be absorbed through skin over a period of hours.

Thus, absorption of a medication depends on the formulation of the drug, the route of administration, and the extent of blood supply to the site of administration. The term **bioavailability** indicates the degree to which the unchanged drug molecule reaches systemic circulation.

DISTRIBUTION

Once a drug has been absorbed into the bloodstream, it is transported throughout the body by the circulatory system. This process is called **distribution**. Drug molecules eventually diffuse out of the bloodstream to the site of action. Because drugs are carried to all parts of the body, their effects can be seen in locations other than the intended area. The amount of drug reaching the site of action depends on the general condition of the patient's circulatory system, effective blood flow to the intended area (tissue perfusion) and on the extent of **plasma protein binding**. For example, bone has very limited blood flow, so intravenous antibiotics often have little effect in treating bone infections. In addition, two barriers exist that limit the distribution of certain drug molecules to particular sites. The placental barrier allows some molecules to pass to the fetus, while restricting others. The blood–brain barrier also limits passage of certain molecules into brain tissue.

Plasma Protein Binding

Not all drug molecules in the bloodstream are available to bind at the site of action. Some drug molecules bind to proteins contained in plasma—the liquid portion of blood—via a process known as plasma protein binding. Both the amount of plasma protein in the blood and the binding characteristics of the drug determine the extent to which a drug is bound. Some drugs are highly bound (up to 99%), some are only minimally bound, whereas others are not bound at all. Highly bound drug molecules have a longer duration of action, because they stay in the body longer, and a lower distribution to the site of action. The only drug molecules available to exert effects on the body are unbound molecules.

Plasma protein binding is usually nonspecific; that is, plasma proteins can bind with many different drug molecules. It is also competitive in that drug molecules also compete with other drug molecules for protein-binding sites, changing the amount of available drug significantly. Potential hazards arise if patients are taking different drugs that compete for the same binding sites. For instance, if a patient taking warfarin sodium (Coumadin), a highly bound anticoagulant, takes aspirin, the aspirin will bind with the same plasma protein sites, making more warfarin available than

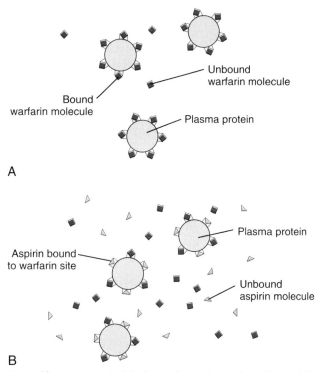

Figure **1–12.**   Plasma protein binding of aspirin and warfarin. **(A)** Warfarin binds to specific receptor sites on plasma proteins. **(B)** Aspirin binds to the same receptor sites, making more warfarin available.

is needed (Fig. 1–12). If more than the expected amount of warfarin is available, overmedication and excessive anticoagulation may occur.

Plasma protein binding is reversible. When the concentration of unbound drug in blood is lowered, either by metabolism or excretion, bound molecules are released from binding sites. The extent of plasma protein binding can prolong a drug's effects and contribute to drug–drug interactions.

METABOLISM

The circulatory system also distributes drugs to the liver, the major structure of the biliary system. In the liver, the chemical composition of a drug is changed by a process called **metabolism** or **biotransformation.** Liver cells (hepatocytes) contain enzymes that break down some drug molecules into other molecules called

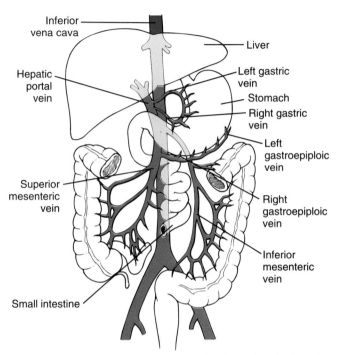

Figure **1–13.** Drugs administered orally are distributed to the liver for metabolism by the hepatic portal circulation.

metabolites. Metabolites are usually less toxic and more easily excreted than the original drug. The effectiveness of liver enzymes depends on several factors, including patient age, concurrent drug therapy, organ disease (e.g., cirrhosis), and nutritional status. Only unbound drug molecules can be metabolized. Whereas some drugs are completely metabolized and some are not metabolized at all, most drugs are at least partially metabolized. Some drugs are really *prodrugs;* this means they are administered in an inactive form, which is metabolized into an active drug to produce the needed effect.

All drugs taken orally enter the liver through the hepatic portal circulation (Fig. 1–13) prior to entering systemic circulation. The hepatic portal circulatory system is the venous drainage of the gastrointestinal tract, carrying molecules absorbed by the gut into veins leading to the liver. Many drugs undergo a first-pass effect, which means they may be altered or nearly inactivated when passing through the liver, potentially reducing the drug's effectiveness. Once liver enzymes begin to metabolize drug molecules, however, the enzymes are less able to metabolize additional drug;

thus, repeated dosing may be used to overcome the first-pass effect.

EXCRETION

Medications taken into the body are eliminated in the process called **excretion.** Some drug molecules are eliminated in the bile, feces, or skin, but most unchanged drugs and metabolites are excreted by the kidneys and eliminated in urine (Fig. 1–14). The circulatory system carries blood to the kidneys, where it is filtered and returned to general circulation. Two renal processes remove drug molecules and metabolites from the body: glomerular filtration and tubular secretion. Only drug molecules *not* bound to

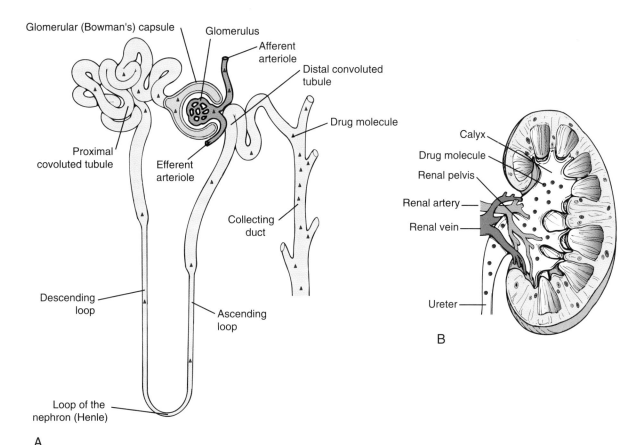

Figure **1–14.** Most drugs are excreted by the kidneys. **(A)** Drugs are removed in the nephrons and **(B)** eliminated by the kidneys.

plasma proteins will be filtered out of blood plasma reaching the glomerulus. How much unbound drug is filtered out depends on the glomerular filtration rate (GFR), which depends on blood pressure and blood flow to the kidneys. Tubular secretion uses cellular energy to force drugs and their metabolites from the bloodstream for elimination. Some drugs, depending on their characteristics and the pH of urine, may be reabsorbed and returned to circulation by tubular reabsorption. Factors influencing renal elimination of drug molecules include presence of kidney disease, such as renal failure, the pH of urine, and the concentration of drug molecules in the plasma.

PHARMACODYNAMICS

As stated previously, pharmacodynamics is the study of how drugs exert their effects on the body, at both the molecular and physiological levels. The human body responds to different drugs in varying degrees and at various rates. Drugs must be able to reach the site of action and interact with cells to produce therapeutic effects. In most cases, drugs bind to specialized proteins, or receptors, on cell membranes. Some drugs are specific in action and some are nonspecific. Interaction with the target site produces the intended effect, whereas interaction with other cells may produce what are called side effects.

Drug molecules with specific mechanisms interact with specific receptors sites on cell membranes. This specificity has been described by the lock-and-key analogy; the lock is the receptor site on the cell membrane (usually a protein complex), and the drug molecule is the key that fits in that specific lock. Very few drugs are exactly specific to a certain receptor; instead, most drug molecules will react with several types of receptors.

Agonists are drugs that bind to or have an affinity (attraction) for a receptor and cause a particular response (Fig. 1–15). Natural agonists include neurotransmitters, such as acetylcholine, and hormones. Some drugs such as succinylcholine act as chemical agonists. Drugs that bind to a receptor and prevent a response are called **antagonists** (Fig. 1–15). Antagonists are also called receptor blockers. Antagonists may be competitive, that is, bind to sites and prevent the agonist from reaching the site, or noncompetitive in that the antagonist alters the target site, preventing the agonist from causing the intended effect.

Drug antagonism is responsible for many drug interactions, some of which are not desired. Many patients are on multiple drug therapy, so potential exists for several drug–drug interactions.

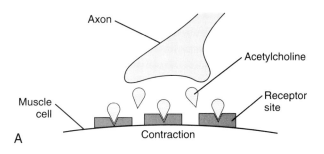

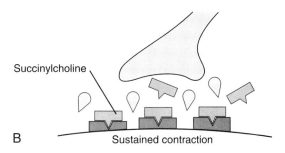

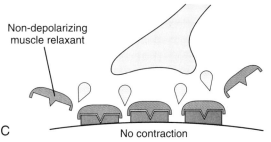

Figure **1–15.   Receptor site agonist and antagonist action: (A)** Acetyl-choline is a natural agonist. **(B)** Succinylcholine is a chemical agonist. **(C)** Nondepolarizing muscle relaxants act as antagonists.

Multiple drugs may cancel each other out or reduce each other's effects. A drug that enhances the effect of another drug is called a **synergist.** Some drug–drug interactions may cause a dramatic increase in the intended effect of the primary drug, as seen in aspirin–warfarin interactions.

Not all drug actions are receptor-type interactions. Antibiotics, for example, may interfere quite specifically with certain aspects of bacterial cell metabolism, such as penicillin inhibiting the formation of bacterial cell wall (see Chapter 5). Some drugs interact specifically with certain enzymes rather than receptor sites on a cell. A drug molecule may bind with a particular enzyme and either inhibit or stimulate the enzyme's activity to produce the desired effect.

An example of a nonspecific (i.e., not a drug–receptor complex) interaction is a drug molecule's ability to change the chemical environment surrounding the target cell. For example, mannitol—an osmotic diuretic—increases the osmotic pressure of urine; this means it reduces the reabsorption of water and produces large amounts of dilute urine. Antacids such as sodium bicarbonate chemically neutralize acid in the stomach. The anticoagulant heparin neutralizes the electric charge on a plasma protein that is needed to initiate blood clotting.

Several terms are used to clarify aspects of pharmacodynamics and the surgical technologist should become familiar with the common terms as applied to the surgical patient. The reason or purpose for giving a medication is called the **indication**, while reasons against giving a particular drug are called **contraindications.** For example, a particular antibiotic may be indicated for a bacterial infection, but is contraindicated when the patient has a known hypersensitivity to that antibiotic.

Some important terms should be understood regarding the timing of expected drug effects. The time between administration of a drug and the first appearance of effects is called the **onset.** The time between administration and maximum effect is called the time to peak effect. Steady state, or equilibrium, is achieved when the amount of drug entering the body is equal to the amount of drug being eliminated. The time between onset and disappearance of drug effects is called the **duration.**

A number of terms are used to describe the body's response or reaction to medications. A **side effect** is an expected but unintended effect of a drug. Side effects are rarely serious, but usually unavoidable. An example of a side effect is the drowsiness that often occurs when antihistamines are used.

Adverse effects are undesired, potentially harmful side effects of drugs. Adverse effects include drug toxicity, hypersensitivity, and idiosyncratic (unusual) reactions. Drug toxicity may be the result of accidental overdosing or failure of the body to process the drug properly, as seen in patients with kidney or liver dysfunction. In cases of drug toxicity, the primary effect of the drug may be exaggerated, such as excessive anticoagulation when taking coumarins. Some drugs may be particularly toxic to a specific organ, such as the liver, kidney, or even the ear. For example, some antibiotics are known to be ototoxic in high doses; that is, they have the potential to damage the hearing mechanism.

Drug **hypersensitivity** is an adverse effect resulting from previous exposure to the drug or a similar drug. A patient may become sensitized to a drug after one or more doses, then exhibit an allergic response on subsequent administration of the drug. An allergic response may be immediate, with symptoms ranging from mild to severe. Mild allergy symptoms include the appearance of raised patches on the skin (wheals) with itching, commonly known as hives. A severe allergic reaction, called anaphylaxis, can result in swollen bronchial passages and possible circulatory collapse (see Chapter 16). Delayed allergic reactions can occur days or weeks after a drug is taken and can include fever and joint swelling.

Another type of adverse effect is called **idiosyncratic.** Idiosyncratic drug effects are rare and unpredictable adverse reactions to drugs. Most idiosyncratic drug reactions are thought to occur in people with some genetic abnormality, causing either an excessive or an inadequate response to a drug. For example, malignant hyperthermia (see Chapter 16) is a life-threatening response to certain drugs, attributable to a genetic defect.

In the fascinating science of pharmacodynamics, some specific mechanisms of drug actions are known, but much remains to be discovered regarding many physiologic interactions involved in drug therapy.

ADVANCED PRACTICES FOR THE SURGICAL FIRST ASSISTANT
Chapter 1 — Basic Pharmacology

KEY TERMS

drug dependence   therapeutic levels
tachyphylaxis   tolerance

MEDICATION ORDERS

As a physician extender, one of the surgical first assistant's duties is to write out the physician's prescriptions and medication orders. Then the physician will clarify, verify, and sign them. It is imperative for the surgical first assistant to have a working knowledge of commonly accepted and

(continued on following page)

ADVANCED PRACTICES FOR THE SURGICAL FIRST ASSISTANT   *(continued)*

approved medical abbreviations and the basic components of a medication order. (See abbreviations in this chapter, and see Table 2–3 for the current listing of "do not use" abbreviations.)

A physician's medication orders and prescriptions, in addition to his or her signature, consist of the same components: *name* of the patient, *medication* name, medication *dosage,* the *route* of administration, the *frequency* or *time* of administration, and the *date* the order was written. For some orders, usually those found in the clinical setting, the *time* the order was written must also be included as well as any special notations. Notice the first five components are essentially the five rights of medication administration. (See the six "rights" and additional information in Chapter 4). To assure patient safety, these are closely checked every time a medication is prepared and administered. It is very important to include all components of the prescription or medication order; if any are omitted, the order is considered invalid and is not a legal order.

 CAUTION

All prescription pads must be secured in a safe location, no matter if they are in the clinical or office setting. The physician should never sign prescription blanks in advance.

The surgical first assistant may be involved in routine preoperative, immediate postoperative, and dismissal orders and/or prescriptions. For example, preoperative orders may include shaving the operative site and verifying the patient has had prophylactic antibiotics; immediate postoperative orders address monitoring vital signs, intravenous fluids, antibiotics, pain medications, and wound management such as bleeding, drains, and tubes. Dismissal orders may include pain medications, antibiotics, follow-up appointments, and wound care at home.

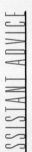 Traditionally there have been four clinically accepted vital signs: temperature, pulse, respirations, and blood pressure. To more accurately and efficiently assess the patient's needs, pain has been added to this group as a fifth vital sign.

 CAUTION

The international system of units (SI) abbreviations is used in this text. Note that milligram is abbreviated as mg, and milliliter as mL. These appear similar, but are *not* interchangeable.

ADVANCED PRACTICES FOR THE SURGICAL FIRST ASSISTANT   *(continued)*

Milligram (mg) is a unit of weight, whereas milliliter (mL) is a unit of volume. Confusing the two can have serious consequences in dosage calculations.

Medication Effects on the Patient

Medication **tolerance** is a phenomenon in which the body develops decreased responsiveness to a medication through repeated exposure to the agent. Many medications can produce tolerance but it is most commonly seen in opiates, and various other central nervous system (CNS) depressants. Tolerance can develop not only through the use of the medication but also to a medication with similar pharmacological properties (particularly those which act on the same receptor sites). Tolerance levels vary from person to person, and to maintain **therapeutic levels,** the physician may have to increase the dosage. Medication tolerance can be reversed by discontinuing the agent.

Another type of tolerance is termed **tachyphylaxis.** In this unique situation tolerance may occur after only one or two doses. Tachyphylaxis can develop very quickly; thus, the patient's initial response to the medication cannot be reproduced, even with a larger dose of the agent.

Drug Dependency

Because of a suggestion from the World Health Organization (WHO), the terms *addiction* and *habituation* have been replaced with the term **drug dependence.** This general term avoids the social stigma associated with drug abuse. Drug dependence is defined as a physiological and psychological compulsion to take medication periodically or continuously.

KEY CONCEPTS

- Knowledge of basic principles of pharmacology can provide the surgical technologist with a solid foundation on which to build an understanding of the many drugs used in surgery.
- Drug sources include natural sources such as plants, animals, and minerals, as well as drugs developed in the chemistry and molecular biology laboratory.
- Drug classification subcategories are helpful in identifying the purpose or use of a drug. Medication orders may be in various forms in surgery, and must be interpreted precisely. The surgical technologist should also be able to use different drug distribution systems, depending on the system in use at the clinical facility.
- Drugs come in many forms or preparations, and surgical technologists must be able to recognize the type needed for the intended purpose.

- Pharmacokinetics is the study of the four basic steps the body uses to process drugs: absorption, distribution, metabolism, and excretion.
- The study of how drugs exert their effects is called pharmacodynamics. Most drugs interact with receptors on target cell membranes to produce the desired effect.
- Many important terms are used to describe aspects of pharmacodynamics.

2

MEDICATION DEVELOPMENT, REGULATION, AND RESOURCES

Medications Covered in Chapter 2		
Generic Name	*Brand or Trade Name*	*Category*
alfentanyl	Alfenta	Opioid analgesic
cocaine	N/A	Narcotic and topical anesthetic
codeine	codeine	Narcotic
morphine	Astramorph	Narcotic
diazepam	Valium	Sedative
lorazepam	Ativan	Sedative
barbiturate	Solfoton	Barbiituate
zidovudine	ZVT, AZT	Anti-viral
laminvudine	3TC	Anti-viral
stavudine	d4T	Anti-viral
didanosine	ddl	Anti-viral
indinavir	IDV	Anti-viral
saquinavir	SQV	Anti-viral
cephalothin sodium	Keflin	Antibiotic
heparin sodium	heparin sodium	Anticoagulant
neomycin and polymixin B sulfates and hydrocortisone	Cortisporin	Antibiotic and steroid
furosemide	Lasix	Loop diuretic

OBJECTIVES

After completing this chapter, you should be able to:

1. Discuss federal and state roles in regulating drugs.
2. Define medication development and testing.
3. Discuss pharmacogenetics and pharmacogenomics.
4. Distinguish brand, generic, and chemical medication names.
5. List information found on medication labels.
6. Obtain medication information from pharmacology resources.

KEY TERMS

American Hospital Formulary
   Service (AHFS) drug
   information
contraindication
controlled substances
Drug Enforcement
   Administration (DEA)
Drug Facts and Comparisons

Food and Drug
   Administration (FDA)
indication
Joint Commission on
   Accreditation of
   Healthcare Organizations
   (JCAHO)
narcotics

over-the-counter (OTC)
PDR
pharmacogenetics/
   pharmacogenomics
prescription drugs
*United States Pharmacopoeia
   and National Formulary
   (USP/NF)*

A s a surgical technologist, you should be aware of federal, state, and local roles in regulating drugs and their administration. In this chapter, then, we'll present a broad overview of federal drug legislation and federal agencies and a general discussion of state and local regulations. Because new medications are approved for use regularly, we'll also briefly consider the process that leads to this approval—testing, study, and using genetic technology. Finally, we'll look at available medication references, which will help you obtain information useful to your practice as a surgical technologist.

MEDICATION REGULATION

Before the 20th century, medications of all kinds were sold freely in the United States, both to physicians and consumers. Thus, neither physician nor consumer had any real proof of the medication's safety or effectiveness. There was also no legal requirement for a physician's prescription. This situation began to change early in the 1900s, when the federal government stepped in to protect consumers and to regulate the pharmaceutical industry. The states, too, established practice acts to regulate the dispensing and administration of medications.

FEDERAL LAWS

Federal regulation of medications was initially intended to protect consumers from harmful, impure, untested, and unsafe medications. Thus, when the Pure Food and Drug Act was passed in 1906, it set standards for quality and required the proper labeling of medications. In 1938, the federal government began to address drug effectiveness. It passed the Food, Drug, and Cosmetic Act, which required animal testing of medications. Now prior to selling a new medication, pharmaceutical companies had to apply for approval to market the medication, and that approval was contingent on proof that the medication was effective on animals. The Durham-Humphrey Amendments to the Food, Drug, and Cosmetic Act were passed in 1952. These amendments required a physician's order to dispense certain medications, called **prescription drugs,** and established an **over-the-counter (OTC)** category of medications that did not require a prescription. Then, in 1970, the Controlled Substance Act was passed. It designated certain medications as **controlled substances.** See Table 2–1 for a summary of federal drug laws.

The Controlled Substances Act of 1970 established classifications, known as schedules, of medications that had potential for abuse. Five schedules (Table 2–2) were determined, based on the level of abuse and dependence potential and on appropriate medical uses for the medication. Drugs such as LSD are listed on the C-I schedule; they have high abuse potential and no accepted medical use. Controlled substances from the C-II schedule have high abuse potential, but also have accepted medical uses, as in the surgical setting. C-II controlled substances that are frequently used in surgery include alfentanyl, cocaine, and morphine. Medications listed as C-III have moderate abuse potential, while medications on schedules C-IV and C-V have low abuse potential.

In 1983, the **Drug Enforcement Administration (DEA)** of the Department of Justice was established to enforce the Controlled Substances Act. It sets standards for handling controlled substances and has the legal authority to enforce those standards. Institutional policies and procedures for storing and handling controlled substances must comply with DEA standards, and documentation requirements must be strictly followed. When hospitals administer **narcotics,** for example, they must keep careful records of the amount of medication used as well as the date, the patient, the person administering the medication, and the person obtaining it.

Table 2–1 Federal Drug Laws

Pure Food and Drug Act of 1906

- Required all drugs marketed in the United States to meet minimal standards of uniform strength, purity, and quality
- Required that preparations containing morphine be labeled
- Established two references of officially approved drugs: the *United States Pharmacopoeia* (*USP*) and the *National Formulary* (*NF*)*

Federal Food, Drug, and Cosmetic Act (1938; amended in 1952 and 1965)

- Established the Food and Drug Administration (FDA)
- Established specific regulations regarding warning labels on preparations, e.g., cautions about a drug's capacity to cause drowsiness or become habit-forming
- Stated that both prescription and nonprescription drugs must be effective and safe
- Stated that all labels must be accurate and include the generic name
- Required FDA approval of all new drugs
- Designated which drugs could be sold over the counter, i.e., without a prescription

Controlled Substances Act of 1970

- Established the Drug Enforcement Agency (DEA)
- Set tighter controls on drugs capable of being abused (controlled substances), e.g., depressants, stimulants, and narcotics
- Required stricter security controls for anyone (physicians, pharmacists, hospitals) who dispenses, receives, sells, or destroys controlled substances
- Set limits on the use of prescriptions, established guidelines for the number of times a drug can be prescribed in a period of time, and set rules on which preparations may be prescribed over the telephone to the pharmacy
- Required that each prescriber register with the DEA, obtaining a DEA number to be used on prescriptions
- Identified abusable and addicting drugs, classifying them into schedules according to the degree of danger

*These two publications have since been combined and are referred to as the *USP/NF*.

Table 2–2 Schedules of Controlled Substances

Schedule	Examples	Description
C-I	Heroin, LSD, PCP, marijuana	Drugs with high abuse potential. No accepted medical use.
C-II	Alfentanyl, opium, cocaine, codeine, morphine	High potential for drug abuse. Accepted medical use, but can lead to physical and psychological dependency.
C-III	Anabolic steroids, products with low amounts of codeine	Potential for drug abuse less than previous categories. Medically accepted for use.
C-IV	Diazepam, lorazepam, Phenobarbital	Potential for dependency. Medically accepted for use.
C-V	Many antitussive and antidiarrheal agents	Very limited potential for dependence. Medically accepted for use. Many are over-the-counter medications.

Federal Agencies

Two federal agencies contribute policies for the safety of health care workers (and of the public), and these policies can influence drug regulation in the health care field. The Occupational Safety and Health Administration (OSHA) is an agency within the U.S. Department of Labor. OSHA's mission is to assure the safety and health of American workers by setting and enforcing standards. An example of how OSHA interacts with surgical technologists is the Occupational Exposure to Bloodborne Pathogens Standard, which went into effect in 2001. OSHA estimates that between 590,000 and 800,000 needle sticks and sharps injuries occur annually, which put people (including surgical technologists) at risk for contracting hepatitis B, hepatitis C, and the human immunodeficiency virus (HIV). This standard states each employer must have a plan that ensures immediate and confidential postexposure treatment and follow-up procedures in accordance with current CDC guidelines. The CDC, or the Centers for Disease Control and Prevention, is an agency under the U.S. Department of Health and Human Services. The CDC is recognized as the leading federal agency for protecting the health and safety of people and for providing credible information to enhance health decisions. It serves as the national focus for developing and applying disease prevention and control. In 1995, the CDC issued a report of a study recommending prophylactic medication treatment as soon as possible after a needle stick or sharps injury (less than 2 hours from the time of exposure). This report and policy are of importance to surgical technologists. Although these medications are not found in the surgical setting, they should be familiar to those who are health care workers at risk. The policy recommends a regimen of zidovudine (ZDV, previously called AZT) in divided doses and laminvudine (3TC). Two other medication regimens are also suggested: laminvudine (3TC) and stavudine (d4T), or didanosine (ddl) and stavudine (d4T). In addition, a third medication may be added to the regimen, indinavir (IDV) or saquinavir (SQV), for exposures with the highest risk of HIV transmission.

☞ **Note:** You must be familiar with and strictly follow needle stick/sharps injuries protocol as set forth by your surgical technology program and also all policies relating to these incidents at your clinical sites.

STATE PRACTICE ACTS

State laws known as *practice acts* govern ordering, dispensing, and administration of medications. Such laws vary from state to state. For example, state laws regulate who—physicians, physician assistants, nurse practitioners—may prescribe drugs. They also regulate pharmacy practices, specifying how medications are to be dispensed and by whom (usually a licensed pharmacist). Drug substitution laws, for example, specify if a pharmacist may automatically substitute a generic equivalent for a prescribed medication if not indicated otherwise.

Physicians can "lend" or delegate some of their functions to others. For example, the surgical technologist functions as a "physician extender"—an extra pair of hands, so to speak. As such, he or she performs medication-handling duties under the delegatory power of the physician. Each state controls the limits of this delegatory power through the Medical Licensing Board.

☞ **Note:** As a surgical technologist, you should be knowledgeable about the medication handling and administration laws in your state. State practice acts are public information; thus to be correctly informed, you can read these acts yourself. This is important because the delegatory power and its interpretations differ from state to state. For instance, many people believe that only nurses may administer medications to patients. However, in many states, credentialed allied health professionals such as perfusionists, respiratory therapists, and medical assistants routinely administer medications legally. Surgical technologists must have direct knowledge of, and function within, the legal standards of medication administration determined by the state in which they practice.

LOCAL POLICIES

When state laws do not specifically address the practice of surgical technology, published institutional policies should be used to determine the scope of practice. The role of the surgical technologist in drug handling is usually specified in institutional policies, which have local authority. The surgical technologist must be thoroughly familiar with medication administration policies and closely adhere to the stated limits. If current policies are outdated or do not reflect the scope of practice appropriate to the education and expertise of the surgical technologist, the institution should revise or update them as appropriate. The surgical technologist's job description may also contain relevant information regarding medication handling and administration.

⚠ CAUTION

Under no circumstances should a surgical technologist exceed the limits of the facility's published job description. These job descriptions are subject to revision as needed to reflect current practice standards.

JCAHO

The **Joint Commission on Accreditation of Healthcare Organizations (JCAHO)** evaluates and accredits approximately 16,000 health care organizations and programs in the United States. These organizations include general and rehabilitation hospitals, critical access hospitals, ambulatory care providers such as outpatient surgery centers and office-based surgery facilities. Thus JCAHO is the predominant standards-setting organization, and facilities that obtain its accreditation demonstrate their commitment to meeting certain performance standards.

Among JCAHO's standards are National Patient Safety Goals. These goals are established annually and address issues such as infection control, Universal Protocol for Preventing Wrong Site, Wrong Procedure, Wrong Person Surgery™, and medical errors. Beginning January 1, 2004, these goals were expanded to include a list of "dangerous" abbreviations, acronyms, and symbols that should not be used in the clinical setting. This is an effort to improve the effectiveness of communication among caregivers and to address the many inherent problems associated with misread abbreviations that contribute to medication errors. This list applies to all handwritten, patient-specific documentation, computer, and preprinted forms. Accredited facilities are required to develop a "do not use" list and must include terms as specified by JCAHO (Table 2–3). Many facilities not only include these required terms but have expanded their lists. It is important to check at your facility for its "do not use" list.

DRUG DEVELOPMENT

Prior to legal regulation, drugs could be manufactured, sold, and administered without scientific proof of safety, quality, or effectiveness. Today, all drugs must undergo stringent testing and provide proof of safety and effectiveness before release. The federal **Food and Drug Administration (FDA)** regulates the pharmaceutical industry, ensuring that basic standards are followed. To do this, the FDA inspects the facilities where drugs are made, reviews new drug applications, investigates and removes unsafe drugs from the market, and requires proper labeling of drugs.

Table 2–3 JCAHO's "Do Not Use" List of Abbreviations and Symbols

Dangerous Abbreviations	Potential Problem	Preferred Term
U for unit	Mistaken for zero, 4, or cc	Write "unit"
IU for international unit	Mistaken for IV (intravenous) or 10	Write "international unit"
Q.D., Q.O.D. (Latin abbreviations for once daily and every other day)	Mistaken for each other	Write "daily" and "every other day"
Trailing zero (as $X.0$ mg) or lack of a leading zero (.X mg)	Decimal point is missed leading to a 10-fold overdose	Never write a single zero after a decimal point (X mg), and always use a zero before a decimal point (0.X mg)
MS, MSO$_4$, MgSO$_4$	Confused for one another. Can mean morphine sulfate or magnesium sulfate	Write "morphine sulfate" or "magnesium sulfate"

JCAHO's Recommended Terms to Add to the "Do Not Use" List

μ for microgram	Mistaken for mg (milligrams) resulting in 1000-fold overdose	Write "mcg"
H.S. (for half strength, or the Latin abbreviation for sleep at bedtime)	Mistaken for either half strength or hour of sleep	Write "half strength"
q.H.S.	Mistaken for every hour	Write "at bedtime"
c.c. (for cubic centimeter)	Mistaken for U (units) if poorly written	Write "mL" for milliliters
A.S., A.D., A.U. (Latin abbreviations for left, right, and both ears)	Mistaken for each other	Write "left ear," "right ear," or "both ears"
O.S., O.D., O.U. (Latin abbreviations for left, right, and both eyes)	Mistaken for each other	Write "left eye," "right eye," or "both eyes"
S.C. or S.Q. for subcutaneous	Mistaken for SL for *sublingual* or "5 every . . ."	Write "Sub Q" or "subcutaneously"
T.I.W. (for three times weekly)	Mistaken for three times a day, or twice weekly	Write "3 times weekly" or "three times weekly"
D/C (for discharge)	Interpreted as discontinue (typically used for discharge medicines)	Write "discharge"

FDA PREGNANCY CATEGORIES

The FDA has developed a classification system related to medication effects on the unborn child, or fetus. This classification is useful for surgical medications in some medical situations: for example, a pregnant woman who develops acute appendicitis and requires surgery. In medication literature and reference books, most medications have a pregnancy category listed. Categories A and B are considered to be within safe limits for medication use during pregnancy, with special attention given to the first trimester of the pregnancy (the first three months) (Table 2–4).

Pharmaceutical companies are continually developing new medications, and each must undergo required testing prior to FDA approval. This testing is an extensive process. All new medications are first tested on animals to determine if it is safe to administer to humans. At least two species of mammals of both genders, must be used for this initial stage of drug testing. During this process, researchers look for toxic effects and determine safe dosage levels. Once the medication has proven safe in animals, the drug company applies to the FDA for permission to begin human testing, which consists of four phases (see Insight 2–1).

Table **2–4**   FDA Pregnancy Categories

Category	Description
A	No risk to fetus per studies.
B	No risk in animal studies, and well-controlled studies in pregnant women not available. It is assumed there is little or no risk.
C	Animal studies a risk to the fetus. Controlled studies on pregnant women not available. Risk versus benefit of the drug must be determined.
D	A risk to the human fetus has been proved. Risk versus benefit must be determined.
X	A risk to the human fetus has been proved. Risk outweighs the benefit, and drug should be avoided during pregnancy.

Source: www.fda.gov.

Insight 2–1   **Phases of Human Medication Testing**

Phase I: Clinical pharmacology—In the clinical pharmacology phase, the new medication is given to healthy volunteers, usually males between the ages of 18 and 45. This phase is used to determine the dose level for symptoms of medication toxicity in humans.

Phase II: Clinical investigation—In the clinical investigation phase, the medication is given to limited numbers of patients with the disease or condition the medication was developed to treat. The clinical investigation phase is used to establish medication effectiveness and to determine optimum dosage and dose range.

Phase III: Clinical trials—In the clinical trial phase, researchers continue to note medication effectiveness, safety, and side effects in large studies. In this phase, which begins only if no serious side effects occur in Phase II, the new medication is given to hundreds or thousands of patients, usually in large medical research facilities. The medication's effectiveness is verified and its actions are characterized by various types of scientific studies. Several kinds of studies may be conducted. For instance, in *double-blind studies,* half of the testing group receives the medication and the other half receives an inactive substance called a placebo. Neither the subject patients nor the prescribing physicians know which group received the placebo until the study has been completed. The results of these and other studies must be thoroughly documented.

Phase IV: Postmarketing study—The postmarketing study phase occurs after the medication is released for use in treatment of the specified condition. In this phase the drug company continues to monitor the medication, gathering results from prescribing physicians. This continuing evaluation of the medication includes results from those patients excluded from the previous phases, such as pregnant patients and the elderly. To document the medication's safety and effectiveness comprehensively, these data must be gathered, analyzed, and reported to the FDA.

Technology in the 21st century is allowing scientists and pharmaceutical companies to test medications in a different way. **Pharmacogenetics** is the study of genetic factors in predicting a medication's action and how it could vary from its intended response. The term combines *pharmaceuticals* and *genetics*. Pharmacogenetics is vital technology, because people have different genetic makeups and do not respond identically to medication dosage or intended therapy. Genetic factors can alter the metabolism of a medication and either enhance or diminish its action. Thus, a patient can have a positive response, a negative response, or no response at all to a medication. **Pharmacogenomics** is the general study of all genes that determine medication behavior. However, the distinction between these two terms is so slight that they are used interchangeably. As technology allows scientists to catalog more genetic variations found within the human genome, pharmaceutical companies can create medications based upon this knowledge. This could facilitate new medication discovery, develop "drug markers" to target specific diseases, revive previously failed medication candidates and match them with a specific population, and facilitate the medication approval process which would lower the costs and risks of clinical trials. The drawbacks to pharmacogenetics are the complexity and cost of genetic research, and educating health care providers in the use of this technology.

MARKETING

During development, the drug company assigns a generic name to the new medication. Later, it selects a company trade name, which it uses for marketing purposes once the medication gains FDA approval. The ***United States Pharmacopoeia and National Formulary (USP/NF)*** assigns an official name to the new medication; this is usually the generic name. Once a drug has been approved for release, the pharmaceutical company responsible for the medication's development has exclusive rights to market that medication under its trade name for 17 years. This process allows the drug company to recover development costs. After these exclusive rights have expired, other companies may begin to market a generic equivalent with a different trade name.

MEDICATION LABELING

As previously mentioned, the Federal Pure Food and Drug Act of 1906 established guidelines for proper labeling of medications. It is important to correctly obtain (read) the information found on medication labels. Clearly, surgical technologists do not directly administer medications to the patient. However, you will be obtaining medications for the sterile field and will play an important part in correct medication identification and avoiding medication errors. Medication labels display pertinent information that the surgical technologist must read and interpret accurately.

Brand and generic names of the medication: The manufacturer's name for a medication is called the brand, trade, or proprietary name. It is selected by the pharmaceutical manufacturer and used to market the medication. It is usually the most prominent word on the label. It may be in large or bold type and is very visible to promote the product. The name is followed by the ® sign, which means that the name and the formula are registered. Directly under the brand name is the generic, or nonproprietary, name in lowercase letters. The generic name is not owned by any one company, so it is not capitalized. On some labels the generic name may be placed inside parenthesis. By law, the generic name must be identified on all medication labels. On the Keflin® label, the brand name appears in large letters set off in a black background. The generic name is *cephalothin sodium* and is printed underneath the brand name.

☞ **Note:** Each medication has several names—usually its brand name, its generic name, and its chemical name. The chemical name has meaning for chemists. It is a precise, systematic description of the chemical composition and molecular structure of the medication. Chemical names can be found in references such as the *Physician's Desk Reference,* but are not normally found on medication labels.

⚠ CAUTION

On some medication labels, only the generic name appears. Be sure to cross-check medication names if you are unsure of their generic equivalents. Many generic spellings are very similar, yet the medications are vastly different and an error could be fatal to the patient. Also, it is important to recognize that some variations may exist between generic medications produced by different manufacturers.

Manufacturer's name: This is also displayed on the label to advertise the company. See the word "Lilly" on the Keflin® label.

Dosage strength: This number on the label refers to dosage weight or the amount of the medication in a specific unit of measurement. On the Keflin® label, the dosage strength of medication in the bottle is given as 1 gram (1 g).

Form: This identifies the composition of the medication. As discussed in Chapter 1, solid forms are tablets and capsules. Some are in powdered or granular form and can be combined with

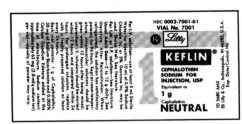

Figure **2–1.**   Keflin label. *(From Ogden SJ: Calculation of Drug Dosages, 7th ed. St Louis, Mosby, 2003.)*

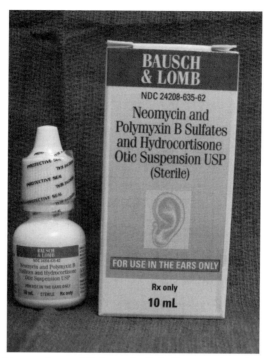

Figure **2–2.**   Neomycin and Polymyxin B Sulfates and Hydrocortisone Otic Suspension USP label.

food or beverages. This is usually found in the medical rather than the surgical setting as for postoperative pain medications that the patient can take at home. Other medications must be reconstituted, or liquefied by being dissolved in a solution such as sterile water or sterile normal saline. These medications are then measured in an exact liquid volume such as milliliters (mL) or cubic centimeters (cc). They may be crystalloid (a clear solution) or a suspension (solid particles in a liquid that separate in the container). On the neomycin and polymyxin B label, the word *suspension* tells us the solution must be shaken to distribute the particles before it is administered to the patient (as discussed in Chapter 1). Other medication forms include creams, patches, and suppositories.

Supply dosage: This refers to dosage strength and medication form. Read it as "x measured units per quantity." For liquid medications, the supply dosage is the same as the medication's concentration. On the heparin sodium label, there are 1000 units per milliliter of solution. Note also that heparin sodium

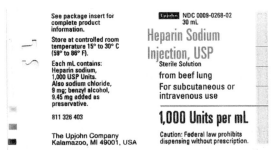

Figure **2–3.**   Heparin sodium label. *(From Morris DG: Calculate with Confidence, 3rd ed. St Louis, Mosby, 2002.)*

is the generic name of the medication and so has no ® registration mark.

Total volume: This is the full quantity contained in the bottle or vial, or its total fluid volume. For solids it is the total number of individual items in the package. On the heparin label, there is a total volume of 30 mL, because this medication is in liquid form.

Administration route: This refers to the method of medication delivery to the patient or body site. Refer to Chapter 4 for further information on medication administration. On the neomycin and polymyxin B label, it states for use in the ears only. The Keflin® label states for injection and the heparin lists subcutaneous or intravenous use.

Label alerts: Manufacturers may print warnings on the packages such as "refrigerate" or "protect from light." Suspension medications would carry the warning to "shake well before use" as found on the neomycin and polymyxin B label.

Expiration date: Medications should be used, discarded, or returned to the pharmacy by this date. This is very important information as is usually presented as a month/year (as 5/05 on the Lasix® label), which would indicate the medication can be used until the last day of May 2005. If this medication were obtained from pharmacy for a procedure, it should not be used, because it is outdated. It should be returned to the pharmacy and another obtained with a date that is not past.

Lot or control numbers: Federal law requires all medication packages to be identified with a lot or control number. If a medication is recalled this number identifies the specific group of packages to be removed from shelves. The Lasix® label gives the lot number as 44570.

Barcode symbols: Used in sales, barcodes document medication dosing for recordkeeping. They may have future use to auto-

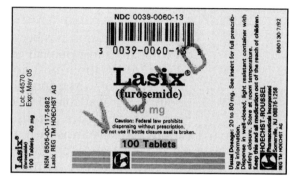

Figure **2–4.**   Lasix label. *(From Ogden SJ: Calculation of Drug Dosages, 7th ed. St Louis, Mosby, 2003.)*

mate medication documentation to the patient's bedside, much like the scanners are used in stores today. You can see a barcode on the Lasix® label.

National Drug Code (NDC): Federal law requires every prescription medication to have an identifying number. It must appear on every manufacturer's label and is printed as NDC ●●●●-●●●●-●●. Note the code on the top of the Keflin® label as NDC 0002-7001-01.

United States Pharmacopeia (USP) and National Formulary (NF): These codes are found on manufacturer-printed labels. These are two official national lists of approved medications. Each manufacturer follows special guidelines that determine when to include these initials on the label. Initials are placed after the generic drug name. Note the initials on the heparin sodium and Keflin® labels.

Insight 2–2   **Medications Under the Labels**

The medications used as examples in the medication-labeling section are ones you will see used in the surgical setting, or for the surgical patient. The first medication, Keflin®, is an antibiotic. It may be used preoperatively, intraoperatively, or postoperatively to help fight infections. Refer to Chapter 5 for more on antibiotics. The next medication, neomycin and polymyxin B sulfates otic drops, is also an antibiotic with other medications mixed in, that is hydrocortisone. Hydrocortisone is a steroid used to decrease the body's inflammatory response. Refer to Chapter 5 and also Chapter 8. The next, heparin sodium, is an anticoagulant that is used on vascular procedures. Refer to Chapter 9 for more on medications that affect the vascular system. The last medication mentioned is Lasix®, a diuretic. It is used in neurosurgery to decrease intracranial pressure. Refer to Chapter 7 for more on diuretics and their actions.

MEDICATION REFERENCES

When a medication has been approved for use, the pharmaceutical company must publish comprehensive information regarding it. This information must appear in package inserts and in compiled reference works. In addition, many medication information resources are available to medical, nursing, and allied health professionals. There are dozens of textbooks on pharmacology and various specialty areas within that science. Moreover, several pharmacology resources are expressly designed for use in clinical practice. Each surgery department should have such references readily available to the staff.

PHYSICIAN'S DESK REFERENCE

One of the most frequently used pharmacology resources is the *Physician's Desk Reference,* or **PDR.** It provides easy access to information on several thousand medications used in medical and surgical practice. The *PDR* is published annually and contains color-coded sections:

1. A list of drug manufacturers
2. An index of brand and generic drug names
3. A list of drugs by prescribing category
4. A photographic identification section
5. A product information section
6. A section on diagnostic agents.

The product information section, which is the largest part of the book, contains manufacturer's information on approximately 3000 medications. Medications are listed alphabetically by manufacturer. Each entry includes data on **indications**, effects, dosage, administration routes, methods, and frequency. It also includes warnings regarding side effects and **contraindications.** The *PDR* also publishes separate references for nonprescription medications and ophthalmic medications. Its website at http://www.pdr.net/pdrnet/librarian refers readers to a free patient resource at http://www.pdrhealth.com/ and also offers subscribers a MobilePDR®.

☞ **Note:** The information presented in the *PDR* is the same as that found in the manufacturer's package insert. Students may easily obtain package inserts for medications used in surgery. You can get them as medications are opened or from the pharmacy at your clinical site.

UNITED STATES PHARMACOPOEIA AND NATIONAL FORMULARY

The *USP/NF* is the official medication list recognized by the U.S. government. It is actually two publications—the *Pharmacopoeia* and the *Formulary*—combined into one volume. The *USP/NF* lists standards for medication quality, safety, and effectiveness; it also contains information on the physical and chemical characteristics of listed medications. Used primarily by drug companies and pharmacists, the *USP/NF* is revised every five years. It is prepared under the supervision of a national committee of pharmacists, pharmacologists, physicians, chemists, biologists, and other scientific professionals. The *United States Pharmacopeic-Drug Information (USP-DI)* is a related clinical reference divided into three volumes—volumes IA and IB provide medication information for health care providers. These include pharmacology, precautions to consider, side and adverse effects, and general dosing information. Volume II gives medication information directed to the patient (client). It is written in understandable language and includes administration of medications, medication effects, indications, adverse reactions, guidelines for dosages, and what to do for missed doses. It should be noted there is also an *International Pharmacopeia,* which is revised every five years. It was first published in 1951 by the World Health Organization (WHO) and appears in English, Spanish, and French.

AMERICAN HOSPITAL FORMULARY SERVICE (AHFS) DRUG INFORMATION

This reference is published annually by the American Society of Health-System Pharmacists in Bethesda, Md. The **AHFS** provides accurate information on almost all prescription medications marketed in the United States. Medications are listed according to therapeutic medication classification. The information includes chemistry and stability, pharmacologic actions, pharmacokinetics, uses, cautions and precautions, contraindications, drug interactions, acute toxicity, dosage and administration, and preparation of the medications. This text is considered unbiased because as it does not contain information supplied only by the pharmaceutical company that manufactures the medications.

THE MEDICAL LETTER

The *Medical Letter,* on medications and therapeutics, is published biweekly by the Medical Letter, Inc. in New York. This is a nonprofit publication for physicians and other allied health professionals. Each issue covers one of two topics: medications for the treatment of diseases such as HIV or two to four new medications recently approved by the FDA. The information includes pharmacokinetics, clinical studies, dosage, adverse effects and interactions.

DRUG FACTS AND COMPARISONS

Drug Facts and Comparisons is a loose-leaf reference book that contains thousands of prescription and OTC medications and thousands of comparison charts and tables. It is a reference for drug actions, indications, warnings and precautions, dosage and route of administration, adverse reactions, overdosage, interactions, contraindications, and patient (client) information. Medications are grouped by therapeutic category, and the resource also includes information on investigational medications. *Drug Facts and Comparisons* is available with an annual subscription that includes monthly updates via a newsletter.

HOSPITAL PHARMACIST

Another valuable source of information on drugs is the clinical pharmacist. Consulting and educating has become an important part of pharmacy practice. The pharmacist is consulted when any question arises regarding medications, especially those which are newly approved.

DATABASES

A vast amount of information regarding medications, their proper use, possible drug side effects and interactions, and other important clinical considerations is available via computer. Databases, such as Micromedex and CliniSphere, are helpful tools that medical professionals use to access current pharmacologic information. The Internet also allows you to access medication information. Helpful Internet sites include the following:

- American College of Clinical Pharmacy
- American Heart Association
- American Medical Association
- Centers for Disease Control and Prevention
- Drug Facts and Comparisons
- Drug Store News
- Internet Drug Index
- National Cancer Institute (CancerNet)
- National Institute of Health (NIH)
- National Library of Medicine
- Occupational Safety and Health Administration
- Pharm Web
- Pharmaceutical Information Network
- Pharmacy Times

- RX List
- RX Med
- U.S. Pharmacist
- U.S. Pharmacopeia
- World Health Organization

Keep in mind that medication information can be posted on the Internet by anyone, so the information may not always be accurate. It is a good idea to check reliable sources such as governmental websites, and always verify information from two different sources. Other drug resource material is easily accessible by computer, including the *USPDI, PDR,* current journal articles, and manufacturers' bulletins.

KEY CONCEPTS

- Federal regulations of medications protect consumers.
- The Federal Pure Food and Drug Act set standards for quality and proper medication labeling.
- The Food, Drug, and Cosmetic Act requires animal testing of medications.
- The Controlled Substances Act established schedules for medications.
- The Drug Enforcement Administration (DEA) enforces the Controlled Substances Act.
- The Food and Drug Administration (FDA) developed a classification system related to medications' effects on the unborn child.
- State practice acts govern the ordering, dispersal, and administration of medications.
- The role of the surgical technologist in medication handling may be specified by institutional policy.
- The Joint Commission on Accreditation of Health Organizations (JCAHO) evaluates and accredits health care facilities and sets policies such as National Patient Safety Goals.
- Genetic factors are being used to predict a medication's action on patients, thus being useful in medication development.
- Medications must undergo testing that involves several phases (including animal testing) before being given FDA approval.
- Numerous medication references and databases that include the Internet can be accessed for information.

3

PHARMACOLOGY MATH

OBJECTIVES

After completing this chapter, you should be able to:

1. Convert civilian time to military time.
2. Define terminology, abbreviations, and symbols used in basic mathematics and measurement systems.
3. Use fractions in conversions and calculations.
4. Read and write decimals accurately.
5. Use decimals in conversions and calculations.
6. Convert between fractions and decimals.
7. Define percentages.
8. Convert between percentages and decimals and between percentages and fractions.
9. Define ratios and proportions.
10. Use ratios and proportions to solve problems.
11. Convert temperatures between the Fahrenheit and Celsius scales.
12. Define the metric system of measurement and explain how it is used as the international standard.
13. Identify other systems of measurement and their medical applications.
14. Identify symbols of measurement and measurement equivalents.

KEY TERMS

Celsius scale   metric system
civilian time   military time
decimal point   percent
exponent   proportion
Fahrenheit scale   ratio
fraction

In this chapter we look at basic mathematics, including military time, fractions, decimals, percents, and ratios and proportions. We review how to solve simple problems, perform fundamental calculations, and make important conversions. Many surgical technology students are familiar with these principles; this chapter is designed as a refresher for students who need to practice their mathematical skills. Each rule is explained, and then examples are given to illustrate its principle. In addition there are exercises, including specific surgical technology story problems, for students to practice the mathematical operations in the accompanying study guide. This chapter also introduces students to measurement systems and how they are used in the medical setting. Students use basic mathematical skills to perform conversions in the systems of measurement. Knowledge of metric measurements and basic mathematical skills are necessary in pharmacology as they are used during surgical procedures, particularly when using implants, grafts, and assisting the surgeon as he or she administers medications from the sterile field.

MILITARY TIME

Hospitals and other medical institutions, along with law enforcement and the military, use a precise method of expressing time called international or **military time**. Military time uses a 24-hour scale without AM or PM designations. It is similar to **civilian time** in the morning hours from midnight until noon. After noon, it increases in one-hour increments from 12, whereas civilian time starts over again with 1.

To convert military time to civilian time after noon, subtract 12. For example, 1900 hours becomes 7 PM (19 − 12 = 7). To convert civilian time to military time after noon, add 12. For example, 1 PM becomes 1300 hours (1 + 12 = 13).

Military time is pronounced differently from civilian time. For example, 5 AM in civilian time, or 5 o'clock in the morning, is

Table **3–1** Military and Civilian Times			
Civilian Time	*Military Time*	*Civilian Time*	*Military Time*
Midnight*	0000	Noon	1200
1:00 AM	0100	1:00 PM	1300
2:00 AM	0200	2:00 PM	1400
3:00 AM	0300	3:00 PM	1500
4:00 AM	0400	4:00 PM	1600
5:00 AM	0500	5:00 PM	1700
6:00 AM	0600	6:00 PM	1800
7:00 AM	0700	7:00 PM	1900
8:00 AM	0800	8:00 PM	2000
9:00 AM	0900	9:00 PM	2100
10:00 AM	1000	10:00 PM	2200
11:00 AM	1100	11:00 PM	2300

*Midnight can be written two ways in military time: 2400 and read as "twenty-four hundred," or 0000 and read as "zero hundred."

0500 in military time and is pronounced "oh-five-hundred" or "zero-five-hundred." In surgery, a procedure scheduled for 4 o'clock in the afternoon would be "sixteen hundred hours" (1600) in military time. If the incision for this 4 o'clock case is made at 4:46 PM, it would be written as 1646 and pronounced "sixteen forty-six hours" in military time. Table 3–1 provides conversions between civilian and military times.

What if an event occurs at 9 minutes after midnight? In civilian time it would be written as 12:09 AM. In military time, it would be written as 0009 and pronounced "zero-zero-zero-nine hours." If the event occurs at 9 minutes after noon, in civilian time it would be written as 12:09 PM. In military time, it would be written as 1209 and pronounced "twelve-oh-nine hours."

☞ **Note:** Midnight can be written two ways in military time: 2400 and pronounced "twenty four hundred," or 0000 and pronounced "zero hundred hours."

FRACTIONS

A **fraction** is a number that represents one or more equal parts of a whole. The word comes from the Latin *fractio*, which means "to break into pieces." A fraction is a quotient—a number that can be written in an a/b or $\frac{a}{b}$ form, where b is never equal to 0. We say that a and b are the terms of the fraction where a is the numerator and b is the denominator.

EXAMPLE
_____

One half = 1/2 = $\frac{1}{2}$ =

$\frac{1}{2}$ $a = 1$ is the numerator
     $b = 2$ is the denominator

Five sixths = 5/6 = $\frac{5}{6}$ =

$\frac{5}{6}$ $a = 5$ is the numerator
     $b = 6$ is the denominator

Five eighths = 5/8 = $\frac{5}{8}$ =

$\frac{5}{8}$ $a = 5$ is the numerator
     $b = 8$ is the denominator

We use fractions to express division of a whole into equal parts:
- The denominator tells how many equal parts into which the whole is divided.
- The numerator tells how many equal parts we are interested in.

EXAMPLE
_____

Imagine a pie divided into 6 equal parts, and 5 of those equal parts are eaten.

$\frac{5}{6}$ number of eaten parts
     number of equal parts into which the whole pie is divided

So
- $\frac{5}{6}$ of the pie is eaten
- $\frac{1}{6}$ of the pie remains

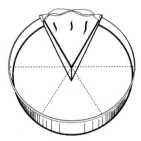

Figure 3–1.

The larger the denominator, the smaller the pieces (fractions) in the whole.

☞ Note:

    $\frac{1}{2}$ greater than $\frac{1}{3}$
    $\frac{1}{3}$ is greater than $\frac{1}{4}$
    $\frac{1}{4}$ is greater than $\frac{1}{5}$
    $\frac{1}{3}$ is greater than $\frac{1}{6}$

and so on.

EXAMPLE
_____

Imagine a circle divided into 8 equal parts, and 5 of those equal parts are shaded:

$\frac{5}{8}$ number of shaded equal parts

number of equal parts into which the whole circle is divided

So
- $\frac{5}{8}$ of the circle is shaded
- $\frac{3}{8}$ of the circle is not shaded

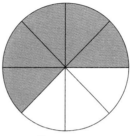

Figure **3–2.**

If the numerator and the denominator are equal to each other, the fraction is equal to 1.

EXAMPLES
_____

$\frac{1}{1} =$ $\frac{2}{2} =$ $\frac{5}{5} =$ $\frac{100}{100} =$ $\frac{3569}{3569} = 1$

If the numerator is less than the denominator, the value of the fraction is less than 1. Then the fraction is a proper fraction.

EXAMPLES
_____

$\frac{2}{3}$ $\frac{3}{4}$ $\frac{3}{5}$ $\frac{99}{100}$

If the numerator is greater than the denominator, the value of the fraction is more than 1. Then the fraction is an improper fraction.

EXAMPLES
_____

$\frac{3}{2}$ $\frac{4}{3}$ $\frac{12}{6}$ $\frac{15}{10}$

A mixed number is a combination of a whole number with a fraction.

EXAMPLES

$1\frac{1}{2}$ $2\frac{1}{3}$ $5\frac{3}{7}$ $8\frac{49}{50}$

☞ **Note:** Anytime the numerator of a fraction is zero, the value of the fraction is zero.

You can change a mixed number to an improper fraction in three steps. Given the mixed number $2\frac{1}{2}$,
Step 1: Multiply the denominator of the fraction by the whole number:

$$\text{Whole number} \times \text{denominator} = 2 \times 2 = 4$$

Step 2: Add the numerator to the result obtained in Step 1:

$$\text{Numerator} + (\text{Step 1 result}) = 1 + 4 = 5$$

Step 3: Use the result obtained in Step 2 as the numerator of the new fraction; use the original denominator as the new denominator:

$$\frac{\text{Step 2 result}}{\text{Original denominator}} = \frac{5}{2} = 2\frac{1}{2}$$

Thus, the mixed number of $2\frac{1}{2}$ is the same as the improper fraction $\frac{5}{2}$. You can change an improper fraction to a mixed number in four steps. Given an improper fraction $\frac{8}{5}$,
Step 1: Divide the numerator by the denominator:

$$\frac{\text{Numerator}}{\text{Denominator}} = \frac{8}{5} = 1\,R3 \quad (\text{i.e., 1 with 3 left over})$$

Step 2: Use the whole number obtained in Step 1 as the whole number of the mixed fraction:

$$\text{Whole number} = \text{Step 1 whole number} = 1$$

Step 3: Use the remainder (R) obtained in Step 1 as the numerator of the new fraction; use the original denominator as the new denominator:

$$\text{Fraction} = \frac{\text{Step 1 remainder}}{\text{Original denominator}} = \frac{3}{5} = \frac{3}{5}$$

Step 4: Put the whole number and the fraction together to get the mixed number:

$$1 \quad \text{and} \quad \frac{3}{5} = 1\frac{3}{5}$$

Thus, the improper fraction $\frac{8}{5}$ is the same as the mixed number $1\frac{3}{5}$.

If you multiply or divide the numerator and the denominator of a fraction by the same nonzero number, you get an equivalent fraction.

EXAMPLE
_____

$$\frac{3}{4} = \frac{3 \times 2}{4 \times 2} = \frac{6}{8}$$

$$\frac{6}{8} = \frac{6 \div 2}{8 \div 2} = \frac{3}{4}$$

Thus, $\frac{3}{4}$ and $\frac{6}{8}$ are equivalent fractions.

A fraction is in its *lowest terms* when no nonzero number except 1 can be evenly divided into both the numerator and the denominator. Reducing fractions to their lowest terms is *always* the last step in mathematical problem solving.

EXAMPLE
_____

In the fraction $\frac{10}{12}$, both the numerator and the denominator can be evenly divided by 2. When this is accomplished, the resulting fraction, $\frac{5}{6}$, is an equivalent fraction to the original and also its lowest terms.

ADDITION AND SUBTRACTION OF FRACTIONS

To add (or subtract) fractions whose denominators are the same, just add (or subtract) the numerators and keep the denominators the same.

EXAMPLE
_____

$$\frac{2}{5} + \frac{1}{5} = \frac{2+1}{5} = \frac{3}{5} \qquad \frac{2}{5} - \frac{1}{5} = \frac{2-1}{5} = \frac{1}{5}$$

To add (or subtract) fractions whose denominators are not the same, first convert the fractions to equivalent fractions with the lowest common denominators, then add (or subtract) the numerators. This can be done in three steps. Given the problem $\frac{1}{2} + \frac{1}{3} = ?$

Step 1: Find the lowest common denominator of $\frac{1}{2}$ and $\frac{1}{3}$. The lowest number divisible by both 2 and 3 is 6, so six is the lowest common denominator.

Step 2: Change the fractions to equivalent fractions using 6 as the new denominator:

$$\frac{1}{2} = \frac{1 \times 3}{2 \times 3} = \frac{3}{6}$$

and

$$\frac{1}{3} = \frac{1 \times 2}{3 \times 2} = \frac{2}{6}$$

Step 3: Now perform your operation. Add the two new fractions as they have the same denominators (remember to always reduce to lowest terms):

$$\frac{3}{6} + \frac{2}{6} = \frac{5}{6}$$

In this example, $\frac{5}{6}$ is in lowest terms.

EXAMPLES

$$\frac{1}{2} - \frac{1}{3} = \frac{3}{6} - \frac{2}{6} = \frac{1}{6}$$

$$\frac{3}{4} + \frac{1}{8} = \frac{6}{8} + \frac{1}{8} = \frac{7}{8}$$

To add (or subtract) mixed numbers, convert the mixed numbers to improper fractions, find the lowest common denominator, and add (or subtract) as usual. Then convert the answer, if it is an improper fraction, to a mixed number. This can be done in four steps.

Given the problem $4\frac{2}{3} + 1\frac{1}{6} = ?$

Step 1: Convert the mixed numbers to improper fractions.

$$4\frac{2}{3} = \frac{14}{3} \quad \text{and} \quad 1\frac{1}{6} = \frac{7}{6}$$

Step 2: Find the lowest common denominator of $\frac{14}{3}$ and $\frac{7}{6}$. The lowest number divisible by both 3 and 6 is 6, so 6 is the lowest common denominator.

Step 3: Change the fractions to equivalent fractions using 6 as the new denominator.

$$\frac{14}{3} = \frac{14 \times 2}{3 \times 2} = \frac{28}{6} \quad \text{and} \quad 7/6 \text{ already has 6 as its denominator}$$

Step 4: Now perform your operation and add the two new fractions as they have the same denominators (and convert back to a mixed number because that is the lowest term for this fraction):

$$\frac{28}{6} + \frac{7}{6} = \frac{28+7}{6} = \frac{35}{6} = 5\frac{5}{6}$$

EXAMPLES

$$9\frac{3}{4} - 2\frac{1}{3} = \frac{27}{4} - \frac{7}{3} = \frac{81}{12} - \frac{28}{12} = \frac{53}{12} = 4\frac{5}{12}$$

$$2\frac{1}{5} + 2\frac{1}{10} = \frac{11}{5} + \frac{21}{10} = \frac{22}{10} + \frac{21}{10} = \frac{43}{12} = 4\frac{3}{10}$$

MULTIPLICATION AND DIVISION OF FRACTIONS

To multiply two fractions, multiply the numerators by the numerators and the denominators by the denominators. The results are the new fraction/answer. Remember to always reduce to lowest terms.

EXAMPLES

$$\frac{2}{3} \times \frac{1}{4} = \frac{2 \times 1}{3 \times 4} = \frac{2}{12} = \frac{1}{6}$$

$$\frac{1}{7} \times \frac{1}{8} = \frac{1 \times 1}{7 \times 8} = \frac{1}{56}$$

To divide two fractions, invert the divisor, then multiply.

EXAMPLES

$$\frac{1}{5} \div \frac{3}{8} = \frac{1}{5} \times \frac{8}{3} = \frac{8}{15}$$

$$\frac{5}{12} \div \frac{1}{3} = \frac{5}{12} \times \frac{3}{1} = \frac{15}{12} = 1\frac{3}{12} = 1\frac{1}{4}$$

☞ **Note:** To remember the rule for division of fractions:
The number you are dividing by
Turn upside down and multiply.

To multiply or divide mixed numbers, first convert them to improper fractions, then multiply or divide.

EXAMPLES

$$1\tfrac{1}{4} \times 2\tfrac{1}{8} = \frac{5}{4} \times \frac{17}{8}$$
$$= \frac{85}{32}$$
$$= 2\tfrac{21}{32}$$

$$2\tfrac{1}{2} \div 3\tfrac{1}{3} = \frac{5}{2} \div \frac{10}{3}$$
$$= \frac{5}{2} \times \frac{3}{10}$$
$$= \frac{15}{20}$$
$$= \frac{3}{4}$$

DECIMALS

Decimal numbers are written by placing digits (0, 1, 2, 3, 4, 5, 6, 7, 8, 9) into place value columns that are separated by a **decimal**

Table **3–2** Decimal Place Values			
Ten thousands			10^4
Thousands			10^3
Hundreds			10^2
Tens			10^1
Ones			10^0
Decimal point			
Tenths			10^{-1}
Hundredths			10^{-2}
Thousandths			10^{-3}
Ten thousandths			10^{-4}
Hundred thousandths			10^{-5}
Millionths			10^{-6}
or			
Ten thousands	10,000.	=	10^4
Thousands	1,000.	=	10^3
Hundreds	100.	=	10^2
Tens	10.	=	10^1
Ones	1.	=	10^0
Decimal point	.	=	
Tenths	0.1	=	10^{-1}
Hundredths	0.01	=	10^{-2}
Thousandths	0.001	=	10^{-3}
Ten-thousandths	0.000 1	=	10^{-4}
Hundred-thousandths	0.000 01	=	10^{-5}
Millionths	0.000 001	=	10^{-6}

point, as shown in Table 3–2. The place value columns are read in sequence from left to right as multiples of decreasing powers of 10:
- Numbers to the left of the decimal point represent values greater than 1.
- Numbers to the right of the decimal point represent values less than 1.
- The number sequence is added.

The number 652.345 is represented as

decimal point

hundreds   tens   ones   ↓   tenths   hundredths thousandths

$(6 \times 100) + (5 \times 10) + (2 \times 1) \bullet (3 \times 1/10) + (4 \times 1/100) + (5 \times 1/1000)$

600   +   50   +   2   •   3/10   +   4/100   +   5/1000

☞ **Note:** Notice that each place value is a power of 10. This can also be written using **exponents.** These are shortcuts to showing multiplication of a number times itself. For example, 10×10 can be written as 10^2. Any number with an exponent of 0 is equal to one. So, $10^0 = 1$. The preceding multiples of 10 can be written as

$$(6 \times 10^2) + (5 \times 10^1) + (2 \times 10^0) + (3 \times 10^{-1}) + (4 \times 10^{-2}) + (5 \times 10^{-3})$$

Remember:

$$10^2 = 10 \times 10 \text{ or } 100$$
$$10^1 = 10$$
$$10^0 = 1$$
$$10^{-1} = 1/10$$
$$10^{-2} = 1/100$$

The decimal 652.345 can be read as "six hundred fifty-two point three four five." It can also be read as "six hundred fifty-two and three hundred forty-five thousandths." Notice that

- The word "and" is used for the decimal point.
- The decimal fraction is named for the rightmost place in the place column sequence.
- The suffix *-th* is used to signify fractions.

EXAMPLES

5.45 is read as "five and forty-five hundredths"
7.0 is read as "seven" or "seven and no tenths"

ADDITION AND SUBTRACTION OF DECIMALS

To add or subtract decimal numbers, line up the decimal points and carry out the calculations.

EXAMPLES

24.531 + 2.798 =
┌──── Align the decimal points
↓

    24.531
     2.798
    ──────
    27.329

5.04 − 1.213 =
    5.040 ← add a zero as a place holder
   −1.213
   ──────
    3.827

☞ **Note:** Adding zeros to the right of a number on the right side of the decimal point does not change its value. Adding zeros to the left of a number on the left side of the decimal point does not change its value.

MULTIPLICATION AND DIVISION OF DECIMALS

To multiply two decimals, carry out the multiplication, then add the number of decimal places from the right of the decimal point in the original two numbers. This total is the number of decimal places from the right of the decimal point in the product (answer).

EXAMPLES

```
   0.07        2 decimal places
 × 2.1        +1 decimal place
 ─────
   007
   014
 ─────        ──
   0.147       3 decimal places
```

```
   0.00051      5 decimal places
 × 0.04        +2 decimal places
 ─────────
 0.0000204      7 decimal places
        └─┬─┘   Add zeros
```

To divide decimals by whole numbers, carry out the long division. Align the decimal point of the quotient directly above that of the dividend.

EXAMPLES

```
         Align decimal points in
   ↓     quotient and dividend
   3.09
5)15.45
  15
  ───
   045
    45
   ───
     0
```

```
   3.3
3)9.9
  9
  ───
   9
   9
  ───
   0
```

If the divisor is a decimal, convert it to a whole number before dividing. To do this, move the decimal point of the divisor and that of the dividend the same number of places to the right.

EXAMPLES

$$2.5\overline{)6.25} \;=\; 2.5.\overline{)6.2.5}$$

$$\begin{array}{r} 2.5 \\ \underline{50} \\ 125 \\ \underline{125} \\ 0 \end{array}$$

One place value

Divisor ⟶   ⌐‾⌐   ⟵ Whole number

(1)   2.5 × 10 = 25
(2)   6.25 × 10 = 62.5

Dividend ⟶

$$0.25\overline{)5} \;=\; 0.25.\overline{)5.00.}$$

$$\begin{array}{r} 20. \\ \underline{50} \\ 00 \end{array}$$

Two place values

Divisor ⟶   ⌐‾⌐   ⟵ Whole number

(1) 0.25 × 100 = 25
(2)   5 × 100 = 500

Dividend ⟶

When more than one operation (addition, subtraction, multiplication, division, exponents) must be carried out, use the order of operations:

Parentheses
Exponents
Multiplication
Division
Addition
Subtraction

☞ **Note:** To remember the order of operations, use the phrase "Please excuse my dear Aunt Sally" or the initials PEMDAS.

To convert fractions to decimals, divide the numerator by the denominator.

EXAMPLES

$$\tfrac{1}{4} = 4\overline{)1.00}$$

$$\begin{array}{r} 0.25 \\ \underline{8} \\ 20 \\ \underline{20} \\ 0 \end{array}$$

$$\tfrac{2}{3} = 3\overline{)2.0000} \;= 0.\overline{66}$$

$$\begin{array}{r} 0.666... \\ \underline{18} \\ 20 \\ \underline{18} \\ 20 \end{array}$$

☞ **Note:** When the answer is a nonterminating, repeating number, you may show this with a line over the repeating numerals.

To convert decimals to fractions, the decimal numeral expressed becomes the numerator and the decimal place (tenth, hundredths) becomes the denominator.

EXAMPLES

0.97 97 is the decimal expressed and becomes the numerator. 1/100 or hundredths is the decimal place expressed and becomes the denominator. thus, .97 = $\frac{97}{100}$

0.05 05 is the decimal expressed and becomes the numerator. 1/100 or hundredths is the decimal place expressed and becomes the denominator. thus, .05 = $\frac{5}{100}$ = $\frac{1}{20}$ (Always reduce to lowest terms.)

☞ **Note:** To round to the nearest tenth, carry the division out to the next decimal value after tenths, which is hundredths. If this number is 5 or greater, round the number in tenths up. If this number is less than 5, the number in tenths place remains the same.

To compare the values of two or more decimals to determine which is larger (or smaller), place the decimals in a column and align the decimal points. Fill in with zeros to the *right* of the decimal point so all decimals have the same number of digits. The larger decimal will have the largest digit in the greatest column (the decimal place farthest left).

EXAMPLES

Compare 0.000350 with 0.000082.
0.000350
0.000082

Align them with equal numbers of digits. Because the 3 is in the ten-thousandths place and the 8 is in the hundredth-thousandths place, the 3 is larger. Thus, 0.000350 is the larger decimal.

Compare 0.012 with 0.0045.
0.0120
0.0045

Align them with equal numbers of digits. As the 1 is in the hundredths place and the 4 is in the thousandths place, the 1 is larger. Thus, 0.012 is the larger decimal.

PERCENTAGES

Percents are special types of fractions that mean "per every hundred." Thus the denominator of a percent is always understood to be 100 and is shown by the symbol % rather than being written.

A percent can be written as a fraction by putting the number expressed as the numerator and the denominator as 100. It can be written as a decimal by putting down the number expressed and moving the decimal point two places to the left, thus signifying hundredths.

EXAMPLES

$25\% = \frac{25}{100}$ or $\frac{1}{4}$
$25\% = .25$
$56\% = \frac{56}{100} = \frac{14}{25}$
$56\% = .56$

In other words, when you drop the % sign, either replace it with a denominator of 100 or a decimal place of hundredths. When you add the % sign, either drop the denominator of 100 or move the decimal point two places to the right.

EXAMPLE

$0.33 = 33\%$
$0.33 = 33/100$
$0.17 = 17\%$
$0.17 = 17/100$

To find the percent of a number, change the percent to a decimal or fraction, replace the "of" with the times (×) sign, and multiply.

EXAMPLES

10% of 100 =
$0.10 \times 100 = 10$

or 0.10 can be expressed as {10/100}, which is reduced to {1/10} × 100 = 10

50% of 10 =
$0.50 \times 10 = 5$

or 0.50 can be expressed as {50/100}, which is reduced to {1/2} × 10 = 5
Try these:

9 is what percent of 27?
$\frac{9}{27} = \frac{1}{3} = 0.333$ or 33.3%

5 is what percent of 25?
$\frac{5}{25} = \frac{1}{5} = 0.20$ or 20%

Table 3–3 Common Fractions, Decimals, and Percents

Fraction	Decimal	Percent
$\frac{1}{2}$	0.5	50%
$\frac{1}{4}$	0.25	25%
$\frac{3}{4}$	0.75	75%
$\frac{1}{3}$	0.333*	$33\frac{1}{3}$%
$\frac{2}{3}$	0.666*	$66\frac{2}{3}$%
$\frac{1}{5}$	0.2	20%
$\frac{2}{5}$	0.4	40%
$\frac{3}{5}$	0.6	60%
$\frac{4}{5}$	0.8	80%
$\frac{1}{10}$	0.1	10%
$\frac{1}{1}$	1.0	100%

*0.333 and 0.666 are *nonterminating* decimals. This means the number patterns 0.333 . . . and 0.666 . . . go on forever.

RATIO AND PROPORTION

A **ratio** is a comparison of two numbers, *a* and *b,* expressed as

$$a{:}b \text{ or } a/b \text{ or } \tfrac{a}{b}$$

EXAMPLES

A two-to-one ratio is expressed as

$$2 : 1 \text{ or } 2/1 \text{ or } \tfrac{2}{1}$$

Insight 3–1

You will see a ratio expressed on a split-thickness skin graft procedure with the skin graft mesher. The mesher uses plates or special rollers to cut slits into the donor skin graft. This meshing allows the graft to be enlarged when it is stretched. The graft can then cover a greater area of the recipient site, and epithelial tissue will grow in between the slits. Meshers are available in a variety of expansion ratios such as 1:2, 1:3, and even 1:9.

A one-to-one thousand ratio is expressed as:

$$1 : 1000 \text{ or } 1/1000 \text{ or } \tfrac{1}{1000}$$

A **proportion** is a statement of equality between ratios: $a/b = c/d$ or $a : b = c : d$
In any proportion, the product of the means must equal the product of the extremes:

$$a \times d = b \times c$$

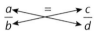

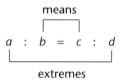   where a and d are the *extremes*
and b and c are the *means*

or

means

$$a \ : \ b \ = \ c \ : \ d$$

extremes

EXAMPLES

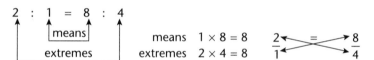

Proportions can be used to solve for an unknown term when the other three terms are known. This can be done in four steps:
Step 1: Let x be the unknown.
Step 2: Set up the proportion with the terms that are given (known).
Step 3: Multiply the means and the extremes.
Step 4: Solve for x.

EXAMPLE

Given $2 : 3 = x : 9$, what is x?

$\dfrac{2}{3} = \dfrac{x}{9}$ Let x be the unknown; set up the proportion.

$3x = 2 \times 9$ Multiply the means and the extremes.

$3x = 18$

$x = 18/3$ Divide both sides of the proportion by the same number (3) to have x alone on one side.

$x = 6$ Answer

Given $4 : 16 = 1 : x$

$\dfrac{4}{16} = \dfrac{1}{x}$ Let x be the unknown; set up the proportion.

$1 \times 16 = 4x$ Multiply the means and the extremes.

$16 = 4x$ Divide both sides of the proportion by the same number (4) to have x alone on one side.

$4 = x$ Answer

You can use ratios and proportions to calculate the quantities of medications. To do this, you must know that strength is a ratio—it is always expressed as units of substance per unit or units of volume—for example, the strength of Demerol may be 100 mg (milligrams) of Demerol per 1 mL (milliliter) of solution. And sometimes we express strength as strength per hundred units of another substance. For example a 5% saline solution is 5 grams of sodium chloride (NaCl) per 100 grams of water.

☞ **Note:** 1 cubic centimeter (cc) of water weighs 1 gram, so a 5% solution of saline is also 5 grams per cubic centimeter (g/cc).

EXAMPLE

The doctor prescribed 50 milligrams of Demerol. The Demerol solution that the anesthesia provider has is a strength of 100 milligrams per milliliter (mg/mL). How many milliliters of that solution are needed?

This relationship can be expressed in the proportion $100 : 1 = 50 : x$, or

$\dfrac{100\,\text{milligrams}}{1\,\text{milliliter}} = \dfrac{50\,\text{milligrams}}{x\,\text{milliliters}}$ x is the unknown amount of solution needed; set up the proportion.

$100 \times x = 50 \times 1$ Multiply the means and the extremes.

$100x = 50$ Solve for x by dividing both sides of the proportion by 100 so x stands alone on one side.

$x = 50/100$ or $\frac{1}{2}$ milliliter   Answer

You can also use proportions to solve other calculation problems. For example, the doctor will be giving the patient medications that are prescribed according to weight in kilograms (kg). You know the patient weighs 150 pounds (lbs), but how many kilograms is this?

First you must know three parts of the proportion, so you research and find that 1 kilogram is equal to 2.2 pounds.

This relationship can be expressed in the proportion $1 : 2.2 = x : 150$

$\dfrac{1\,\text{kg}}{2.2\,\text{lbs}} = \dfrac{x\,\text{kg}}{150\,\text{lbs}}$ x is the unknown; set up the proportion.

$1 \times 150 = x \times 2.2$ Multiply the means and the extremes.

$150 = 2.2x$ Divide both sides of the proportion by 2.2 to leave x alone on one side

$x = 68.18$ kg   Answer

Sometimes we can think of ratios in terms of parts of a whole. In this case, it is easy to think about percents.

EXAMPLE

You want to make up a 3 : 3 : 4 solution of saline, Lincocin, and Garamycin. (1) What percentage of the solution does each ingredient represent? (2) If you wanted to make up 200 milliliters of this solution, how many milliliters of saline would you use? Of Lincocin? Of Garamycin?

(1) A 3 : 3 : 4 solution means there are three parts to three parts to four parts. That is, you need a total of $3 + 3 + 4 = 10$ parts of whole solution.

By convention, the parts are listed in the same order as the ingredients, so you have

3 parts of saline in 10 parts of solution = 3/10 = 30/100 = 30%
3 parts of Lincocin in 10 parts of solution = 3/10 = 30/100 = 30%
4 parts of Garamycin in 10 parts of solution = 4/10 = 40/100 = 40%
Total parts of solution = 100%

(2) You want 200 milliliters of solution, so you multiply each ingredient's percentage by 200:

Saline (30%) .30 × 200 milliliters = 60 milliliters
Lincocin (30%) .30 × 200 milliliters = 60 milliliters
Garamycin (40%) .40 × 200 milliliters = 80 milliliters
Total = 200 milliliters

You want to make up a 1 : 1 : 3 solution of saline, antibiotic a, and antibiotic b. What percentage of the solution does each ingredient represent?

1 : 1 : 3 solution means one part to one part to three parts. That is, $1 + 1 + 3 = 5$ total parts in the solution

The parts are listed in the same order as the ingredients, so you have

1 part of saline in 5 parts of solution = 1/5 = 20/100 = 20%
1 part of antibiotic a in 5 parts of solution = 1/5 = 20/100 = 20%
3 parts of antibiotic b in 5 parts of solution = 3/5 = 60/100 = 60%
Total parts of solution = 100%

Another way to use proportions for calculations is to use the standard dilution equation. This is expressed as

$$\frac{C_1}{C_2} = \frac{V_2}{V_1} \text{ or } C_1 \times V_1 = C_2 \times V_2$$

where C stands for concentration in percent and V stands for volume. Thus

C_1 = concentration 1
C_2 = concentration 2
V_1 = volume 1
V_2 = volume 2

EXAMPLE

The procedure calls for 60 cubic centimeters (cc) of 1/2% contrast media. How much saline and how much contrast media solution do you need to make the required amount of solution when you have 1% contrast media?

In this problem, you are being asked for a dilution, so you start by sorting out what you know from what you do not know:

$C^1 = \frac{1}{2}$ or .5% asked for contrast media
$C^2 = 1\%$ have on hand contrast media
$V_1 = 60$ asked for volume
$V_2 = x$ unknown volume of saline (solve this unknown first)

Now you can write the standard dilution equation as

$$C_1 \times V_1 = C_2 \times V_2$$
$$\tfrac{1}{2} \times 60 = 1 \times x$$
$$30 = x$$
$$x = 30 \text{ cc of saline are needed}$$

But we are not finished with the problem; it also asks how much of the 1% contrast media solution we need. If you add 30 cc of saline and the amount you want is 60 cc, that means that 60 cc − 30 cc = 30 cc of the 1% contrast media is added.

 CAUTION

Contrast media, radiopaque dye, and dye are often interchangeable terms used in the operating room for the same agents. They are used for diagnostic examinations such as x-rays. However, the term *dye* must not be confused with other "dyes," which are tissue staining agents (see Chapter 6).

TEMPERATURE CONVERSIONS

In medicine we use two scales to measure temperature (Fig. 3–3): the **Fahrenheit scale** and the **Celsius** (centigrade) **scale.** In the Fahrenheit scale, the boiling point of water is 212° F and its freezing point is 32° F. In the Celsius scale, the boiling point of water at 100° C and its freezing point is 0° C. Nine degrees on the Fahrenheit scale corresponds to 5 degrees on the Celsius scale. Using these ratios, the following formulas (Table 3–4) were developed to convert temperatures from one scale to the other.

$$C = 5/9 \ (F - 32)$$
$$F = 9/5 \ C + 32$$

where C is the Celsius temperature and F is the Fahrenheit temperature.

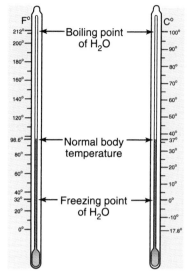

Figure **3–3.** Fahrenheit and Celsius scales.

Table **3–4**	Temperature Conversions	
To Convert From	*Use the Formula*	*The Operation Means*
Fahrenheit to Celsius	$C = \frac{5}{9}F - 32$	1. Subtract 32 from the Fahrenheit temperature. 2. Multiply the Celsius temperature by $\frac{5}{9}$.
Celsius to Fahrenheit	$F = \frac{9}{5}C + 32$	1. Multiply the Celsius temperature by $\frac{9}{5}$. 2. Add 32 to the result.

Temperature is important in many aspects of the surgical setting, and readings may be given in Fahrenheit or Celsius degrees. The surgical patient's body temperature is of vital importance and is constantly monitored. Normal body temperature is 98.6° F or 37° C. Preoperatively, an elevated temperature could signify an infection or other health problem. This could result in the postponement of the surgical procedure. Intraoperatively, the body temperature is monitored by anesthesia personnel. An abnormal body temperature—whether below normal *(hypothermia)* or elevated *(hyperthermia)*—alters the basal metabolic rate, interfering with blood pressure, heart rate, circulation, etc. Hyperthermia can also indicate life-threatening situations such as malignant hyperthermia (see Chapter 16). Postoperatively, temperature is monitored for the same reasons, and an elevated temperature at this time may indicate a wound infection. Another surgical aspect of temperature is the sterilization of instruments and equipment. Here, temperature, along with pressure and time, is monitored for proper sterilization. Temperature is also important for the surgical environment. Each surgical room is kept at 68° to 75° F (20° to 24° C) to discourage the growth of bacteria that can cause surgical site infections. It is also important to keep the room in this temperature range for the comfort of surgical personnel, who are working under surgical lights attired in full scrub apparel. A cool environment decreases the chance that perspiration will drip from a surgical team member onto the sterile field.

MEASUREMENT SYSTEMS

Although the surgical technologist does not administer medications directly to the patient, the technologist is responsible for obtaining medicines and mixing them for use in the sterile field. You may, for example, have to mix antibiotics in an irrigation solution. This may require you to calculate measurements and perform some conversions. Therefore, you'll need to know conversion equivalents and be able to perform the calculations involved in such conversions.

The metric system of measurement is the most commonly used in medicine. However, there are other systems with which the surgical technologist should be familiar. They include the apothecary and household systems; and measurements of some medications are based on their strengths.

THE METRIC SYSTEM

The **metric system** is the *international standard* (used by scientists and engineers everywhere) of weights and measures. Developed by the French in the 18th century, today it is the preferred system for prescribing and administering medications. It is also used extensively in the health care field. The *United States Pharmacopoeia,* for example, uses it exclusively, and all specimens sent to pathology are weighed and measured in metric terms. The metric system allows a way to calculate small drug dosages, and most manufacturers use this system for calibration in the development of new drugs. Most medications used in surgery are dispensed using the metric system of measurement.

In the metric system, length, volume, and weight (mass) are measured against certain defined units called *base units:*

Length—the *meter* (m)
Volume—the *liter* (L)
Weight—the *gram* (g)

Each of these base units is divided into smaller and larger units based on multiples of 10, and these multiples are indicated by prefixes:

Prefix (abbreviation)	Multiply base unit by
micro (μ)	.000001 (or 1/1,000,000)
milli (m)	.001 (or 1/1000)
centi (c)	.01 (or 1/100)
deci (d)	.1 (or 1/10)
UNIT	meter, liter, gram
deka (da)	10.
hecto (h)	100.
kilo (k)	1000.

Any prefix can be used with any base unit to indicate a measurement. For example, 1 **mm** = .001 m, 1 **mL** = .001 L, and 1 **mg** = .001 g; similarly, 1 **km** = 1000 m, 1 **kL** = 1000 L, and 1 **kg** = 1000 g. But you'll be most concerned with just a few of them—particularly, micro, milli, and centi.

Because the metric system is based on the decimal system, conversions are very easy. You just have to recognize the correct multiple of 10. Then you can use the appropriate unit conversion.

Unit Conversion

Length

1 meter = 1000 millimeters	1 m/1000 mm = 1	or	1000 mm/1 m = 1
1 meter = 100 centimeters	1 m/100 cm = 1	or	100 cm/1 m = 1
1 meter = 1,000,000 micrometers (microns)	1 m/1,000,000 μm = 1	or	1,000,000 μm/1 m = 1
1 millimeter = 1000 micrometers (microns)	1 mm/1000 μm = 1	or	1000 μm/1 mm = 1

Volume

1 liter = 1000 milliliters	1 L/1000 mL = 1	or	1000 mL/1 L = 1
1 kiloliter = 1000 liters	1 kL/1000 L = 1	or	1000 L/1 kL = 1

Weight (mass)

1 gram = 1000 milligrams	1 g/1000 mg = 1	or	1000 mg/1 g = 1
1 gram = 1,000,000 micrograms	1 g/1,000,000 μg = 1	or	1,000,000 μg/1 g = 1
1 milligram = 1000 micrograms	1 mg/1000 μg = 1	or	1000 μg/1 mg = 1
1 kilogram = 1000 grams	1 kg/1000 g = 1	or	1000 g/1 kg = 1

Metric Comparisons

The meter is about 39.37 inches, just over a yard (36 inches). It's a linear measure used for lengths, including heights and widths. For example, patient height is measured in meters, whereas tumors, flaps, and defects are measured as lengths and widths—usually in centimeters or millimeters (hundredths or thousandths of meters). Note that when a length measure is multiplied by another length measure, the result is an area, which is a *square measure*. For instance, a defect that is 10 cm by 5 cm has an area of $5 \times 10 = 50$ cm^2.

The meter is related to volume by *cubic measure*. When 1 centimeter is multiplied by itself three times—1 cm × 1 cm × 1 cm—it becomes the volume 1 cubic centimeter (1 cm^3), which is about the same size as a sugar cube. When length, width, and height (or depth) are multiplied together, the result is measured in cubic terms. Thus, a block of tissue that is 5 cm long, 3 cm wide, and 1 cm deep is $5 \times 3 \times 1 = 15$ cm^3.

The liter is a fluid (or liquid) measure approximately equal to a quart (1 L = 1.06 qt). Most medicines in surgery are in liquid form, including intravenous and irrigation solutions (often measured in liters) as well as many antibiotic solutions (usually measured in milliliters or thousandths of liters). In medicine, however, we call a cm^3 a "cc" (short for cubic centimeter, of course). This liquid measure of volume is related to the solid measure by one simple definition: 1 cc = 1 cm^3 = 1 mL. You'll see and hear these terms used interchangeably.

The gram is a small unit of mass (or weight) that is much less than an ounce (30 g is about 1 oz). For a mental picture, consider a paper clip; it weighs about a gram. In this case it's easier to think in terms of kilograms. One kilogram is 2.2 pounds (picture a 2-lb can of coffee). It's worth knowing that 1 cc (1 mL) of water weighs 1 gram, which means that aqueous solutions measured in weight percent (g/100 g) can also be reckoned in grams per milliliter of solution. You'll encounter gram or milligram measures when working with drugs in powder form, such as antibiotics that must be reconstituted (dissolved) in water. And you'll encounter kilogram measures when calculating dosages determined by body weight.

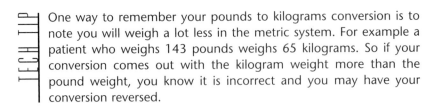

One way to remember your pounds to kilograms conversion is to note you will weigh a lot less in the metric system. For example a patient who weighs 143 pounds weighs 65 kilograms. So if your conversion comes out with the kilogram weight more than the pound weight, you know it is incorrect and you may have your conversion reversed.

The metric system is, by far, the most important measuring system in the world—and the most important to you. It lets you measure—and calculate with—small and large quantities of any kind without having to multiply by such ill-behaved conversion factors as 12 inches per foot, 2 pints in a quart (and 4 quarts in a gallon), and 16 ounces per pound. All you have to do is multiply and divide by 10, which is mostly a matter of moving the decimal point the correct number of places in the proper direction. Eventually, you'll find yourself thinking in it. But if you aren't already used to it, you'll find it helpful to compare metric measures with common measures. If, for example, you already know how long an inch is, you can easily picture that length as about 2.5 cm. Table 3–5 lists some of the more common equivalents, giving approximate conversions.

☞ **Note:** One cubic centimeter (cc) is the amount of space occupied by one milliliter (mL) of liquid. Thus, 1 cc = 1 mL.

Table **3–5**   Approximate Measurement Equivalents

Weight

1 kilogram = 2.2 pounds
1 gram = 15 grains
1 ounce = 30 grams
1 grain = 60 milligrams

Volume

1 kiloliter = exactly 1000 liters
1 liter = 1 quart
1 milliliter = 1 gram = 1 minims = 1 cubic centimeter
1 fluid ounce = 8 fluid drams = 30 milliliters
1 gallon = 4 liters
1 pint = 500 milliliters
1 quart = 2 pints = 1000 milliliters
1 gallon = 4 quarts = 4000 milliliters
1 teaspoon = 60 drops
1 minim = 1 drop

Length

1 meter = 39.37 inches = approx. 1 yard
1 yard = 3 feet = 36 inches
1 inch = 2.54 centimeters

Insight 3–2

The apothecary system was the system of weights and measures used for writing medication orders in ancient Greece and Rome and in Europe during the Middle Ages. It is rarely used today. The apothecary system is based on everyday items (such as the weight of a grain of wheat) and uses lowercase Roman numerals. For example, 4 grains would be written as "gr. $\overline{iv}$ " Some medications continue to use this system, as do pharmacists, so it is important to recognize the basic units of measure of the apothecary system:

Volume—the *minim* (fluid)
Weight—the *grain*

A minim is approximately equal to one drop. (As drops vary according to the dropper used, this measurement is not always accurate. For accuracy, a calibrated dropper should be used.) Larger quantities are multiples of the minim:

60 minims – 1 fluid dram
8 fluid drams – 1 fluid ounce
1 pint – 16 fluid ounces
2 pints – 1 quart
4 quarts – 1 gallon

The grain was based on the average weight of a grain of wheat. Larger quantities are multiples of the grain:

20 grains ("xx") = 1 scruple
3 scruples   = 1 dram
60 grains   = 1 dram
12 ounces   = 1 pound
8 drams   = 1 ounce

Note that in the apothecary system, 12 ounces equals 1 pound rather than 16 ounces (as in avoirdupois weight).

Although household measurements are used primarily for administering over-the-counter medications—and never in surgery—it's useful to see how they compare with more accurate standard measures. (See the following chart.)

Household Conversions

1 teaspoon = 5 milliliters = 5 cubic centimeters = 1 fluid dram
1 tablespoon = 1/2 fluid ounce = 4 fluid drams = 15 milliliters = 15 cubic centimeters
2 tablespoons = 1 fluid ounce = 30 milliliters = 30 cubic centimeters

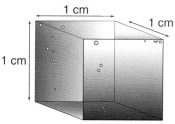

Figure **3–4.**   A cubic centimeter filled with water (1 cc = 1 mL here).

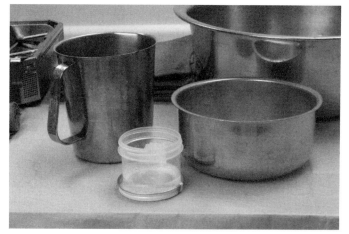

Figure **3–5.**   Measuring equipment in surgery.

☞ **Note:** The apothecary and the household systems were used more in the past. It is not necessary to learn conversions from these measurement systems because medications are prepared and administered primarily from the metric system. These systems can be used for comparisons as measurements we are more familiar with until we are proficient with the metric system.

OTHER STANDARDIZED MEASUREMENTS (DOSES)

Some medications are measured directly by their strengths—that is, they are measured in *units* (u.) based upon their potency. A common medication measured in units is insulin. There are special insulin syringes calibrated to these units. In surgery, several antibiotics, including penicillin and Bacitracin, are also measured in units. These medications are used in antibiotic irrigation solutions during surgical procedures. Another medication measured in units is heparin, an anticoagulant administered intravenously to

Table **3–6**   Symbols of Measurement

Metric System		Apothecary System		Household System	
meter	m	minim	m, min, ♍	teaspoon	tsp
liter	L	grain	gr	tablespoon	tbsp
cubic centimeter	cc	dram	dr, ʒ	ounce	oz
centimeter	cm	fluid dram	fl dr, ℨ	pint	pt
millimeter	mm	drop	gtt	quart	qt
gram	g	ounce	oz	gallon	gal
kilogram	kg	pint	pt	inch	in
milligram	mg	quart	qt	yard	yd
milliliter	mL	gallon	gal		
kiloliter	kL	pound	lb		
microgram	mcg, μg	scruple	scr, ℈		
micron (micrometer)	μm				
unit	U				
international unit	IU				
milliunit	mU				
milliequivalent	mEq				

Note: As discussed in Chapter 2, some symbols are not being used with medication orders in an effort to decrease medication errors. However, the surgical technologist should be familiar with symbols as hospital policies on their use vary.

the patient by anesthesia personnel during vascular cases. Heparin is also used diluted in saline on the backtable.

Other measurements used to indicate quantity of medicine prescribed are the international unit (IU) and the milliunit (mU). The international unit is used to measure vitamins and chemicals. The milliunit, which is one-thousandths (.001 or 1/1000) of a unit, is used for dosages of Pitocin. Pitocin is used in childbirth to stimulate the uterus to contract (see Chapter 8). Another measurement of medications according to their strength is the *milliequivalent* (mEq.) A milliequivalent is equal to 1/1000 (0.001) of a chemical equivalent, a measurement associated with electrolytes. Concentrations of electrolytes are often expressed as milliequivalents per liter. Electrolytes are essential for metabolic activities in the body and for normal function of body cells. A common electrolyte administered to the surgical patient is potassium chloride (KCl), which is necessary for the transmission of nerve impulses, control of heart rhythm, and fluid balance. Low potassium levels can pose a risk to the surgical patient undergoing general anesthesia. Potassium chloride is administered in milliequivalents preoperatively or by anesthesia personnel.

See Table 3–6 for symbols of measurement.

KEY CONCEPTS

- Military time is used by hospitals and other medical institutions, and it uses a 24-hour scale without AM or PM designations.
- Surgical technologists may use fractions, decimals, and percents, together with ratios and proportions, to solve problems and perform calculations and conversions.
- A fraction is a number that represents one or more equal parts of a whole and can be written as a quotient *a/b.*
- Fractions may be proper, improper, or expressed as mixed numbers.
- Decimals are numbers written by placing digits into value columns that are separated by a decimal point.
- Exponents are shortcuts to showing multiplication of a number times itself.
- Percents are special types of fractions that mean "per every hundred" and are shown by the symbol %.
- A ratio is a comparison of two numbers expressed as *a:b, a/b,* or $\frac{a}{b}$
- A proportion is a statement of equality between ratios expressed as a:b = c:d or a/b = c/d
- Two temperature scales are used in medicine, the Fahrenheit and the Celsius.
- Conversion from one temperature scale to the other can be accomplished by using one of the following formulas: C = 5/9(F-32) or F = 9/5C + 32.
- The metric system is the international standard of weights and measures.
- In the metric system the base units are represented by the following: length—meter, volume—liter, weight—gram.
- Other measurements include medications measured by strength such as units, international unit, milliunit, and milliequivalent.

MEDICATION ADMINISTRATION

Medications Covered in Chapter 4

Generic Name	Brand or Trade Name	Category
lidocaine	Xylocaine	Local anesthetic
epinephrine 1:100,000	N/A	Vasoconstrictor
epinephrine 1:1000	N/A	Potent vasoconstrictor
phenylephrine	Neosynephrine	Vasoconstrictor
heparin	N/A	Systemic anticoagulant
bupivacaine with epinephrine 1:100,000	Marcaine, Sensorcaine	Local anesthetic
thrombin	Thrombin	Topical hemostatic
absorbable gelatin	Gelfoam	Topical hemostatic
cocaine	N/A	Topical anesthetic

OBJECTIVES

After completing this chapter, you should be able to:

1. Describe the role of the surgical technologist in medication administration.
2. Explain the six "rights" of medication administration.
3. Describe the steps of medication identification.
4. Discuss aseptic techniques for delivery of medications to the sterile field.
5. State the procedure for labeling drugs on the sterile back table.
6. Identify supplies used in medication administration in surgery.

KEY TERMS

asepsis   diluent
carpule   hypersensitivity
contamination   reconstitute

The role of the surgical technologist in medication adminis-tration varies from state to state and differs from facility to facility. As a surgical technologist, you should have firsthand knowledge of medication administration legislation in your state.

> **TECH TIP**
> Do not depend on hearsay or someone else's understanding or opinion regarding the limits of your practice. Use your computer competence and the easy availability of the Internet to read the pertinent legislative statutes for yourself. Ask for assistance at your facility's medical library or from the reference librarian at any public library. Remember, professional surgical technologists should be highly knowledgeable regarding their own practice.

Institutional policies and procedures regarding medication handling and administration should be clearly understood as well. All staff members have a duty to know and adhere to established medication policies and procedures. Handling medications is a critical function in the surgical technologist's job description. Several different types of medications are obtained and passed to the surgeon routinely during a procedure, and the surgical tech-nologist must be knowledgeable regarding such drugs.

☞ **Note:** The limits of legal authority for the surgical technologist to perform the indicated roles described in this text are controlled by each state through its statutes, case law, regulatory law, attor-ney general opinions, and medical licensing boards. Discussion of these sources of law is beyond the scope of this text. Except as otherwise noted, this book describes the general practice of surgical technology in the United States, not the legal authority for such practice. It is the surgical technologist's responsibility to consult the limitations in his or her area on acts described in this book.

SURGICAL TECHNOLOGIST'S ROLES IN MEDICATION ADMINISTRATION

Administration of drugs from the sterile field is a team effort. Each team member has a particular role in the process (Table 4–1). Most

Table **4–1**   The Surgical Technologist's Roles in Medication Administration

Circulator Role

Obtain correct medication.
Deliver medication to the sterile field using aseptic technique.
Document all medications used from sterile field.

Scrub Role

Identify medication.
Accept medication into the sterile field.
Label the medication immediately.
Pass the medication to the surgeon as requested.

commonly, medications used from the sterile field are obtained by the *circulator* and delivered to the *scrub,* who is responsible for passing the medication to the surgeon for administration. Each team member is responsible for accurately identifying all medications used from the sterile field during a surgical procedure.

CIRCULATING ROLE

The surgical technologist in the circulating role obtains medications as specified on the surgeon's preference card, delivers those medications to the sterile field as needed, and documents the medications used from the sterile field during an operation. The circulator must be sure that the medication obtained is the exact drug and strength specified on the preference card. The circulator must also inspect the container for integrity and expiration date. The circulator must maintain strict **asepsis** when transferring medications to the scrub person. All medications must be properly identified, both by the scrub and by the circulator. The circulator is responsible for documenting all medications used from the sterile field according to institutional policy.

SCRUB ROLE

The surgical technologist in the scrub role correctly identifies and accepts medications from the circulator, immediately labels (Fig. 4–1) those medications, and passes medications to the surgeon as requested. Accurate identification and immediate labeling of all drugs accepted onto the sterile field is crucial. If medications are

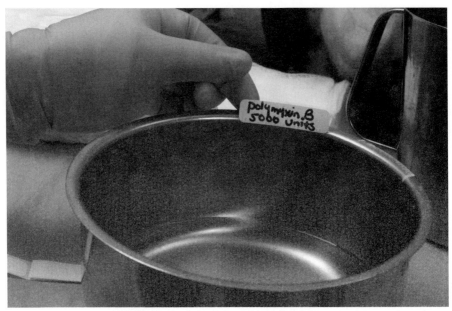

Figure **4–1.** The scrubbed surgical technologist labels medications immediately.

Table **4–2** Six "Rights" of Medication Administration
• Right Drug—**What** drug is required?
• Right Dose—**How much** of the drug is required in **what concentration?**
• Right Route—**How** will the drug be administered?
• Right Patient—**Who** will receive the drug?
• Right Time—**When** will the drug be administered?
• Right Documentation—**How and when** will the drug be recorded?

not clearly identified, they should be discarded immediately and a new dose should be obtained. This practice is essential to avoid possible drug administration error. The surgical technologist will clearly state the name and strength of a medication when passing it to the surgeon.

THE SIX "RIGHTS" OF MEDICATION ADMINISTRATION

To help prevent medication errors, the six "rights" of medication administration have been established (Table 4–2). Team members

Surgeon: Dr. Ferguson	Procedure: Excision skin lesions (local)
Glove size: $7\frac{1}{2}$	Position of patient: According to lesions
Skin prep: Betadine	Drapes: Towels–drape sheets If face, split sheet and turban drape
Sutures and needles	**Instruments and equipment**

Ties:
 	
Peritoneum:
 	
Fascia:
 	
Sub-cu:
      5-0 Dermalon P-3   > have in room
Skin: 6-0 mild chromic SH-1 > do not open
 	
Retention:
 	
Other:
	Basic: Small dissecting set
	
	Special:
	
	      4×8 Raytec sponges
	      cautery pencil c̄ needle tip
	      #11 knife blade
	      5cc syringe
	      #18 g. and #25 g. needles $1\frac{1}{2}$"

Dressings: Steri-strips $\frac{1}{4}$"	Local anesthetic: 1% lidocaine c̄ epinephrine 1:100,000

Figure **4–2.**   A surgeon's preference card showing medication needed for procedure.

must work together to ensure that the right drug is given in the right dose, by the right route, to the right patient, at the right time and that it is accurately documented.

RIGHT DRUG

Drugs that are routinely needed on the sterile field during a procedure should be clearly specified on the surgeon's preference card (Fig. 4–2). The information is initially obtained directly from the surgeon and entered on the preference card by a member of the surgery department staff (surgical technologists, registered nurses). The information stated on the preference card must be accurate, including correct spelling and strength. Handwritten preference cards must be written legibly to avoid confusion. Preference cards should be updated as needed to reflect any changes in routine medications. Additional drugs are obtained in response to verbal orders by the surgeon during the procedure.

When any medication is delivered to the sterile back table, it must be carefully identified by both the circulator and scrub, and labeled immediately and accurately by the scrubbed surgical technologist.

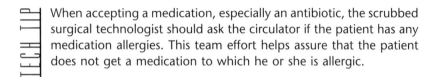

When accepting a medication, especially an antibiotic, the scrubbed surgical technologist should ask the circulator if the patient has any medication allergies. This team effort helps assure that the patient does not get a medication to which he or she is allergic.

The scrub person always states the name and strength of the drug aloud as he or she hands it to the surgeon; this practice serves as confirmation that the medication is correct. All empty medication vials and bottles should be kept in the room during the procedure as evidence that the proper medication has been delivered to the field.

RIGHT DOSE

The actual dose of a medication is a factor of both its amount (volume) and its strength (concentration). You might see, for instance, an order for 30 mL (amount) of 0.5% (strength) lidocaine with epinephrine 1:100,000 on a surgeon's preference card. This information must be clearly specified and clearly understood. It's especially important when the drug must be mixed or diluted on the sterile back table. Suppose, for example, a surgeon requests 0.5 mL of 1% phenylephrine (Neosynephrine) diluted in 20 mL of saline. Further suppose that phenylephrine is available in 1 mL vials. If the entire 1 mL vial (instead of the 0.5 mL specified) is mixed with the correct amount (20 mL) of saline and dispensed to the sterile field, the dosage of phenylephrine administered will be *twice* the desired dose.

Written protocols may be instituted and posted to eliminate common confusions about some medications. Heparin (a systemic anticoagulant) is an excellent example of a medication that is available in a number of different strengths, yet in the same volume (see Chapter 9). During insertion of a venous access port, different strengths of heparin may be needed from the sterile back table: 100 units per milliliter and 10 units per milliliter may be used, each concentration with a specific purpose. Given the 10-fold difference in heparin concentration, immediate labeling is crucial. In addition, the scrubbed surgical technologist must understand the reasons or purposes for the various strengths of heparin required to know which concentration to hand at the appropriate time. In this case, a department routine or protocol for heparin dosages in venous access procedures may be established and posted to minimize the potential for error.

The surgical technologist serves a key role in the prevention of administration of the wrong dosage of a medication from the sterile field. In addition to correct identification and labeling, the scrubbed surgical technologist provides the final safety check by stating out loud and clearly the name and strength of the medication as it is handed to the surgeon.

RIGHT ROUTE

Most medications administered in surgery are given intravenously, usually by the anesthesia provider. However, many other medications may be injected or applied topically by the surgeon at the surgical site. Different administration routes may require different preparations and concentrations of a medication. The preference card should clearly state administration route or form, so that the proper form of the drug for a particular route may be obtained. For example, the preference card for cystoscopy may state that 1% lidocaine jelly is needed for local anesthesia. Although the preference card should clearly state "for topical application," it may also be safely assumed that properly educated surgical team members know that jelly, a semisolid form of the drug, is intended for topical application, not injection. In a situation of a novice practitioner or a person with a knowledge deficit, careful reading of the medication label will reveal that this form of lidocaine is intended for topical use only. This situation also provides an excellent example of the importance of always carefully reading the medication label. When in doubt, always clarify the information stated on the preference card.

Another common example demonstrating the use of the right form of a drug for the right route is 1% lidocaine with epinephrine 1:100,000 for local anesthesia for procedures such as breast biopsy. Again, the administration route may not be stated clearly on the preference card, because the drug specified is formulated for injection. If for some unusual reason, a team member does not know that a local anesthetic agent is *injected* for breast biopsy, careful reading of the medication label will provide the necessary information.

RIGHT PATIENT

Although the possibility of administering a drug to the wrong patient in surgery is remote, it is not unknown. Thus caution must be exercised to avoid errors. All surgical patients must be accurately identified before being transported into the operating room. This identification should also include relevant information about the patient. For example, any history of drug allergies or **hypersensitivity** should be noted. In addition, the surgical procedure and operating surgeon should be verified, and the preference card containing medication orders for that specific procedure should be kept available in the operating room. In addition, the recent institution of a universal policy for a "time out" final check prior to incision will further verify that the intended surgical procedure is being performed on the correct patient.

RIGHT TIME

In surgery, the surgeon (or as delegated to the surgical first assistant) administers all medications at the surgical site. This practice prevents the vast majority of medication timing errors during surgery. The purpose of the drug, when stated on the preference card, often indicates the timing of administration. If, for example, 1% lidocaine with epinephrine 1:100,000 is listed on the preference card for a local anesthetic, it will be administered prior to incision. In addition, it may be administered periodically throughout the procedure as needed (PRN) for patient comfort. If 0.5% bupivicaine with epinephrine 1:100,000 is listed on the preference card for postoperative pain control, it will usually be administered at the time of wound closure. Some routine medications (e.g., contrast media for cholangiography, antibiotics for irrigation, heparinized saline) are obtained and labeled during case setup and passed to the surgeon at the appropriate time. Other medications may be obtained, passed to the surgeon from the sterile back table, and administered by the surgeon as soon as requested.

RIGHT DOCUMENTATION

It is crucial that medications given from the sterile table be accurately recorded in the operative record. The circulator will record all medications delivered to the field, and the scrubbed surgical technologist will verbally provide a final total of the amount of each medication administered for the circulator to note in the record. When a medication is repeatedly administered during a procedure, such as a local anesthetic, the scrubbed surgical technologist must also maintain an accurate ongoing total of the amount of medication being used throughout the procedure.

MEDICATION IDENTIFICATION

Both the scrub and the circulator are responsible for correctly identifying medications delivered to and used from the sterile

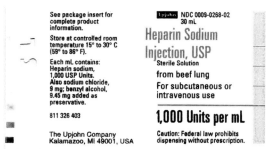

See package insert for
complete product
information.

Store at controlled room
temperature 15° to 30° C
(59° to 86° F).

Each mL contains:
Heparin sodium,
1,000 USP Units.
Also sodium chloride,
9 mg; benzyl alcohol,
9.45 mg added as
preservative.

811 326 403

The Upjohn Company
Kalamazoo, MI 49001, USA

[Upjohn] NDC 0009-0268-02
30 mL

**Heparin Sodium
Injection, USP**
Sterile Solution

from beef lung

For subcutaneous or
intravenous use

1,000 Units per mL

Caution: Federal law prohibits
dispensing without prescription.

Figure **4–3.** A label for heparin sodium. *(From Morris DG: Calculate with Confidence, 3rd ed, St. Louis, Mosby, 2002.)*

Table **4–3**   Steps for Medication Identification
Circulator reads label.
Circulator reads label aloud to scrub.
Circulator shows label to scrub.
Scrub states medication information aloud.
Scrub accepts medication.
Scrub labels medication containers immediately.

---

field. This dual responsibility minimizes the potential for errors in medication administration, as does following a logical series of steps (Table 4–3) to properly identify drugs. The first step in medication identification is to carefully read the label on the medicine container (Fig. 4–3). The team member obtaining the drug reads the label initially and checks the container for cracks or discolored contents. If there is any doubt as to the integrity of the container, the medication should not be used. Rather, it should be returned to the pharmacy with a note indicating the specific concern. The medication label contains important information about the drug, as Table 4–4 shows. The most crucial information is the drug name (both generic and trade), the strength, the amount, and the expiration date. Special handling instructions (such as refrigeration, or keeping medication from direct light), the drug form and intended administration route are also key pieces of drug information contained on the label (for more detail see Chapter 2). The circulator reads vital label information aloud just prior to delivery to the sterile field, and shows the label to the scrub person (Fig. 4–4). Finally, the scrub repeats the label information aloud to confirm the correct drug. The drug should be delivered to the sterile field only after the steps described have

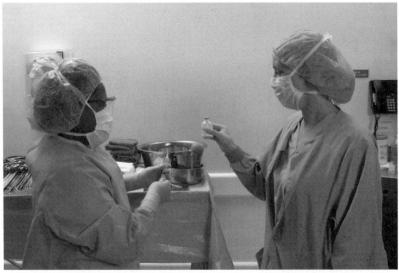

Figure **4–4.**   The circulator shows a drug label to the scrub.

Table **4–4** Sample Information Contained on a Medication Label	
Type of Information	**Example**
Name (brand and generic)	Sensorcaine (bupivacaine HCl)
Strength	0.5%
Amount	50 mL
Expiration date	01/08
Administration route	Injection
Manufacturer	Astra
Storage directions	Store at room temperature
Warnings or precautions	Federal law prohibits dispensing without prescription
Lot number	1234567
Schedule (C-I to C-V)*	

*Only if drug is a controlled substance.

been completed. Alternately, both scrub and circulator may read the information aloud together prior to delivery of the medication to the sterile field.

 CAUTION

All medications delivered to the sterile field must be labeled immediately.

DELIVERY TO THE STERILE FIELD

Principles of asepsis must be followed when delivering and receiving medications into the sterile field. Medications frequently used from the sterile back table are packaged in different types of containers including vials and ampules (Fig. 4–5) and aseptic delivery method varies by type of container. One of the most common containers is a glass or plastic vial with a rubber stopper encased in a metal cap. The metal cap is peeled away, so that the circulator can draw up the drug (if in liquid form) with a syringe and hypodermic needle and then empty the contents of the syringe into a sterile medicine cup held by the scrub (Fig. 4–6). The circulator should handle only the outside of the vial and should not touch the rubber stopper unless it is being removed. Alternatively, the circulator may hold the vial in an inverted position while the scrub withdraws the drug from the vial with a syringe and needle (Fig. 4–7). The scrubbed surgical technologist should first draw some air into the syringe, then puncture the rubber stopper with the needle and inject air into the vial, which will allow the contents of the vial to enter the syringe rapidly. In addition, the hypodermic needle used to puncture the vial should be a larger needle, such as an 18-gauge, to permit rapid filling of the syringe. After the medication is in the syringe, the 18-gauge needle is removed and replaced with the correct gauge needle for injection (such as a 25-gauge).

If a drug is in powder form in a vial, the circulator must **reconstitute** it with an appropriate liquid, such as saline (NaCl) solution, withdraw the resulting liquid, and deliver it to the sterile field as described earlier. If a syringe is used to draw up and inject the recon-

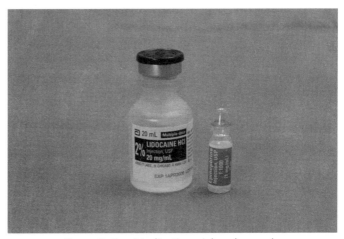

Figure **4–5.** Medication vial and ampule.

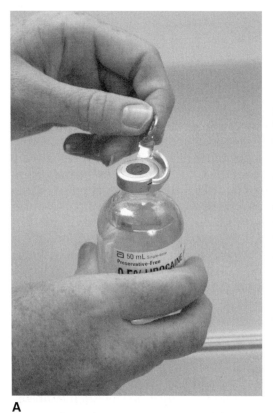

A

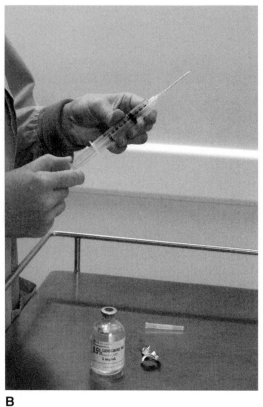

B

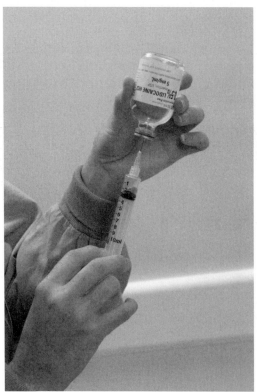

C

Figure **4–6. Drawing medication from a vial.**
(A) Peel off the metal cap and remove plastic cover.
(B) Aspirate air into a syringe. **(C)** Inject air into the vial
to displace the medication, drawing medication into the
syringe.

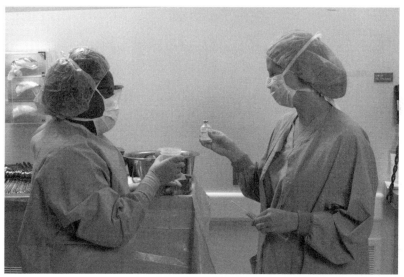

D

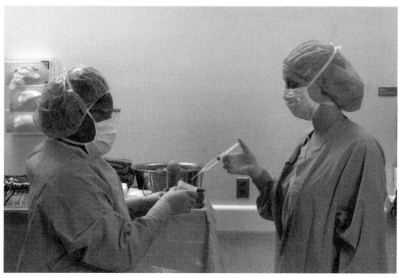

E

Figure **4–6, cont'd.**   (**D**) Show the label to the scrub. (**E**) Squirt the medication into a medicine cup held by the scrub person.

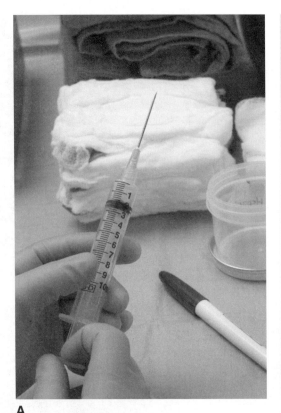 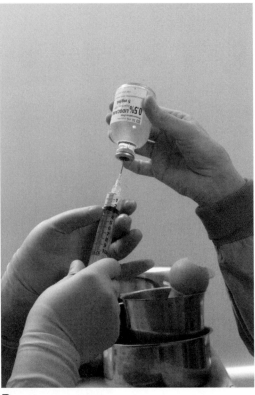

A   **B**

Figure **4–7.** The scrubbed surgical technologist may draw up medication from a vial held by the circulator. **(A)** Air is drawn into the syringe. **(B)** Air is injected into the vial to facilitate removal of medication.

stituting agent and to withdraw the mixture, care must be taken not to touch the sides of the plunger (Fig. 4–8). If unsterile hands touch the plunger, the plunger contaminates the inside of the barrel as it moves down the barrel when injecting. If the drug mixture is then drawn into the syringe barrel, it too becomes contaminated.

In some cases, the rubber top of a vial may be removed aseptically and the solution poured directly into a medicine cup (Fig. 4–9). If the stopper is removed for pouring, care must be taken to avoid contact with the lip of the vial, which must remain sterile. Sterile disposable spouts are commercially available to facilitate sterile delivery of medications contained in vials and in bags of intravenous solution. Medications may be added to a bag of intravenous solution, such as a gram of an antibiotic into 1000 mL of normal saline, and disposable spouts called bag decanters may be used to deliver the solution to the sterile field aseptically (Fig. 4–10).

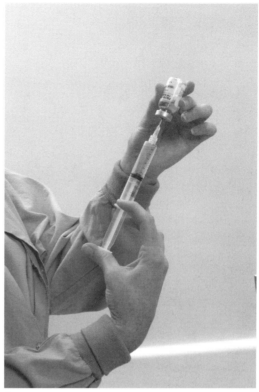

Figure **4–8.**   Unsterile hands must not touch the syringe plunger.

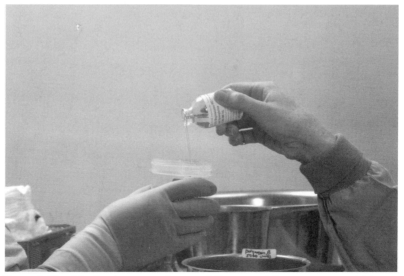

Figure **4–9.**   Medications may be carefully poured from an open vial into a medicine cup or other container.

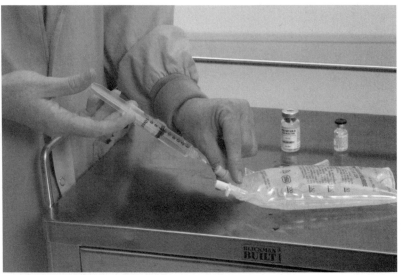

A

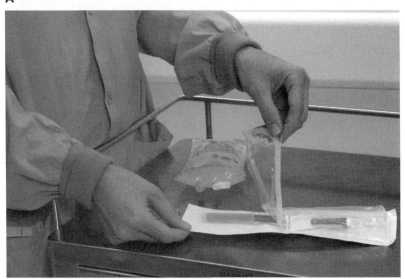

B

Figure **4–10.**   A sterile, disposable pour spout (decanter) is used to deliver medication contained in a bag of intravenous fluid. The metal cap and plastic cover are removed from the medication vial. **(A)** The medication is injected into an injection port on the bag. **(B)** The bag decanter is opened.

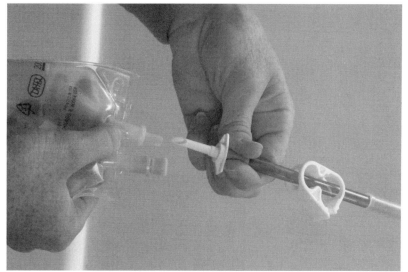

C

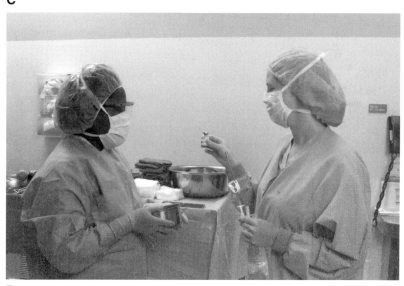

D

Figure **4–10, cont'd.**   **(C)** The bag decanter is grasped by the hub and the prong is inserted into injection port on the bag. **(D)** The label is shown to the scrubbed surgical technologist.   *Continued*

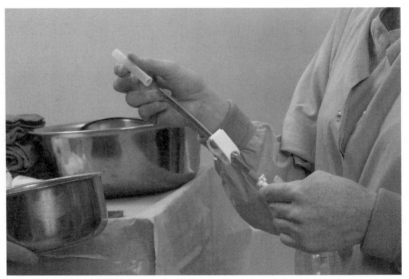

E

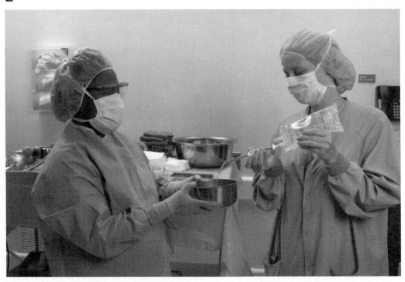

F

Figure **4–10, cont'd.**   **(E)** The protective cover on the decanter pour spout is removed. **(F)** The bag and decanter are inverted to pour medication into a container held by the scrubbed surgical technologist.

Some medication vials and ampules are available in sterile packages, which can be opened directly onto the sterile field. The scrub is responsible for showing the medication label and expiration date to the circulator prior to opening the vial and drawing up the contents.

Some medications are available in an ampule, a sealed glass container with a narrowed neck. The top of an ampule is broken off at the neck and a sterile needle attached to a syringe is inserted to aspirate and withdraw the medication. Special care should be used when breaking the glass ampule, because glass may cut unprotected hands (Fig. 4–11) or fly into unprotected eyes. Thus, the glass ampule should always be "snapped" away from the face and eye protection is required. Some ampules come with a plastic protective cap that is used to prevent injury during opening. If the ampule does not come with a protective device, a gauze sponge may be placed over the narrowed area of the ampule for protection. Some glass ampules also come packaged sterile for use on the back table, such as the liquid component used to make polymethyl methacrylate (bone cement). Once again, care must be taken to protect the gloved hands. After the ampule is broken, the item used to protect the hands should be discarded from the sterile field to avoid accidental transfer of glass particles into the surgical wound.

If medication is contained in a pour bottle (as seen in antibiotic irrigation prepared in the pharmacy), the cap should be lifted straight up and off (Fig. 4–12), and the entire contents poured

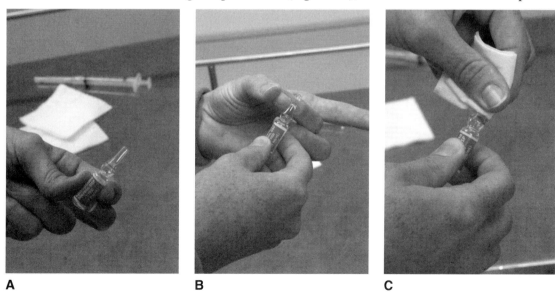

A   **B**   **C**

Figure **4–11. Caution must be taken to protect the hands when breaking a glass ampule.**
(A) Grasp ampule firmly. **(B)** Tap ampule to get entire contents into lower portion of ampule. **(C)** Using protective mechanism, break ampule at narrowed area.

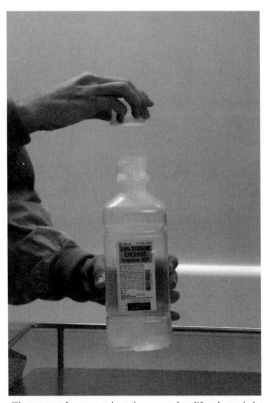

Figure **4-12.**   The cap of a pour bottle must be lifted straight up and off.

immediately. Unused portions should not be saved for later use, as sterility cannot be assured. If the bottle is recapped, its contents are considered unsterile due to potential contamination of the bottle lip during replacement of the cap.

To avoid potential **contamination**, the circulator must take care not to lean over the sterile field when delivering medications or solutions. The scrub should hold containers away from the sterile table or place containers at the table edge.

Several different types of containers are available to store medications and solutions on the sterile back table (Fig. 4–13). Medicine cups, pitchers, basins, or syringes may be used, depending on the volume of medication needed.

CAUTION

Medications intended for topical administration (such as Thrombin or epinephrine 1:1000) should *never* be kept in a syringe on the back table. Syringes are used to inject medications. Some topical medications are *fatal* if injected. Use a labeled shallow container, such as a petri dish, to

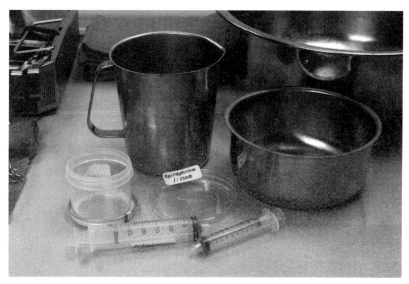

Figure **4–13.** A variety of medication containers, such as pitchers, basins, medicine cups, petri dishes, or syringes, may be used on the sterile back table.

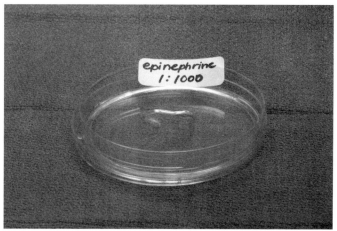

Figure **4–14.** A medication intended for topical application, such as epinephrine 1:1000, should be kept in a shallow container, such as a petri dish, rather than a syringe. For example, Gelfoam pledgets are dipped into topical epinephrine (1:1000) for hemostasis in the middle ear.

store topical medications. The use of a shallow container will make it more difficult to accidentally draw up a topical medication into a syringe. In addition, a shallow container provides easy access to the medication when needed, for example when dipping pieces of Gelfoam® into the medication for topical application (Fig. 4–14).

MEDICATION LABELING ON THE STERILE BACK TABLE

Once a medication has been delivered to the sterile back table, it is no longer in its original container, so it must be labeled immediately. Most drugs used from the sterile field are clear in color; thus, they are easily confused if not clearly marked. There are different methods of labeling medications on the sterile back table, but the most important point is that each medication must be labeled—in the intermediate storage container (such as pitcher or medicine cup) and in any delivery vehicle (such as a syringe). The most accurate method is the use of preprinted medication labels available from sterile supply manufacturers. If preprinted labels are not available, a sterile skin marking pen may be used to write on blank labels (Fig. 4–15). If blank labels are not available, sterile skin adhesive strips may be used. Regardless of the labeling method employed, proper identification of all medications on the sterile field is an absolutely crucial step in preventing medication administration errors.

Occasionally, the scrubbed surgical technologist may be replaced during a procedure (e.g., for shift change or lunch relief). All medications must be plainly labeled and reported to the new scrub. If there is any doubt as to the identity of a solution, it must be discarded and new medication must be obtained.

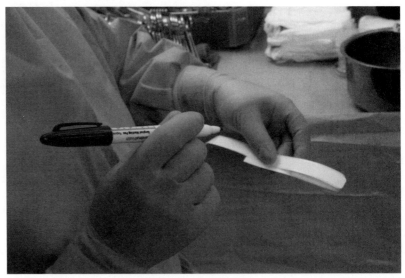

Figure **4–15.** A marking pen may be used to complete a label for a medication on the sterile back table.

There is no acceptable excuse for the presence of unlabeled (unidentified) medications on the sterile back table. Improper or inadequate labeling of drugs may be considered negligent. Negligence is defined in the Miller-Keane *Encyclopedia and Dictionary of Medicine, Nursing and Allied Health* as "failure to do something that a reasonable person of ordinary prudence would do in a situation or the doing of something that such a person would not do." By this definition, it is "reasonable" to expect that the correct medication will be obtained, identified, and passed to the surgeon and that a "prudent" person will perform these duties. This means that reason and prudence are everyone's responsibility, whatever the situation. This isn't always easy. The rapid pace of events in surgery often pressures team members to accomplish difficult tasks in a hurry. However, the process of medication identification should never be compromised. nor should staff become complacent about routine medications. If a question or doubt arises regarding a medication, it must be clarified and resolved. If the medication seems wrong or the dose appears to be incorrect, verify it with the physician before using it. It is better to be certain about the drug—even if it means provoking the surgeon—than to make an error and thus cause harm to the patient.

Do not be embarrassed to admit ignorance or confusion, and always admit an outright error. Honesty and integrity are vital characteristics in health care professionals. If you make a medication error, acknowledge it at once so that corrective measures may be taken. Notify the surgeon immediately. Then follow institutional policy. Usually, when a medication error occurs, the unit supervisor is notified and an incident or occurrence report is completed. Above all, immediate action is taken to correct the error, thus ensuring patient safety.

Special caution is required when handling controlled substances in surgery. Local policies regarding handling of controlled substances must be in compliance with federal law (see Chapter 2); thus, they must be understood and followed by all staff members. For example, cocaine is a schedule C-II drug frequently used for topical anesthesia in surgery. If needed for a particular procedure, cocaine is obtained immediately prior to use and is never left unattended. Any cocaine remaining at the end of the procedure must be rendered useless—usually by dilution with large amounts of water—and then discarded. The dilution and disposal of any controlled substance should be witnessed by at least two team members.

HANDLING MEDICATIONS

When medications have been delivered to the sterile field and labeled, some additional handling may be necessary. Occasionally, the surgeon may order that two medications be mixed for concurrent administration. For example, an anti-inflammatory agent and a long-acting local anesthetic agent may be mixed for injection into a joint at the conclusion of an arthroscopy. Some medications may be diluted prior to use, such as Hypaque, which may be diluted with equal parts of injectable saline as ordered on the preference card. It is vital that the surgical technologist read the preference card carefully and use basic math skills (see Chapter 3) to assure the correct mixture or dilution of medications at the sterile back table. All containers (such as medicine cups) must be labeled for the original medications, and a separate container must be clearly labeled indicating the mixture or diluted medication. The administration container, usually a syringe, must be labeled with complete information on the mixture or dilution. The final check for accuracy is performed when the scrubbed surgical technologist states the complete mixing or dilution information when handing the medication to the surgeon.

Other medications may require reconstitution prior to use (Insight 4–1). An example is topical thrombin, which is available in a sterile kit with a pump spray bottle. The kit contains a vial of thrombin, a vial of **diluent**, and a spray bottle. The scrub draws the diluent into a syringe and injects it into the thrombin vial. The mixture is shaken until the thrombin is dissolved and trans-

---

Insight 4–1   **Reconstituting**

Medications are not the only agents that may need to be reconstituted for a surgical procedure. Orthobiologic implants (Restore™), derived from porcine small-intestine submucosa that has been processed, disinfected, and sterilized, are designed as a tissure scaffold that is resorbable by the body. The implant helps to reinforce weakened or damaged soft tissue and is a less invasive alternative to allograft. Examples of surgical procedures that may use an orthobiologic implant are rotator cuff repair and Achilles tendon repair. The implant must be kept refrigerated until needed and then soaked for 7 to 10 minutes (or reconstituted) in sterile saline/buffer or water prior to use.

ferred to the pump spray bottle for administration to large, oozing surfaces such as the liver.

SUPPLIES

Syringes and hypodermic needles are used frequently in surgery to draw up, measure, and administer medications. Disposable syringes are made of plastic, but reusable glass syringes may be indicated for specific situations. The most common sizes of syringes routinely used in surgery range from 1 mL to 60 mL. A syringe has three basic parts: the barrel (or outer portion), the plunger (inside portion), and the tip. The barrel of the syringe is marked or calibrated to indicate the amount of medication contained in the syringe. The amount of medication in the syringe is measured from the innermost edge of the rubber tip on the end of the plunger. Some syringes have a finger-control attachment on the barrel and plunger to provide ease of motion and more precise control when injecting (Fig. 4–16). The most common type of syringe tip used in surgery is the Luer-loc tip, which has a screw-type locking mechanism used to securely attach a hypodermic needle. Plain-tip or slip-tip syringes are also available, but these are used for specific purposes. For example, a plain-tip syringe may be attached to a spinal needle for subclavian

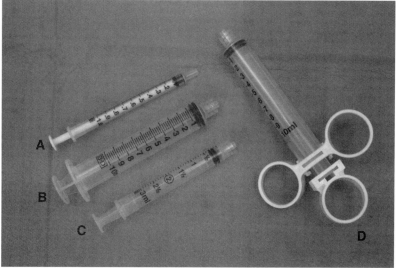

Figure **4–16. Types of syringes.** (A) 1-mL plain-tip tuberculin syringe. (B) A 10-mL Luer-loc syringe. (C) A 3-mL Luer-loc syringe. (D) A 10-mL finger-control Luer-loc syringe.

venipuncture during a venous access procedure. Various sizes of syringes are used for various purposes, so consult the surgeon's preference card for specific information. Generally, 1-mL (called TB or tuberculin) and 3-mL syringes are used to inflate the tiny balloon on the end of an embolectomy catheter. A 5-mL syringe is used to fill the balloon on a 5-mL Foley catheter. By far the most common syringe size used in the operating room is a 10-mL syringe, used for a number of purposes, including inflating the cuff on a tracheostomy tube and injection of a local anesthetic agent throughout a surgical procedure. 30-mL syringes are most frequently used to inject saline irrigation and contrast media into the common bile duct, inflate a 30-mL balloon on a Foley catheter, or administer heparinized saline through an arterial irrigation catheter.

Special syringes are available for particular purposes. For example, a tubex syringe has a metal or plastic device used to accommodate a **carpule** of medication for injection (such as lidocaine or heparin). The glass medication carpule has a rubber cap that is penetrated by a special needle attached to the tubex syringe (Fig. 4–17).

Hypodermic needles are used to draw up and administer drugs. A hypodermic needle has three basic parts: the hub (which fits onto a syringe), the shaft, and the tip (the beveled end of the shaft). Needles vary in diameter (gauge) and length (measured in inches). The larger the gauge of a needle, the smaller the diameter of the lumen (inside channel). So, an 18-gauge needle has a

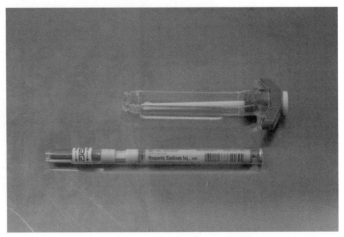

Figure **4–17.**   A tubex syringe, glass carpule, and needle.

much larger lumen than a 25-gauge needle. Most needles used in surgery are disposable and are color-coded by size at the plastic hub for ease in identification. Sizes of hypodermic needles routinely used in surgery range from 27-gauge needles (used in ophthalmology) to larger 18-gauge needles (used to draw up medications). The most common needle length used in surgery is $1\frac{1}{2}$ inches. Shorter, $\frac{5}{8}$-inch needles may be used for superficial injections, whereas longer needles (3-inch), called spinal needles, may be used for specific purposes, such as aspiration of cysts (Fig. 4–18).

⚠ CAUTION

Standard precautions state that used needles must never be recapped, because most needle puncture injuries are the result of attempting to recap a used needle. However, it is also dangerous to leave an unsheathed hypodermic needle exposed on the sterile table. If a needle must be recapped for protection between repeated uses during a surgical procedure, you should use a one-handed technique (Fig. 4–19) or a recapping device intended for that purpose.

Several new products are becoming available to help improve needle (sharps) safety, including syringes preloaded with retractable one-time-use needles. After injection, the needle is automatically withdrawn into the syringe. The design is intended to prevent accidental injury from the needle tip and effectively prevents reuse of the needle and syringe. These items are most

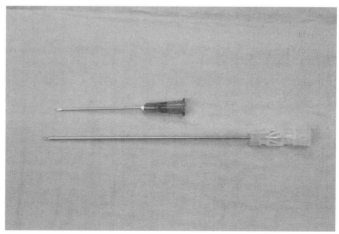

Figure **4–18.**   Hypodermic needles, $1\frac{1}{2}$-inch and 3-inch.

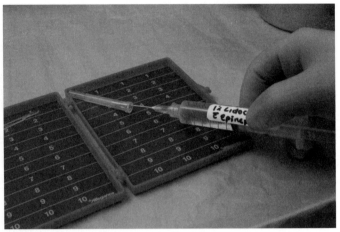

Figure **4–19.**   If a needle must be recapped for protection for reuse during an operation, such as the periodic injection of local anesthetic for patient comfort, use a one-handed recapping technique.

appropriate for use by the anesthesia provider when administering a medication through the intravenous line, but have limited use at the sterile field where multiple injections of a medication may be given with the same syringe and needle (as seen in the use of a local anesthetic agent).

ADVANCED PRACTICES FOR THE SURGICAL FIRST ASSISTANT
Chapter 4—Medication Administration

KEY TERMS

half-life   systemic effect

MEDICATION ADMINISTRATION FROM THE STERILE FIELD

Intraoperative administration of medications to the surgical patient presents a unique situation unlike any other medical environment, especially for the advanced practitioner functioning as a surgical first assistant. Different personnel administer medications to the patient through several routes, often at the same time. Although the surgical first assistant might not perform the actual administration of medications, it is important that he or she be aware of the effects any medication can have on the patient.

ADVANCED PRACTICES FOR THE SURGICAL FIRST ASSISTANT   *(continued)*

Personnel who fulfill the role of the surgical first assistant will have different educational and clinical backgrounds ranging from medical school to physician's assisting, nursing, and surgical technology. These different backgrounds and employment disciplines dictate the different regulatory agencies under which each professional practices in regard to administration of medications. State statutes will supercede any other regulatory agency in regard to limitations of practice; however, when there is no statute regulating specific personnel, it is usually the individual facility that regulates the practice. All personnel practicing as surgical first assistants should be aware of the policies or bylaws regulating their practice. For example, the surgical first assistant functioning as an independent practitioner may be regulated by the medical staff bylaws of the facility. However, the surgical first assistant employed by the facility may be regulated by that facility's policies and procedures.

The process of administering medications at the sterile field requires a team effort. Medications pass through at least two other people, the circulator and the scrub person, before being delivered to the surgeon. The medication is almost always in a container different from its original; usually a syringe, medicine cup, basin, or pitcher. To prevent medication errors, strict policies and procedures have been developed for delivery of medications onto the sterile field (as described in this chapter). The surgeon and the surgical first assistant may be the last line of defense to avoid medication errors; therefore, each should be aware of and follow all these procedures. The person who administers the medication *always* has the right to question the procedure and decide if the medication will be given or a new medication obtained. It is always in the best interest of the patient to discard any questionable medication (Table A).

Table **A**   Guidelines for Administering Medications from the Sterile Field

- Always be aware of the process of delivering medications to the sterile field.
- Always read the label on the device you receive that contains the medication.
- Always confirm name and strength of the medication with the scrub person.
- Always inform anesthesia personnel when administering medications.
- Always be aware of any patient allergies.
- Always be aware of the amount of the medication administered.
- Never administer medications that are discolored or contain sediment.
- Never administer medications that are contaminated with other materials from the sterile field.
- Never administer a medication from any unlabeled container.
- Never administer a medication when there is any doubt about its identification or strength.

(continued on following page)

ADVANCED PRACTICES FOR THE SURGICAL FIRST ASSISTANT   *(continued)*

☞ **Note:** When medications are administered from the sterile field, it is important to communicate to the anesthesia provider the name of the agent and amount given. For example, when a local anesthetic agent is administered that contains epinephrine, the anesthesia provider should be notified immediately and verbally advised as to the amount of the medication ultimately injected (which is also noted on the operative record). This is important because epinephrine acts as a vasoconstrictor and can affect the patient's blood pressure.

DOSE–TIME–EFFECT RELATIONSHIP

All medications have **systemic effects** on the patient. It is important for the surgical first assistant to be aware of these effects as well as the duration of medications and safe dosages. This pharmacological principle is known as the dose-time-effect relationship. Drug effects are a result of the dose administered and the time from absorption to elimination. Medication dosage, time the medication is absorbed by the body, and the duration of action are all interrelated and interdependent. The duration of a medication's effect is based on the **half-life** of the medicine. Half-life is the time it takes a certain medicine to be eliminated by the body. Certain conditions such as decreased liver or renal function alter the half-life of medications. It is important to note that a medication may go through many half-lives before it no longer has a therapeutic effect on the body. This must be recognized when calculating subsequent doses of the same medication to maintain a therapeutic level of its desired effects. A common example in the surgical setting is the administration of sodium heparin to achieve anticoagulation during vascular surgery (Table B).

Table **B**   Half-Life of Sodium Heparin, 5000 u

Time from Dosage (in hours)	Remaining Serum Amount in Body
1	2500 u
2	1250 u
3	625 u
4	312 u
5	156 u

KEY CONCEPTS

- The role of the scrubbed surgical technologist in medication administration is to identify, label, and clearly state the medication while passing it to the surgeon.
- Each facility's established policies and procedures should always be understood and scrupulously followed.
- In addition, the surgical technologist must be aware of state regulations regarding specific practices.
- Application of the six "rights" of medication administration will reduce the potential for drug errors.
- The surgical technologist in the scrub role must never accept a medication without properly identifying it.
- Aseptic technique must be used when delivering or accepting drugs into the sterile field. Accurate and immediate labeling of drugs on the sterile back table is required to minimize potential for errors.

Unit Two

Applied Surgical Pharmacology

Many medications are used in surgery each day. This unit provides an introduction to the medications you will frequently encounter as a surgical technologist. We'll look at antibiotics, diagnostic agents, diuretics, hormones, fluids, and antineoplastic chemotherapy agents. We'll also examine medications that affect blood coagulation and medications used as ophthalmic agents. To understand these agents, you'll need to be familiar with some basic anatomy and physiology, so we'll review some of those principles as well. Once you know the generic and brand names of common surgical medications and their categories, you'll be better able to recognize their purposes, action, administration, routes, and proper handling in order to provide safe patient care.

5

ANTIBIOTICS

Medications Covered in Chapter 5

Generic Name	Brand or Trade Name	Category
amikacin	Amikin	Aminoglycoside
gentamicin	Garamycin, Jenamicin	Aminoglycoside
streptomycin	N/A	Aminoglycoside
tobramycin	Nebcin	Aminoglycoside
neomycin	Neobiotic	Aminoglycoside
kanamycin	Kantrex	Aminoglycoside
cefazolin	Ancef, Kefzol, Zolicef	1st-generation cephalosporin
cefadroxil	Duricef, Ultracef	1st-generation cephalosporin
cephalexin	Keflex, Keflet	1st-generation cephalosporin
cephalothin	Keflin	1st-generation cephalosporin
cephapirin	Cefadyl	1st-generation cephalosporin
cephradine	Anspor, Velocef	1st-generation cephalosporin
cefoxitin	Mefoxin	2nd-generation cephalosporin
cefaclor	Ceclor	2nd-generation cephalosporin
cefamandole	Mandol	2nd-generation cephalosporin
cefmetazole	Zefazone	2nd-generation cephalosporin
cefonicid	Monocid	2nd-generation cephalosporin
cefotetan	Cefotan	2nd-generation cephalosporin
cefuroxime	Ceftin, Zinacef	2nd-generation cephalosporin
cefotaxime	Claforan	3rd-generation cephalosporin
cefixime	Suprax	3rd-generation cephalosporin
cefoperazone	Cefobid	3rd-generation cephalosporin
ceftazidime	Ceptaz, Fortaz, Tazicef, Tazidime	3rd-generation cephalosporin

(continued on following page)

Medications Covered in Chapter 5   *(continued)*

Generic Name	Brand or Trade Name	Category
ceftizoxime	Cefizox	3rd-generation cephalosporin
ceftriaxone	Rocephin	3rd-generation cephalosporin
cefepime	Maxipime	4th-generation cephalosporin
erythromycin	E-mycin, ERYC	
erythromycin ethylsuccinate	EES, Ery Ped	
azithromycin	Zithromax	
clarithromycin	Biaxin	
penicillin G	Pentids, Pfizerpen	Natural penicillin
benzathine penicillin G	Bicillin L-A, Permapen	Natural penicillin
penicillin V	Beepen-VK, Betapen-VK	Natural penicillin
methicillin	Staphcillin	Penicillinase-resistant penicillin
cloxacillin	Cloxapen	Penicillinase-resistant penicillin
dicloxacillin	Dycill, Pathocil	Penicillinase-resistant penicillin
nafcillin	Nafcil, Unipen	Penicillinase-resistant penicillin
oxacillin	Bactocill	Penicillinase-resistant penicillin
ampicillin	Omnipen	Aminopenicillin
amoxicillin	Amoxil, Polymox	Aminopenicillin
bacampicillin	Spectrobid	Aminopenicillin
carbenicillin	Geocillin	Broad-spectrum penicillin
mezlocillin	Mezlin	Broad-spectrum penicillin
piperacillin	Pipracil	Broad-spectrum penicillin
ticarcillin	Ticar	Broad-spectrum penicillin
tetracycline hydrochloride	Achromycin-V, Sumycin	Tetracycline
minocycline	Minocin	Tetracycline
oxytetracycline	Terramycin	Tetracycline
doxycycline	Vibramycin	Tetracycline
chlortetracycline hydrochloride	Aureomycin	Tetracycline
linezolid	Zyvox	Oxazolidinone
ciprofloxacin	Cipro	Quinolone
ofloxacin	Floxin	Quinolone
norfloxacin	Noroxin	Quinolone
enoxacin	Penetrex	Quinolone
silver sulfadiazine	Silvadene	Sulfonamide
sulfisoxazole	Gantrisin	Sulfonamide
sulfamethoxazole	Gantanol	Sulfonamide
Sulfamethoxazole with trimethoprim	Bactrim, Septra	Sulfonamides
sulfasalazine	Azulfidine	Sulfonamide
sulfacetamide sodium	Sodium Sulamyd	Sulfonamide
aztreonam	Azactam	Monobactam
chloramphenicol	Chloromycetin	Antibiotic
clindamycin	Cleocin	Antibiotic
imipenem	Primaxin	Antibiotic
metronidazole	Flagyl	Antibiotic

OBJECTIVES

After completing this chapter, you should be able to:

1. Define terminology related to antimicrobial therapy.
2. Discuss the purpose of antibiotic therapy in surgery.
3. Describe various ways in which antimicrobials work.
4. Discuss antibiotic resistance.
5. List categories of antibiotics used in surgery and give examples of each.
6. Identify the category of various antibiotics.
7. Use drug resources to gather pertinent information on antibiotics.

KEY TERMS

antibiotic resistance
bactericidal
bacteriostatic
culture and sensitivity (C&S)
endogenous
eukaryotes
exogenous
Gram's staining
methicillin-resistant *Staphylococcus aureus* (MRSA)

morphology
nephrotoxicity
ototoxicity
polymicrobic infections
prokaryotes
prophylaxis
selective toxicity
vancomycin-resistant enterococci (VRE)

Before the discovery of antimicrobial agents, surgical patients often died from infections of various kinds. Surgical procedures, such as amputations, were quite dangerous in themselves. The most common danger, however, was a postoperative wound infection. Even if patients survived surgery, the resulting wound infection was often fatal. Today, however, many antimicrobial agents are available. They are used (1) to prevent and (2) to treat infections caused by pathogenic (disease-causing) microorganisms. The term *antimicrobial* applies to several categories of agents: These include antivirals, antibacterials, antiprotozoals, antifungals, and antiparasitics. In surgery, however, the only antimicrobial agents routinely used are antibacterials, commonly referred to as *antibiotics*.

Antibiotics are natural chemicals (or *metabolites*) produced by microorganisms that inhibit the growth of other microorganisms. These natural chemicals may be altered in the chemical laboratory to produce semisynthetic antibiotics. Approximately 85% of the antibiotics currently available are produced by actinomycetes—a family of bacteria that resemble fungi because of their filamentous projections. Other antibiotics, such as the penicillins, are derived from fungi.

Antibiotics are given both preoperatively and intraoperatively for **prophylaxis**—that is, prevention—of postoperative wound infections. They may also be prescribed postoperatively. Postoperative wound infections (most commonly referred to as surgical site infection, or SSI) are potential complications of every surgical intervention because any such procedure penetrates the body's first line of defense, the skin. SSIs may range from minor to serious; they may even be deadly, depending on several factors. Antibiotics do not take the place of aseptic technique. Rather, antibiotics are adjuncts that assist the patient's own defenses to prevent—or diminish the severity of—postoperative SSIs.

MICROBIOLOGY REVIEW

SSIs are caused by the introduction of pathogenic microorganisms into a susceptible host (Fig. 5–1) via a route of transmission. The pathogen must have a source, a means of transmission, and a host to cause an infection. The source of pathogenic microorganisms may be **endogenous** or **exogenous**. That is, the infectious microbe may come from the patient's own bacteria (endogenous) or from outside the patient (exogenous). For example, among the most common causative agents of SSIs are bacteria known as *Staphylococcus aureus,* which are normally present on the patient's skin (endogenous source) and may be carried into the surgical site during the course of the operation. Exogenous sources of pathogenic microbes include surgical personnel and the environment. An example of an exogenous source of infectious microbes is various bacteria carried under artificial fingernails when worn by

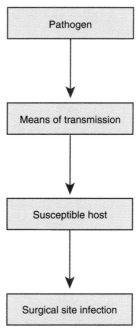

Figure **5–1.**   Infection cycle: source of pathogenic microbe plus transmission route plus susceptible host equals infection.

sterile team members. Such microbes are introduced into the surgical site by glove tears commonly associated with long fingernails.

 CAUTION

Long and/or artificial nails are prohibited in surgery, and team members who wear them are failing to follow policies established to prevent postoperative SSIs.

Another example of an exogenous source of pathogens is improperly cleaned or sterilized instruments, which may carry microbes into the wound. Regardless of the source, many other factors influence the surgical patient's susceptibility to an infection, including general health, nutritional status, operative site, and length of surgical procedure.

If a surgical site infection occurs, treatment requires identification of the causative microorganism and selection of an appropriate antimicrobial agent. Pathogenic microorganisms causing SSIs are identified by several methods. Common methods used to identify pathogens include **culture and sensitivity (C&S) and**

Gram's staining. Culture and sensitivity is the process of growing microbes in culture to determine the infecting pathogen and the exposure of the pathogen to various antibiotics to determine which agent will best inhibit the pathogen's growth. To perform C&S, a fluid or tissue specimen is obtained with a swab from the infection site, and placed in one or more culture tubes for transport to the microbiology laboratory. Note that separate culture tubes are available for aerobic (in oxygen) and anaerobic (lacking oxygen) testing. In the laboratory, the culture swab is used to spread the fluid sample onto nutrient agar and differential (distinguishing) media in petri dishes called *plates*. This process is called *inoculation*. The inoculated plates are incubated for 24 to 48 hours, after which they can be examined for microbial growth. Miniaturized reaction containers allow laboratory personnel to identify causative microbes faster and easier. Once the microbe has been isolated, it is grown in a pure culture and exposed to different antibiotics. This process of successive exposure to antibiotics to determine which agent is most effective against it is called *sensitivity testing*. The conventional Kirby-Bauer disk diffusion method of sensitivity testing takes longer than the newer Rapid Antibiotic Susceptibility Test (RAST).

When the causative microorganism is identified and tested for antibiotic sensitivity, the appropriate therapy can be initiated. Often, however, a broad-spectrum antibiotic is prescribed to begin treatment while awaiting the results of C&S testing. Occasionally during a surgical procedure such as an incision and drainage (I&D), a sample of abscess fluid may be subjected to an immediate Gram's stain process (Insight 5–1).

A Gram's stain is a rapid identification test that assists the physician in prescribing an initial course of antibiotic therapy

---

Insight 5–1   **Gram's Staining**

Gram's staining is a differential staining procedure, which means it is used to distinguish between two types of bacteria. The Gram's stain procedure was developed in 1884 and is still widely used today. A specimen containing the pathogenic microorganism to be identified is swabbed onto a slide and fixed. Crystal violet is applied first, staining all cells a bluish-purple. Gram's iodine is then applied to the slide as a mordant—an agent that increases the cell's affinity for the primary stain. The slide is then rinsed with acetone or alcohol, decolorizing the cells. Next, safranin—a red counterstain—is applied. Only cells that were decolorized pick up the red counterstain. The cell walls of gram-positive bacteria do not decolorize, remaining purple. Gram-negative bacteria lose the purple stain during decolorization, so they appear red or reddish-pink after application of safranin.

Table 5–1 Pathogenic Microorganisms by Gram's Staining and Morphology

Gram-Positive (stain purple)	Gram-Negative (stain pink)
Cocci (round)	
Staphylococcus aureus	*Neisseria meningitidis*
Staphylococcus epidermidis	
Streptococcus pneumoniae	
Streptococcus pyogenes	
Enterococci	
Bacilli (rods)	
Mycobacterium tuberculosis	*Klebsiella pneumoniae*
Listeria monocytogenes	*Bacteroides*
Actinomyces israelii	*Escherichia coli*
	Pseudomonas aeruginosa
	Proteus
	Salmonella
	Serratia
	Haemophilus influenzae

based on the probable pathogen causing the infection. Gram's staining is a way of distinguishing types of bacteria. In combination with **morphology** (the study of shapes), it can be used to identify many common bacteria. Bacteria occur in many shapes, most of which may be placed in three major groups: spirilla (spiral shaped), bacilli (rod or oblong shaped), and cocci (round or spherical). Table 5–1 lists some common microorganisms classified by Gram's stain and morphology.

To be effective, an antimicrobial agent must have **selective toxicity**, that is, it must act against pathogenic microorganisms without harming host cells. Antibiotics must target structures and functions in pathogenic microorganisms that differ from those of host cells. To understand how antimicrobials work, then, we need to know what differences exist between pathogen and host cell structure.

Bacteria are one-celled organisms that don't have a fully developed nucleus. This means they are classified as **prokaryotes**. (A karyote is a nucleus. A *pro*karyote is an early, or "pre" nucleus.) Multicellular organisms, including fungi, plants, and animals, are classified as **eukaryotes** ("true" karyotes). Both prokaryotic and eukaryotic cells have a plasma membrane that encloses the cell and preserves its integrity. Thus it both protects the cell and

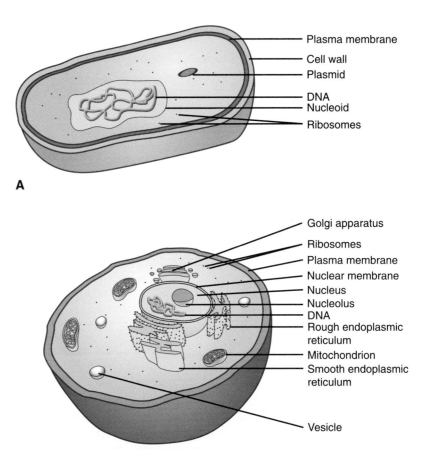

Figure **5–2.** **Eukaryotic cells are encased in a plasma membrane whereas prokaryotic cells have a cell wall in addition to a plasma membrane:** (**A**) Prokaryotic cell; (**B**) eukaryotic cell.

regulates the movement of materials in and out of the cell. Prokaryotes differ from eukaryotes because they have a cell wall in addition to the plasma membrane. This cell wall provides a potential location for antibiotic therapy (Fig. 5–2).

Prokaryotic cells also differ from eukaryotic cells in the structures responsible for protein synthesis—the *ribosomes*. These tiny structures assemble or synthesize proteins from amino acids. Both prokaryotes and eukaryotes have ribosomes, but prokaryotic ribosomes are smaller than eukaryotic ribosomes (Fig. 5–3). This size difference offers another avenue of action for antibiotics. That is, antibiotics that bind to the smaller bacterial ribosomes do not bind to the larger ribosomes of the eukaryotic host cells.

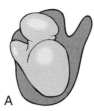 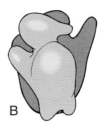

Figure 5–3. Prokaryotic (**A**) and eukaryotic (**B**) ribosomes differ in size.

Table **5–2** Methods of Antimicrobial Action
Inhibit cell-wall synthesis Interfere with protein synthesis Alter cell membrane function Inhibit production of nucleic acids (RNA or DNA) Interfere with cell metabolism

ANTIMICROBIAL ACTION

MECHANISMS AND TYPES

Antimicrobial agents may work against pathogenic microorganisms by five different mechanisms, as summarized by Table 5–2. Some agents, such as cephalosporins, penicillins, vancomycin, and bacitracin, keep bacteria from synthesizing adequate cell walls. They can stop cell walls from forming or inhibit the synthesis process so the walls are too weak to maintain vital functions. Antibiotics such as aminoglycosides, erythromycins, and tetracyclines interfere with protein synthesis. This means they bind to prokaryotic ribosomes, thus preventing the assembly of critical proteins. Polymixins and some antifungal agents work by disrupting the bacterial cell membrane, causing leakage of materials necessary for cell function. A few agents, such as quinolones and some antivirals, inhibit production of the nucleic acids (RNA or DNA) that are necessary for bacterial replication. Still other agents interfere with bacterial cell metabolism. Sulfonamides, for example, take the place of a vital substance needed to produce folic acid.

We classify antimicrobial agents as **bactericidal** or **bacteriostatic**. Bactericidal agents kill bacteria. These include agents such as the aminoglycosides, cephalosporins, and penicillins. Bacteriostatic agents inhibit bacterial growth, relying on the host's own immune system to take over once the pathogenic microorganism is suppressed. Bacteriostatic agents include the erythromycins and tetracyclines. Antimicrobial agents are also classified by their *spectrum* of activity. A *broad-spectrum* antibiotic has a wide range of activity—usually effective against both gram-negative and gram-positive bacteria. *Narrow-spectrum* antibiotics have a smaller range of activity—often effective against only one category of microorganisms, gram-negative or gram-positive. *Limited-spectrum* antibiotics are effective against just one species of microorganism.

ANTIBIOTIC RESISTANCE

Certain pathogenic microorganisms have developed an alarming capacity to resist antibiotics (Insight 5–2). **Antibiotic resistance**

Insight 5–2   **Developing and Sharing Antibiotic Resistance**

Microorganisms grow and divide rapidly, so genetic material (DNA) is constantly replicated (copied). When a microorganism develops a characteristic, such as resistance to an antibiotic, that characteristic is passed to every daughter cell through the DNA. Bacteria obtain antibiotic resistance by mutation (i.e., changes in the sequence of DNA). There are at least four known methods: random mutation, transformation, transduction, and conjugation. Some random mutations are beneficial to the cell, whereas others may be lethal. The addition or deletion of a single nucleotide (the building blocks of DNA) may confer resistance to an antibiotic, a trait crucial to bacterial survival. These changes can cause the production of an enzyme to break down the antibiotic, alter the structure of targeted antibiotic binding sites, or make the bacterial membrane impervious to the agent. Widespread use of antibiotics may actually promote the development and survival of antibiotic-resistant strains of bacteria. Transformation is the transfer of free DNA (probably leaked from destroyed bacteria) into another bacterium. The new DNA is incorporated into the host, transforming the host and subsequent daughter cells by displaying new characteristics, such as antibiotic resistance. Transduction is the transfer of DNA from one bacterium to another bacterium by a viral carrier, known as a *phage* (a virus that infects bacteria). When the virus replicates in the host bacterium, some of the host DNA may be incorporated within the viral capsule (the coat surrounding the virus). When the virus infects another bacterium, the previous host DNA may then be combined with the new host DNA, providing a trait such as antibiotic resistance. Conjugation, or joining together, is another means of transmitting antibiotic resistance. Some types of bacteria have the ability to join and thus share DNA in segments called plasmids. Microorganisms have become adept at changing to survive. As scientists develop agents to kill microbial pathogens, these microorganisms change to resist the antimicrobial agent and pass the trait to the next generation. Antimicrobial resistance is one of the most challenging pharmacologic problems in medicine today.

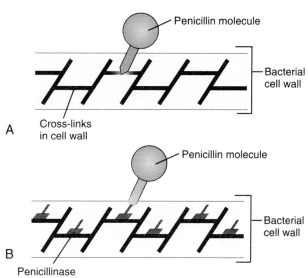

Figure **5–4. Penicillinase inactivates penicillin.** (**A**) Penicillin breaks down crosslinks in bacterial cell wall. (**B**) Penicillinase breaks down a portion of penicillin structure, inactivating it.

is the ability of some strains of pathogenic microbes to prevent or overcome the activity of antimicrobial agents. Antibiotic resistance mechanisms generally fit into three major categories:

- The microorganism may manufacture microbial enzymes that inactivate the antibiotic.
- The cell membrane may be altered to prevent the antibiotic from entering the cell.
- The target area, such as ribosome, may be altered so that the agent is no longer effective.

For example, some bacteria produce an enzyme known as penicillinase. This enzyme breaks down part of the chemical structure of penicillin, making the drug ineffective (Fig. 5–4). Penicillinase is produced by a number of microbes, including two common strains of staphylococci. Thus these microorganisms have become resistant to treatment with penicillin. When antibiotic resistance appears as a bacterial trait, pharmaceutical manufacturers attempt to develop new forms of the antibiotic or to overcome the bacterial resistance mechanism. For example, methicillin (which is not broken down by penicillinase) was developed and remains useful for some strains of pathogenic microbes. However, a strain of *Staphylococcus aureus* has become resistant to methicillin. This strain is known as **methicillin-resistant *Staphylococcus aureus* (MRSA).** This resistant strain of bacteria is difficult to treat with available agents.

Other pathogens are becoming resistant to more than one antibiotic. Scientists have identified a plasmid (a segment of bacterial DNA) that confers resistance to six antibiotics. Multiple antibiotic resistance is found in a number of pathogens including a strain of the tubercle bacillus (TB), the pathogen that causes tuberculosis. This strain of TB resists several powerful antibiotics, including streptomycin and rifampicin. Similarly, one group of enteric (digestive tract) bacteria has developed resistance to vancomycin. These bacteria are known as **vancomycin-resistant enterococci (VRE).** Additional strains of antimicrobial-resistant pathogenic microorganisms are being continually identified.

The major cause of concern in antibiotic resistance is that microbes are capable of developing resistance mechanisms to prevent or inactivate agents much faster than scientists can develop new agents. It is generally accepted that there will be increasing morbidity and mortality due to infections with resistant microbes for a significant time to come.

The rapid development of resistant pathogens has been linked to the widespread practice of prescribing antibiotics for nontreatable viral infections such as colds. When normal host bacteria are frequently exposed to antibiotics, they have many opportunities to develop resistance; this means an antibiotic may be ineffective against a subsequent bacterial infection because the resistant trait has pervaded the host's bacterial population. Similarly, when patients do not take necessary antibiotics as prescribed—regularly and in the right dose—they give pathogens a chance to develop resistance. Weaker pathogens may be destroyed, but stronger, mutated strains may survive and reproduce.

ANTIBIOTIC AGENTS

Many antibiotics are available to treat a wide variety of infectious processes. In this text, however, we focus on the few categories of antibiotics commonly used in surgical procedures (Table 5–3). Antibiotics are usually administered intravenously both before and during a surgical procedure for prophylaxis against surgical site infections. Antibiotics may also be administered topically, often in the form of irrigant solutions or as ointments. Antibiotics are also prescribed for postoperative use, to be administered intravenously or orally, to prevent or treat infection. Here, we look at some common categories of antibiotics, together with their

Table 5–3   Major Groups of Antibiotics

Aminoglycosides
Cephalosporins
Macrolides
Penicillins
Tetracyclines

origins, mechanisms of action, surgical uses, and bacterial resistance mechanisms against the agent.

AMINOGLYCOSIDES

Aminoglycosides, which are derived from various strains of *Actinomyces* bacteria, interfere with protein synthesis by binding to bacterial (prokaryotic) ribosomes. They are bactericidal and relatively narrow in spectrum. Generally active only against aerobic, gram-negative bacteria, aminoglycosides also provide some activity against some gram-positive bacteria such as *Staphylococcus* species, including some methicillin-resistant strains. Otherwise, they are not very active against gram-positive organisms. All aminoglycosides are contraindicated if the patient has a history of hypersensitivity or toxic reactions to any aminoglycoside. Major adverse effects include **ototoxicity** and **nephrotoxicity**; that is, these drugs can damage hearing and balance and kidney cells (nephrons). Irreversible deafness, renal failure, and death have been reported after extensive irrigation of surgical fields with aminoglycosides.

Aminoglycosides are poorly absorbed orally, but are almost completely absorbed when applied topically during surgical procedures. Intramuscular and intravenous injections are the most common administration routes for aminoglycosides.

Aminoglycosides are indicated for short-term treatment of serious infections due to susceptible organisms. Such infections include bacterial septicemia as well as infections of the respiratory tract, bones and joints, central nervous system (meningitis), skin, and soft tissue. Aminoglycosides may also be prescribed for intra-abdominal infections.

Among the drugs in the aminoglycoside category are amikacin (Amikin), gentamicin (Garamycin), streptomycin, tobramycin (Nebcin), neomycin (Neobiotic), and kanamycin (Kantrex), as listed in Table 5–4. Amikacin is often effective even when strains

Table **5–4** Aminoglycosides	
Generic Name	*Trade Name*
amikacin	Amikin
gentamicin	Garamycin, Jenamicin
streptomycin	
tobramycin	Nebcin
neomycin	Neobiotic
kanamycin	Kantrex

of susceptible organisms are resistant to other aminoglycosides. Gentamicin is available in cream and ointment, ophthalmic solution and ointment, and solution for injection. Streptomycin is used in combination with other agents to treat infections caused by *Mycobacterium tuberculosis* (the tubercle bacillus) and is administered intramuscularly only. Neomycin is too toxic for systemic use, so it is applied topically only.

Bacterial resistance to aminoglycosides is conferred by the production of enzymes that modify the chemical structure of the agent, inactivating it.

CEPHALOSPORINS

Cephalosporins are broad-spectrum antibiotics derived from the fungus *Cephalosporium acremonium*. Cephalosporins are bactericidal, targeting cell-wall synthesis. That is, they block an enzyme needed to strengthen the bacterial cell wall, causing cell lysis (rupture). Cephalosporins are classified into four generations based on different ranges of activity:

First-generation cephalosporins are active against many gram-positive and some gram-negative microbes.

Second-generation cephalosporins are effective on a wider variety of gram-negative, but fewer gram-positive organisms.

Third-generation cephalosporins have a wider range of activity against gram-negative microbes than second-generation agents, but are less effective on gram-positive organisms.

Fourth-generation cephalosporins have an expanded spectrum on both gram-positive and gram-negative microorganisms.

Cephalosporins are used as prophylaxis in a variety of surgical procedures and are often indicated when patients are allergic to penicillins (although some cross-reactivity is possible). Administration is oral, intramuscular, or intravenous, depending on the

Table **5–5** Cephalosporins	
Generic Name	*Trade Name*
First-Generation	
cefazolin	Ancef, Kefzol, Zolicef
cefadroxil	Duricef, Ultracef
cephalexin	Keflex, Keflet
cephalothin	Keflin
cephapirin	Cefadyl
cephradine	Anspor, Velocef
Second-Generation	
cefoxitin	Mefoxin
cefaclor	Ceclor
cefamandole	Mandol
cefmetazole	Zefazone
cefonicid	Monocid
cefotetan	Cefotan
cefuroxime	Ceftin, Zinacef
Third-Generation	
cefotaxime	Claforan
cefixime	Suprax
cefoperazone	Cefobid
ceftazidime	Ceptaz, Fortaz, Tazicef, Tazidime
ceftizoxime	Cefizox
ceftriaxone	Rocephin
Fourth-Generation	
cefepime	Maxipime

particular cephalosporin. Some cephalosporins may be used as topical irrigation solutions in surgery. Bacterial resistance to cephalosporins is conferred by the production of an enzyme (cephalosporinase) that changes the chemical structure of the agent, inactivating it. Table 5–5 lists cephalosporins by generation.

MACROLIDES

Macrolides, which include the erythromycins, are a group of broad-spectrum agents that inhibit bacterial protein synthesis by binding to the prokaryotic ribosomal subunit. Bacteriostatic for

Table 5–6 Macrolides	
Generic Name	Trade Name
erythromycin	E-mycin, ERYC
erythromycin ethylsuccinate	EES, Ery Ped
azithromycin	Zithromax
clarithromycin	Biaxin

most bacteria, macrolides are bactericidal for several gram-positive bacteria such as *Legionella*. This cidal activity is explained by the fact that these antibiotics can penetrate the cell walls of gram-positive organisms. Macrolides may be obtained from isolates of *Streptococcus erythreus* or they may be synthesized in the laboratory. Macrolides are only partially metabolized and are excreted almost unchanged in bile. Most macrolides are administered orally; however, erythromycin is available in topical ointment and solution, as well as in an ophthalmic ointment for local infections. Bacterial resistance is primarily due to changes in bacterial cell wall permeability, such as some strains of *Psuedomonas* have developed to erythromycin. Macrolide antibiotics include erythromycin, erythromycin ethylsuccinate, azithromycin, and clarithromycin, as listed in Table 5–6.

PENICILLINS

Penicillin was the first of the antibiotics (Insight 5–3). Originally extracted from the mold *Penicillium*, this antibiotic is now available in many natural and semisynthetic forms effective against a wide variety of gram-positive and gram-negative microbes. Penicillins are bactericidal; they block an enzyme needed to strengthen the bacterial cell wall, so the cell eventually ruptures. Four basic categories of penicillins are available: natural penicillins, penicillinase-resistant penicillins, aminopenicillins, and broad-spectrum penicillins. Penicillins may be given orally or by intramuscular or intravenous injection, depending on the agent. Penicillins are often used preoperatively for prophylaxis against surgical site infections. Allergic reactions to penicillin are common, with cross-reactivity among penicillins and some of the cephalosporins. Some species of bacteria have become resistant to penicillin by producing *penicillinase,* an enzyme that breaks down the drug molecule, inactivating it. Table 5–7 lists some of the penicillins by category.

> **Insight** 5–3   **Yesterday and Today: Vaccines and the Discovery of Penicillin**
>
> Penicillin, discovered by Alexander Fleming in 1928, was the first of the "wonder drugs" known as antibiotics. It revolutionized medicine by fighting bacterial infections, which, at that time, could be deadly complications to any type of wound. A chain of events led to the development of this wonder drug. Prominent in these events were men who would lay the foundations for modern-day bacteriology and immunology.
>
> The first event took place in 1796, more than a hundred years before Fleming's discovery, when Edward Jenner discovered a way to prevent smallpox. An English country doctor, Jenner had observed that dairy maids who contracted a mild infection known as cowpox did not come down with smallpox. So he injected patients with pus from cowpox sores. These injections immunized his patients against smallpox. He knew nothing about the viruses that caused the disease and even less about the antibodies his inoculations stimulated. But his work was the first step toward understanding the disease-causing mechanisms of certain microorganisms. The next step was taken in the 1850s when a French chemist named Louis Pasteur began work with microscopic organisms called bacteria (or germs). By 1870, he had proved that disease in silkworms was caused by germs. He then reasoned that germs could also cause disease in animals, including humans. But as Pasteur was not a physician, he kept his research centered around animals. Next, he worked with chicken cholera. When he accidentally infected some chickens with an old strain of cholera, he found that the inoculated chickens did not develop the full-blown disease. In fact, the chickens recovered from their mild infection and subsequently proved immune to cholera. Pasteur was familiar with Jenner's work, so he deduced that old or weakened germs could be used to protect people from contracting a particular disease. Pasteur called his inoculum a "vaccine," and went on to develop other vaccines for anthrax and rabies.
>
> Another event took place when a highly respected Scottish surgeon named Joseph Lister became interested in Pasteur's work. He reasoned that germs could get into surgical wounds and cause postoperative problems—pus, swelling of tissue, fevers, and (all too often) death. Lister added a surgical link to the chain by using chemicals to kill germs in the operating room. His methods—which included spraying the room with carbolic acid—yielded impressive results. Lister's germ-killing chemicals were the first antiseptics. In the meantime, the chain of events strengthened as a German physician, Robert Koch, worked on the role played by bacteria in disease. It was he who proved that specific germs causing diseases in animals caused them in humans as well. In 1876, Koch identified the germ that causes anthrax, showing that it affects cattle, sheep, and people, too. Then, in 1882, he isolated the tuberculosis germ, a common killer of that time.
>
> In 1893, an influential British Army Medical School physician named Almroth Wright forged another link in the chain when he began the search for a typhoid vaccine. He was concerned that this disease was a serious threat to soldiers in the field. Spread by unsanitary conditions that contaminated water, milk, or food, typhoid killed 10% to 30% of its
>
> *(continued on following page)*

Insight 5–3   **Yesterday and Today: Vaccines and the Discovery
              of Penicillin**   *(Continued)*

victims at that time. Wright took six years to produce a successful vaccine. Then the army authorities refused to use it on a large scale. As a result, thousands of British troops contracted typhoid during the Boer War (1899–1902), and more troops died of this disease than from battle wounds. Shocked and bitterly chagrined, Wright resigned from the Medical School and joined the faculty at St. Mary's Hospital in London. There he created a department to study germs, immunity, and vaccines. In 1910, Wright hired a new research worker—Alexander Fleming.

To develop vaccines, Fleming and the staff of Wright's "Inoculation Department" took blood and pus samples from patients with ulcers, boils, and sores. They kept their samples in petri dishes filled with agar (a gelatin made from seaweed). Fleming was particularly interested in a pus-producing bacterium called *Staphylococcus,* which is commonly found on the skin. He prepared many microscopic slides from these germ samples. One day, Fleming noticed a mold growing on one of his samples. Molds are simple, nonflowering organisms from the fungi family; they can float freely in the air and this one had blown onto his petri dish by accident. But this "spoiled" sample was special: *Around the area of the mold was a wide, clean area—no staphylococci.* Even beyond this clean area, the staphylococci were dissolving. Clearly, something from the mold was killing the disease-causing germs. Fleming found out the killer mold was a common one, often found on ripened cheese, stale bread, and rotting fruit. It was from the group of molds called *penicillia,* so Fleming named his discovery "penicillin." However, when he announced his discovery to the rest of the department, no one was impressed. Even Wright showed little enthusiasm. Fortunately, Fleming continued his research, growing more of the mold and testing it on a variety of bacteria. Some were not affected, but a number of them were destroyed. Among those affected were the germs that cause pneumonia, scarlet fever, meningitis, diphtheria, and gonorrhea. Then Fleming took the next step. He went on to test the mold on human blood and found it did not kill white blood cells. He successfully used it topically on a lab assistant to cure an eye infection. But Fleming was no chemist, so he had problems extracting and purifying the mold. This left him believing the new medicine was good for topical use only. When he presented a paper on penicillin to a medical audience in 1929, he was met with indifference. Fleming's interest waned and his work was directed along other paths.

Ten years later, a team of Oxford medical researchers picked up where Fleming left off. The Oxford team took samples of penicillin to the United States, sought backing, and found manufacturers for the new antibiotic. The mass production of this wonder drug in the United States was to save millions of Allied soldiers' lives during World War II. And after the war, penicillin and its "wonder-full" derivatives were to change the history of medicine forever.

Table **5–7** Penicillins	
Generic Name	**Trade Name**
Natural Penicillins	
penicillin G	Pentids, Pfizerpen
benzathine penicillin G	Bicillin L-A, Permapen
penicillin G	Beepen-VK, Betapen-VK
Penicillinase-Resistant Penicillins	
methicillin	Staphcillin
cloxacillin	Cloxapen
dicloxacillin	Dycill, Pathocil
nafcillin	Nafcil, Unipen
oxacillin	Bactocill
Aminopenicillins (not penicillinase-resistant)	
ampicillin	Omnipen
amoxicillin	Amoxil, Polymox
bacampicillin	Spectrobid
Broad-Spectrum Penicillins	
carbenicillin	Geocillin
mezlocillin	Mezlin
piperacillin	Pipracil
ticarcillin	Ticar

Natural penicillins include penicillin G, penicillin V, and benzathine penicillin G. Advantages of natural penicillins are low cost and low toxicity. Natural penicillins display a relatively narrow spectrum of action, primarily against gram-positive microbes.

Penicillinase-resistant penicillins are semisynthetics that include methicillin, cloxacillin, dicloxacillin, nafcillin, and oxacillin. This class of penicillins was developed to be effective against strains of bacteria that produce penicillinase. However, some bacteria have developed a means of resistance against penicillinase-resistant penicillins. MRSA is actually resistant to all penicillinase-resistant penicillins.

Aminopenicillins have been chemically altered by adding an amino group, which makes them effective against gram-negative species, but they are not penicillinase resistant. These semisynthetics include ampicillin, amoxicillin, and bacampicillin.

*Table **5–8*** Tetracyclines	
Generic Name	*Trade Name*
tetracycline hydrochloride	Achromycin-V, Sumycin
minocycline	Minocin
oxytetracycline	Terramycin
doxycycline	Vibramycin
chlortetracycline hydrochloride	Aureomycin

Broad-spectrum penicillins include carbenicillin, mezlocillin, piperacillin, and ticarcillin. Broad-spectrum penicillins are semi-synthetics that have been chemically altered to be effective against strains of gram-negative microbes.

TETRACYCLINES

Tetracyclines were the first broad-spectrum antibiotics, originally obtained from cultures of *Streptomyces.* Bacteriostatic action against many gram-positive and gram-negative bacteria, tetracyclines bind to the bacterial ribosomal subunit, interfering with protein synthesis. They also exhibit some action on bacterial cell membranes, causing leakage. Many common bacteria have developed resistance to tetracyclines, so their use is now limited. They are used primarily to treat acne and rickettsial infections. Resistance factors are carried in plasmids (pieces of bacterial DNA), which are widely distributed among many bacteria. Tetracycline antibiotics are listed in Table 5–8.

Tetracycline hydrochloride is administered orally, as no parenteral form is available. Minocycline may be administered intravenously if the oral route is not feasible. Oxytetracycline may be administered intramuscularly if the oral route is not feasible; it is also available in an ophthalmic ointment combined with polymixin B sulfate. Doxycycline may be administered orally or intravenously. Chlortetracycline hydrochloride is available only in ophthalmic and topical ointment. In septoplasty or tympanoplasty, packing strips may be saturated with chlortetracycline hydrochloride and used as dressings.

MISCELLANEOUS ANTIBIOTICS

Many other antibiotics are available for prophylaxis and treatment of infections caused by susceptible microorganisms, as listed

Table 5–9   Miscellaneous Antibiotic and Chemotherapeutic Agents

General Categories	Individual Agents	Combination Agents
Oxazolidinone linezolid (Zyvox) **Quinolones** ciprofloxacin (Cipro) ofloxacin (Floxin) norfloxacin (Noroxin) enoxacin (Penetrex) **Sulfonamides** silver sulfadiazine (Silvadene) sulfisoxazole (Gantrisin) sulfamethoxazole (Gantanol) sulfasalazine (Azulfidine) sulfacetamide sodium (Sodium Sulamyd)	aztreonam (Azactam) chloramphenicol (Chloromycetin) clindamycin (Cleocin) imipenem (Primaxin) metronidazole (Flagyl) polymixin B sulfate (Aerosporin) vancomycin (Vanocin)	Coly-mycin S Cortisporin Neosporin

in Table 5–9. Miscellaneous agents presented in this chapter include three additional antibiotic categories, several individual agents, and three combination agents.

Oxazolidinone

Oxazolidinone is an entirely new class of synthetic antibiotics. The first agent in this class is linezolid (Zyvox). Zyvox inhibits bacterial protein synthesis by an entirely different mechanism of action than other agents, targeting a specific ribosomal subunit. It is administered intravenously or orally and is used to treat infections caused by MRSA, VRE, and some streptococci. It is bacteriostatic against enterococci and staphylococci, and bactericidal against the majority of streptococci. Resistance to linezolid is conferred by altering the site of action (ribosomal subunit).

Quinolones

Quinolones are a category of antibiotics that inhibit DNA-gyrase, a protein necessary for bacterial replication. These antibiotics have a relatively low toxicity and a broad spectrum of activity against both gram-positive and gram-negative aerobes, including *Pseudomonas*. Quinolones are given orally or intravenously for systemic infections or for urinary tract infections (UTIs). Agents include ciprofloxacin, ofloxacin, norfloxacin, and enoxacin.

Sulfonamides

Sulfonamides are not really antibiotics; they are antimicrobials, more commonly known as sulfa drugs. Sulfonamides are laboratory-synthesized chemicals that interfere with cell metabolism by inhibiting bacterial synthesis of folic acid. Introduced in 1935 by Gerhard Domagle, sulfonamides are the oldest of the chemotherapeutic agents. They are in limited use today (owing to increasing microbial resistance) but are still prescribed for nonobstructive UTIs, severe burns, and superficial eye infections. Sulfonamides are administered orally, topically, and occasionally intravenously. Resistance is conferred by altering bacterial cell wall permeability, thus preventing the agent from entering the bacterium. Examples of sulfonamides include silver sulfadiazine, sulfisoxazole, sulfamethoxazole, sulfasalazine, and sulfacetamide sodium. Sulfamethoxazole is also combined with trimethoprim (another antibacterial) and is available as Bactrim and Septra.

Individual Agents

Aztreonam (Azactam) is the first drug of a new class of antibacterials called monobactams. Aztreonam is the totally synthetic form of an antibiotic originally isolated from *Chromobacterium violaceum*. It inhibits bacterial cell-wall synthesis and has a wide spectrum of cidal activity against gram-negative aerobic pathogens. It is available for intramuscular or intravenous injection.

Chloramphenicol (Chloromycetin) is the synthetic form of an antibiotic originally isolated from *Streptomyces venezuelae,* and is structurally different from all other antibiotics. It is bacteriostatic, inhibiting protein synthesis, with a wide range of activity against gram-positive and gram-negative microbes. Chloramphenicol has potential for serious toxicity, so it is used only when less hazardous antibiotics are ineffective. Adverse effects include bone marrow depression and various blood disorders; consequently, chloramphenicol is inappropriate for prophylaxis. Chloramphenicol may be taken orally or injected intravenously; it is also available as a topical ointment, an otic solution, and as an ophthalmic solution and ointment.

Clindamycin (Cleocin) is the synthetic analog of the natural antibiotic lincomycin. It is active against gram-positive and anaerobic bacteria. It inhibits protein synthesis by binding to the bacterial ribosomes. Used to treat infections in patients who are allergic to penicillin, clindamycin may be administered orally or intravenously. Its high affinity for bone makes it effective in the treatment of osteomyelitis. In addition, clindamycin may be used to treat serious respiratory, pelvic, and intra-abdominal infections caused by anaerobic bacteria. Resistance is obtained by changes in the ribosomal structure, which prevents the agent from binding.

Imipenem (Primaxin) has the widest spectrum of activity of all antibiotics currently available. It works by inhibiting bacterial cell-wall synthesis and is available in forms suitable for intramuscular and intravenous administration. Primaxin is indicated only for serious infections, especially **polymicrobic infections** (caused by several different microbes) and infections caused by bacteria resistant to other antibiotics.

Metronidazole (Flagyl) is a synthetic antibiotic intended for intravenous administration. It is bactericidal against anaerobic gram-positive and gram-negative bacilli, inhibiting both DNA and RNA synthesis. Often used for prophylaxis in colorectal procedures when contamination from enteric anaerobic bacteria is possible, Flagyl is also used to treat postoperative surgical site infections caused by susceptible anaerobic bacteria. Bacterial resistance is accomplished by the production of enzymes and by changes in cell membrane permeability.

Polymixin B sulfate (Aerosporin) is a bactericidal antibiotic effective against nearly all species of gram-negative bacilli. It works against bacteria by increasing the permeability of the cell membrane. Polymixin B sulfate is available in powder form, which is reconstituted for topical, intravenous, or intramuscular administration. It is measured in units rather than milligrams. Resistance is rare.

Vancomycin (Vanocin) is an antibiotic derived from *Amycolatopsis orientalis* and used to treat infections caused by MRSA. It is bactericidal, only against gram-positive bacteria blocking a reaction needed to form crosslinks in the cell wall. Vancomycin also alters cell-membrane permeability and interferes with RNA synthesis. It is administered intravenously and is active against staphylococci, streptococci, and enterococci. Bacterial resistance occurs by altering the bacterial binding site.

Combination Agents

Several antibiotics are combined with other drugs and used to treat specific conditions. Coly-mycin S Otic is a combination drug used topically to treat bacterial infections of the external auditory canal. It is often administered in surgery after myringotomy and insertion of pressure equalization (PE) tubes. Coly-mycin contains two bactericidal antibiotics, colistin and neomycin, in combination with hydrocortisone (a corticosteroid used as an anti-inflammatory agent).

Cortisporin ophthalmic suspension is a drug used topically when an anti-inflammatory agent is needed in combination with an antibiotic. It contains neomycin and polymixin B sulfate with hydrocortisone. Because Cortisporin is in suspension, it must be shaken prior to administration to distribute the drug particles evenly. It is not intended for injection. Cortisporin is also available combined with bacitracin in an ointment.

☞ **Note:** Otic preparations are intended for use in the ear only. Ophthalmic preparations, while intended for use in the eye, may be used safely in locations such as the ear.

Neosporin G.U. Irrigant is a combination of neomycin and polymixin B sulfate. It is used as a topical bladder irrigant when the presence of an indwelling urinary catheter increases the risk of bladder infection.

ADVANCED PRACTICES FOR THE SURGICAL FIRST ASSISTANT
Chapter 5—Antibiotics

KEY TERMS

peak and trough   sepsis   surgical site infections (SSIs)

ANTIBIOTIC THERAPY

Advanced practitioners functioning as surgical first assistants will encounter the use of antibiotic therapy for the treatment and prevention of infections in the surgical patient. Antibiotics are administered for the treatment of **sepsis**, prevention of **surgical site infections (SSIs)**, and for intraoperative wound irrigation. As there are many classifications of antibiotics, the selection of the appropriate medication relies on several factors. For any specific infection; however, there is usually one antibiotic that research determines to be superior. Some of the factors for medication selection include patient allergy, inability of the antibiotic to reach the site of infection, patient susceptibility to the medication's toxicity, medication efficacy, and medication's

ADVANCED PRACTICES FOR THE SURGICAL FIRST ASSISTANT   *(continued)*

spectrum. Although the physician selects the appropriate antibiotic, to assure that the patient receives the correct dosage of antibiotic at the right time the surgical first assistant must have knowledge of antibiotic usage and actions. The surgical first assistant acts as another line of defense against medication errors and adverse reactions caused by antibiotic therapy.

PEAK AND TROUGH

Antibiotic medications rely on their ability to penetrate the bacteria cell wall and bind with sufficient concentration levels to be effective. The concentration levels depend on the half-life and elimination of the medication. When maintaining a therapeutic dosage of antibiotics, it is important to understand **peak and trough** levels. The time when the medication is at the highest plasma concentration is referred to as its peak level. This peak level depends on the absorption rate and the route of administration. Intravenous administered medications take much less time to reach peak levels than do oral medications. The point of time when the medication is at the lowest level of plasma concentration is referred to as the trough level. Ideally, to maintain a therapeutic response an antibiotic would be redosed before it reaches trough level.

SEPSIS

Antibiotic therapy is essential for the treatment of sepsis. Sepsis is defined as decay and putrefaction of living tissue. It is a life-threatening syndrome that is the leading cause of death in intensive care units, usually resulting from an overwhelming infection. The patient's response to sepsis may be low and short term, to critical and long term or demise. Sepsis can be divided into several categories according to symptoms and certain criteria. Each category has an associated mortality rate (Table A). The clinical management of sepsis is a multifocal approach that includes resuscitation, organ system support, and control of the infection. The control of infection combines the use of antibiotics in addition to drainage or debridement of involved tissues. Most septic patients will be on an antibiotic therapy and it is imperative that therapy be continued throughout the surgical procedure.

ASSISTANT ADVICE

Check the dosage and timing of the antibiotic ordered for the patient. Be sure the next doses are available in the surgical suite if required during the procedure. Also check with the surgeon concerning any extra bolus of medication that may be needed and have it available.

(continued on following page)

ADVANCED PRACTICES FOR THE SURGICAL FIRST ASSISTANT   *(continued)*

☞ **Note:** The antibiotic ordered initially for infection treatment may have been selected due to the Gram's stain and the source of the infection. The exact microorganism may not have been isolated prior to the time of surgery. Cultures will be taken during the procedure that include aerobic and anaerobic. The results of these cultures will help isolate the pathogens, and the antibiotic may be changed to target these specific microorganisms.

PREOPERATIVE ANTIBIOTIC PROPHYLAXIS

The use of prophylactic antibiotics to prevent surgical site infections (SSIs) has proved beneficial in certain procedures. However, in other situations these antibiotics have no benefit to the patient. Prophylactic antibiotics may be beneficial when used before implant procedures and clean-contaminated (surgical wound classification category 3) surgical wounds (category IA). They have no benefit in clean surgical wounds (incised, noninfected) or contaminated wounds. Errors that occur most during prophylactic antibiotic therapy concern the timing of administration and the duration of the therapy. In general, preoperative antibiotics should be administered within 30 minutes of incision and be continued not more than 24 hours postoperatively.

Table **A**   Associated Mortality Rates of Sepsis

Definition	Symptoms and Criteria	Mortality Rate
Systemic inflammatory response syndrome (SIRS)	2 or more of the following: • temperature >36–38° C • heart rate >90 bpm • respirations <30/min or PaCo₂ <32 mm of Hg • WBC >12,000, 4,000 or 10% immature cells	3%–17% depending on the number of symptoms
Sepsis	SIRS with the addition of an infection site confirmed by culture (positive blood cultures are not necessary)	16%
Severe sepsis	Sepsis plus organ dysfunction and tissue hypoperfusion or hypotension	20%
Septic shock	Hypotension induced by sepsis despite fluid bolus or organ and tissue hypoperfusion	46%

ADVANCED PRACTICES FOR THE SURGICAL FIRST ASSISTANT *(continued)*

The administration of the initial dose of preoperative antibiotics presents a challenge to health care providers in today's fast-paced systems. Patients may arrive at the facility within one hour of their scheduled procedure. Most facilities will have a standard protocol for starting pre-operative antibiotics. The surgical first assistant must be familiar with the protocol and make sure that it is followed at all times. The choice of antibiotic will depend on the type, classification, and site of the procedure. The medication will cover against any natural flora in the surgical field. *Staphylococcus aureus* and *Staphylococcus epidermidis* cause most surgical wound infections. Administering a first-generation cephalosporin, as cefazolin, can cover these microorganisms. Another indicator of antibiotic choice is any allergies the patient may have. In patients with an allergy to penicillin, the surgeon may prescribe clindamycin or, in some cases, vancomycin.

INTRAOPERATIVE ANTIBIOTIC WOUND IRRIGATION

Many surgeons choose to use an antibiotic agent in the irrigation fluid to help prevent surgical site infections. This usually will be the final irrigation before closure of the wound. The antibiotic of choice, such as ancef, is mixed in the appropriate volume of irrigation fluid (usually 500 mL). To prevent the irrigation solution from cooling, this should not be mixed in advance. When the irrigation solution is placed into the wound it should remain a short period of time to allow the antibiotic to absorb into the tissues. (Refer to Chapter 11 for more information on irrigation fluids.)

 CAUTION

Cool temperature irrigation fluid may adversely affect the patient's core body temperature.

KEY CONCEPTS

- Antibiotics are antimicrobial agents used in surgery for prophylaxis against wound infections. They are also given to treat postoperative surgical site infections. Despite meticulous aseptic technique, SSIs may arise when pathogenic microorganisms are transmitted to a susceptible host. When that happens, the causative microbe will be identified, and tested for antibiotic sensitivity before a definitive course of antibiotic therapy is selected.
- Antibiotics work against microbes in five major ways. The agent may inhibit bacterial cell wall synthesis, impede protein synthesis, interfere with nucleic acid (RNA or DNA) synthesis, alter bacterial cell wall function, or disrupt bacterial cell metabolism. Antibiotics

may be bacteriostatic or bactericidal and may have a broad, narrow, or limited spectrum of activity. Some bacteria have developed resistance to some leading antibiotics, making treatment protocols difficult. Antibiotics may be administered orally, intramuscularly, intravenously, or topically, depending on the agent.

- Major categories of antibiotics include aminoglycosides, cephalosporins, macrolides (erythromycins), penicillins, and tetracyclines. Several other categories of antibacterials are in use today, as well as several unique agents. Surgical technologists should become familiar with antibiotics used routinely during surgery.

6

DIAGNOSTIC AGENTS

Medications Covered in Chapter 6

Generic Name	Trade or Brand Name	Category
iohexol	Omnipaque	Contrast media
diatrizoate meglumine	Hypaque 30%, 60%	Contrast media
diatrizoate sodium	Hypaque 25%, 50	Contrast media
iodixanol	Visipaque	Contrast media
iopamidol	Iosvue	Contrast media
methylene blue	Methylene blue 1%	Dye
isosulfan blue	Lymphazurin 1%	Dye
indigotindosulfate sodium	Indigo carmine	Dye
gentian violet	Gentian violet	Dye, antifungal
potassium triiodide	Lugol's solution	Staining agent, antihyperthyroid medication
acetic acid	vinegar	Staining agent

OBJECTIVES

After completing this chapter, you should be able to:

1. Define contrast media, dyes, and staining agents.
2. Give examples of contrast media and how each is used in radiographic studies in surgery.
3. Give examples of dyes and how each is used in surgical procedures.
4. Give examples of staining agents and how each is used in surgical procedures.

KEY TERMS

contraindicated	hypersensitivity
contrast media	radiopaque
dye	staining agent

Surgery is a discipline that depends on visualizing the anatomy and the physiological functioning of body organs and systems. It is very dependent on techniques that give insight into the position, activity, and health of these structures. Since the discovery of x-rays at the turn of the 19th century by Carl Roentgen, imaging (or radiographic testing) has played a central role in the management of patients, and this guidance is used for both diagnosis and treatment. Pharmacologic agents called **contrast media** are used in certain diagnostic radiographic tests. To perform these tests, a contrast medium is injected into the circulatory system or instilled into a body cavity; then an x-ray is taken. Many contrast media contain iodine, which is **radiopaque**, the opposite of *radiotransparent*. Thus anatomic structures that take up iodine appear opaque on radiographic examination; this means that such pathologic conditions as tumors, stones, or blockages become visible. In surgery, these agents are often referred to incorrectly as dyes.

Dyes are solutions that color or mark tissue for identification. Dyes may be used to mark skin incisions, delineate normal tissue planes, or enhance visualization of certain anatomic structures during a surgical procedure. Dyes may be applied topically, injected into the bloodstream, or instilled into a body cavity.

Staining agents are used in surgery to help visually identify abnormal cells, most frequently in procedures on the cervix. Staining agents are chemicals in solution that react differently with abnormal cells from the way they react with normal cells.

CONTRAST MEDIA

Contrast media are radiopaque chemicals. Several different contrast media are available for various diagnostic examinations (Table 6–1). Four common contrast media frequently used in surgery are discussed here as examples. The surgical technologist must exercise caution when preparing these agents because the agents are clear in color and may easily be confused with other

Table 6–1 Contrast Media for Radiographic Studies

Name	Purpose
Amipaque	Myelography and CT
Angio-Conray	Arteriography
Barium sulfate	Gastrointestinal studies
Cardiografin	Angiography and aortography
Cystografin	Urography
Dionosil	Bronchography
Hypaque Meglumine, 30%, and Hypaque sodium, 25%	Urography and CT
Hypaque Meglumine, 60%, and Hypaque sodium, 50%	Urography, cerebral and peripheral angiography, aortography, venography, cholangiography, hysterosalpingography and splenoportography
Hypaque-M, 75%	Angiocardiography, angiography, aortography, and urography
Isovue	Myelography, cerebral angiography, peripheral arteriography, venography, angiocardiography, left ventriculography, selective coronary angiography, aortography, selective visceral arteriography, urography, arthrography, and CT
Renografin	Cerebral angiography, peripheral arteriography and venography, cholangiography, splenoportography, arthrography, urography, and CT
Renovist	Aortography, angiocardiography, peripheral arteriography and venography, venacavography, and urography
Cholografin Meglumine	Cholangiography and cholecystography
Omnipaque	Angiography, excretory urography, and myelography
Optiray	Arteriography and CT
Pantopaque	Myelography
Renovue	Excretory Urography
Sinografin	Hysterosalpingography
Visipaque	Cardiography, peripheral, visceral and cerebral arteriography, CT, excretory urography, peripheral venography

CT, Computed tomography.

clear medications on the sterile back table. All containers and syringes containing contrast media must be clearly labeled to avoid administration errors. Most contrast media are sensitive to light, so they should be stored covered and away from direct lighting. However, these agents may be safely exposed to light when on the sterile back table during a procedure. This is because the duration of exposure is not sufficient to cause damage to the contrast medium.

Most contrast media contain iodine; therefore, a thorough patient history of allergies or reactions to iodine must be obtained and noted in the chart (this includes shellfish allergies). The circulator will also check for a history of patient allergies or reactions to iodine during the preoperative assessment. If the patient has a positive history for iodine reaction, and use of contrast media is anticipated during the surgical procedure, the surgeon should be alerted prior to patient transport to the operating room.

OMNIPAQUE

Iohexol (Omnipaque) is a water-soluble iodine-based radiographic contrast medium, containing approximately 45% iodine. Omnipaque is available in various strengths (140, 180, 210, 240, 300, and 350), expressed as milligrams of iodine per milliliter (mg/mL). It comes in glass vials ranging in size from 10 mL to 250 mL. Omnipaque is absorbed from the site of administration into the bloodstream; it undergoes little or no metabolism and is excreted by the kidneys virtually unchanged. It is **contraindicated** (inappropriate) for use in patients with known **hypersensitivity** to iodine. Omnipaque may be injected intrathecally or intravascularly, or it may be instilled into a body cavity prior to radiographic examination. Intrathecal (into the lumbar subarachnoid space) injection of Omnipaque is used for myelography and contrast enhancement of computed tomography (CT) myelography to visualize the spinal cord and nerve roots (Fig. 6–1). For many years, myelography was the standard method used to diagnose a ruptured intervertebral disk. Because myelography involves the injection of contrast media and use of x-ray, it is considered an invasive diagnostic examination. In many instances, traditional myelography is being replaced by magnetic resonance imaging (MRI), a noninvasive diagnostic tool.

When injected into a blood vessel, Omnipaque will opacify that blood vessel—and all other vessels in the path of flow—on radiographic examination (angiography). Angiography is used to demonstrate blockages or anatomic abnormalities of the vascular

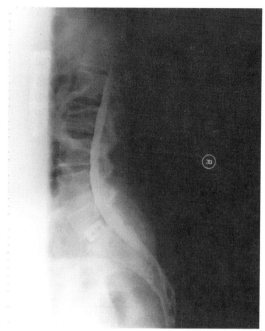

Figure **6–1.** Normal myelogram.

system. Variations of angiography include angiocardiography, aortography, and peripheral arteriography. Angiography may be performed on vessels of the head, neck, abdomen, or kidneys, as well as on peripheral blood vessels. Omnipaque may be used for intraoperative angiography. For instance, it may be used to confirm removal of a blockage in a peripheral vessel, such as after a femoral embolectomy or laser atherectomy.

Retrograde urography (Fig. 6–2) may be performed with intravascular injection of Omnipaque. The contrast medium will reach the kidneys in 1 to 5 minutes, at which time a urogram may be taken to visualize renal structures or detect possible blockage.

HYPAQUE

Diatrizoate meglumine 30% and 60%, and diatrizoate sodium 25% and 50% (Hypaque) are water-soluble radiopaque contrast media. The percentage given in the names refers to the amount of meglumine or sodium per 100 mL of solution, not the amount of iodine. It is supplied in glass vials of 50 mL and 100 mL. Hypaque is *not* intended for intrathecal administration and is

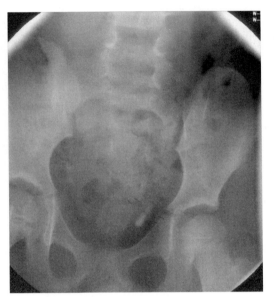

Figure **6–2.**   Retrograde urogram.

contraindicated in patients with known hypersensitivity to iodine. Common uses for Hypaque include excretory urography, cerebral angiography, peripheral arteriography, and cholangiography.

Hypaque is used in surgery for operative cholangiograms— open or laparoscopic—to determine the presence of stones in the common bile duct (Fig. 6–3). Often Hypaque is diluted at the sterile back table with equal parts of normal saline solution. One method of cholangiography involves attaching one 30-cc syringe filled with saline and one 30-cc syringe filled with Hypaque solution to a three-way stopcock adapter connected to a cholangiogram catheter (Fig. 6–4). Saline is injected into the catheter to verify correct placement; then Hypaque is injected and an x-ray is taken. These syringes must be clearly identified to prevent inadvertent injection of saline prior to radiographic exposure. Although saline will not harm the patient, inadvertent injection prior to x-ray will negate the examination and require additional radiographic exposure and extended anesthesia time.

This type of contrast media (containing diatrizoate meglumine) can also be inserted directly into the urinary bladder via a catheter. The bladder is then filled (distended) with the contrast and an x-ray is taken (Fig. 6–5).

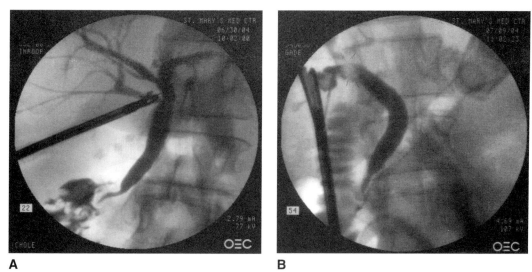

A   B

Figure **6–3.** **Cholangiogram:** (**A**) normal; (**B**) calculus.

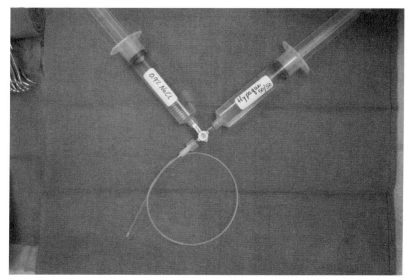

Figure **6–4.** Cholangiogram catheter set for injection.

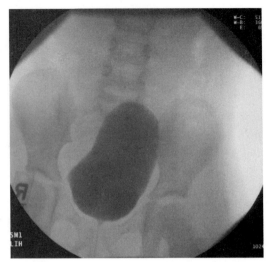

Figure **6–5.** Cystogram showing distended bladder.

VISIPAQUE

Iodixanol (Visipaque) is a water-soluble radiopaque contrast media. It is available in concentrations of 270 and 320 mg of organically bound iodine per mL. It has many of the same properties as Omnipaque: it is absorbed into the bloodstream and excreted virtually unchanged by the kidneys; it is contraindicated in patients with iodine sensitivity; and when injected into a blood vessel it opacifies that vessel and others in the path of flow for radiographic examination. However, Visipaque is not for intrathecal use. It is supplied in 50-mL vials, and 100-, 150-, and 200-L glass and plastic bottles. It is used in cardiography; peripheral, visceral, and cerebral arteriography; contrast-enhanced computerized tomography (CECT) of the head and body, excretory urography, and peripheral venography.

ISOVUE

Iopamidol (Isovue) is a water-soluble contrast media for intravascular, intrathecal, and body cavity administration for radiographic procedures. It is rapidly absorbed into the bloodstream and excreted predominantly via the kidneys. It should be used immediately after opening and any remaining in the bottle should be discarded. Isovue comes in concentrations of 150-, 200-, 300-, and 370 mg/mL. It is used for lumbar and thoracocervical myelogra-

Table **6–2** Dyes Used in Surgery	
Name	**Purpose**
Methylene blue	Cystoscopy: Detect bladder injury
	Tubal dye studies: Verify patency of uterine tubes
	Bladder surgery or exploration: Detect bladder injury
Lymphazurin	Delineation of lymphatic vessels for sentinel lymph node biopsy
Indigo carmine	Kidney or bladder procedures: Detect injury to urinary structures
	Verify kidney function during any surgical procedure: Colored urine will be excreted
Gentian violet	Skin marking

phy, cerebral angiography, peripheral arteriography, venography, angiocardiography, left ventriculography, selective coronary angiography, aortography, selective visceral arteriography, urography, arthrography, and computerized tomography (CT) enhancement. Isovue is supplied in 10-, 20-, 50-, 100-, and 200-mL bottles.

DYES

Dyes have varied uses in surgery. They are used to mark skin incisions and structural positioning of normal body anatomy, and for visual identification of organ injury or pathology. Four of the most common dyes used in surgery are discussed here, with examples of practical applications (Table 6–2).

METHYLENE BLUE

Methylene blue U.S.P. is available in a 1% solution (10 mg/mL of water), packaged in 1-mL and 10-mL vials or 5-mL ampules. It is most often used in surgery during procedures on the urinary bladder or fallopian tubes. Methylene blue is added to a fluid, such as normal saline, to give a deep blue color to the solution. To detect possible injury, the solution is then instilled into the bladder through an indwelling urinary catheter. If the bladder has a leak or tear, blue solution will be obvious in the pelvis and will be visible as it flows out of the damaged area.

In gynecology, a methylene blue solution is used to demonstrate patency of the fallopian tubes. During a procedure called tubal dye study (TDS), or chromotubation, a laparoscope is used to observe the fimbria (ends of the uterine tubes) while

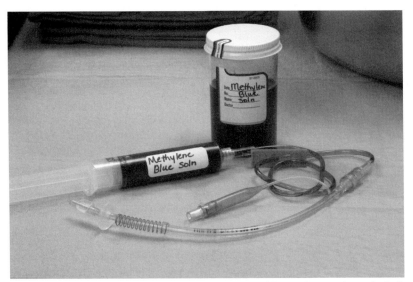

Figure **6–6.** Cervical cannula with methylene blue solution for tubal dye study (TDS).

methylene blue solution is instilled into the uterus through a special cervical cannula (Fig. 6–6). Methylene blue solution enters the fallopian tubes and is observed exiting into the pelvic cavity, verifying patent tubes. If the tubes are blocked, often due to pelvic inflammatory disease, methylene blue solution will not be evident in the pelvis.

Methylene blue may also be used immediately before the surgical procedure begins to outline, or mark, normal body anatomy or position, such as when a tissue flap graft is measured, marked, "cut," then transferred to fill a defect on the body (see Insight 6–1). Methylene blue is commonly used to mark the planned skin incisions for surgical procedures. The solution is poured into a medicine cup, and a sterile toothpick or 25-gauge needle is dipped into the solution and applied to the skin. In many instances, manufactured skin-marking pens are replacing this method.

ISOSULFAN BLUE (LYMPHAZURIN 1%)

Lymphazurin is a sterile, aqueous solution for the delineation of lymphatic vessels. It is administered subcutaneously and is selectively picked up by lymphatic vessels which drain the region of the injection site, making them a bright blue color. This makes the vessels easily discernible from the surrounding tissue. It is

---

Insight 6–1   **Marking the Skin for Breast Surgery**

In the surgical procedure reduction mammoplasty, measurements and markings are made for removing excess breast tissue and skin and transposing the nipples–areola complexes. The marks with a skin-marking pen are made immediately preoperatively by the surgeon with the patient standing or sitting upright, because this is the natural position of the breasts. It is important for the circulator not to remove these markings with the skin prep. Once the patient is positioned on the table and anesthetized, additional markings may be done with a 25-gauge needle dipped into methylene blue and used to "tattoo" breast tissue as additional guides for the surgeon during the procedure.

---

primarily excreted via the biliary route and should not be used on patients with known hypersensitivity to the medication or related compounds. Lymphazurin is supplied as 5-milliliter (mL) single-dose vials.

Lymphazurin is used as an adjunct to lymphography to diagnose primary and secondary lymphedema of the extremities, lymph node involvement by primary or secondary neoplasm, and lymph node response to therapeutic modalities. Lymphazurin is most commonly used in the surgical setting for sentinel node biopsy for breast tumors. Three to 5 mL of the medication are injected by the surgeon before the skin prep. This allows approximately 5 minutes time before the first incision is made, allowing the medication to be carried by the lymphatic system. The surgeon follows the blue path of lymphatic drainage from the breast tumor to the first node of the axillary basin, or sentinel node, which is then dissected for pathological examination (see Insight 6–2).

INDIGO CARMINE

Indigo carmine is a blue dye that is usually given intravenously to color urine for verification of bladder integrity or kidney function. Each 5 mL of indigo carmine contains 40 mg of indigotindisulfonate sodium in water. It is excreted by the kidneys, usually within 10 minutes after intravenous injection, retaining its color in urine. This process allows immediate identification of possible leaks or damage to the ureters or bladder, as well as demonstration of kidney function. Intravenous injection of indigo carmine during cystoscopy may be used to help identify the location of ureteral openings. Indigo carmine is packaged in 5-mL glass ampules and, when stored, should be protected from light.

Insight 6–2   **Sentinel Lymph Node Biopsy**

Sentinel lymph node biopsy is performed following a diagnosis of breast cancer. Within a few hours of the procedure, the patient is taken to the radiology and nuclear medicine departments. The radiologist places a localization wire into the tumor to pinpoint its location. Then the patient goes to nuclear medicine for a mapping of the lymphatic system. This is accomplished with a radioactive isotope (called a tracer), technetium-99, which is injected at or around the tumor site. The tracer enters the lymphatic system and travels to the regional basin and settles in the first, or sentinel lymph node. The radiologist will use a gamma, or scintillation, camera to map this drainage path and a scan, like an x-ray, is taken and sent to surgery. This is called lymphoscintigraphy.

The patient is taken to surgery where the surgeon injects 3 to 5 cc of isosulfan blue (Lymphazurin 1%) approximately 5 minutes before the incision is made. The dye travels through the lymphatic system just as the tracer did. The surgeon may use a gamma probe, which is covered with a sterile sleeve, to find the radioactive "hot spots" and then mark the skin with a skin-marking pencil at the site of the sentinel node. The incision is made and the surgeon follows the Lymphazurin blue's path to excise the node, which is sent to the pathology department for examination. If the pathology report comes back negative for cancer, the breast cancer is considered to have not spread, or metastasized, to the lymph nodes. If the report comes back showing cancer in the node, further lymph node dissection is carried out, with more specimen sent to pathology for diagnosis.

GENTIAN VIOLET

Gentian violet is a purple dye most frequently used in surgery to mark incision lines. Special sterile marking pens containing gentian violet are available from various manufacturers. These pens are particularly useful for plastic and reconstructive procedures involving complicated incisions such as Z-plasty (Fig. 6–7) or tissue flap grafts. Sterile marking pens may also be used to label containers of medications (Fig. 6–8). Gentian violet also belongs to a category of medications called antifungals. Topically, it works to treat types of fungus infections inside the mouth (thrush) and the vagina (yeast infection), and of the skin.

STAINING AGENTS

Staining agents may be used in surgery to help identify abnormal tissue for biopsy or excision. Because of differences in cell metabolism between normal and abnormal cells, some chemicals applied to the suspect area react in a way that more clearly demonstrates the location of tissue changes. In surgery, staining

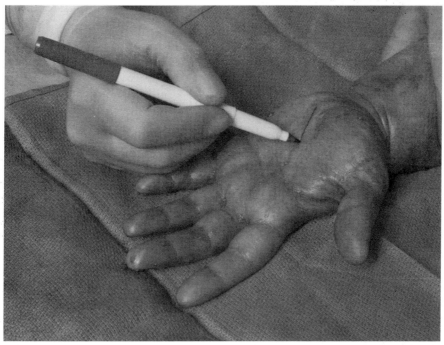

Figure **6–7.**   Use of a commercial marking pen to mark a skin incision.

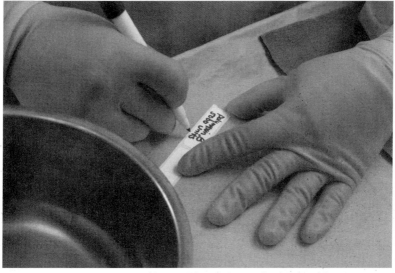

Figure **6–8.**   Marking medications on the back table.

techniques are most often used by gynecologists to locate areas of cervical dysplasia for biopsy or excisional conization.

LUGOL'S SOLUTION

Lugol's solution is a strong iodine mixture used to perform Schiller's test on cervical tissue. For Schiller's test, Lugol's solution is applied topically to the external cervical os with a sponge stick or large cotton-tipped applicator. Abnormal cells will not take up the brown iodine stain as readily as normal cells, visually demonstrating the area of cervical dysplasia to be biopsied. Lugol's solution is contraindicated for use in patients with a history of hypersensitivity to iodine. Lugol's solution is also used to treat overactive thyroid gland function, iodine deficiency, and to protect the thyroid gland from the effects of radiation as a result of radiation therapy treatments with radioactive iodine. (See Chapter 8.)

ACETIC ACID

Acetic acid (commonly known as vinegar) may also be used to help identify areas of cervical dysplasia. Although it is not specifically a colored staining agent, acetic acid causes abnormal tissue to appear whiter than surrounding healthy tissue. Acetic acid may be used as a staining agent when laser is used to excise dysplasia. Laser energy is absorbed by different colors in the spectrum, and tissue stained brown with an iodine solution may interact less effectively with the laser.

ADVANCED PRACTICES FOR THE SURGICAL FIRST ASSISTANT
Chapter 6—Diagnostic Agents

KEY TERMS

acute renal failure (ARF)	iodinated
diaphoresis	nephrotoxicity
hydration	urticaria

RISK FACTORS FOR IODINATED CONTRAST MEDIA

In recent years there has been a dramatic increase in the use of diagnostic agents in the surgical setting, especially **iodinated** contrast media used for radiologic imaging. The advanced practitioner performing as the surgical first assistant should be aware of patient risk factors

ADVANCED PRACTICES FOR THE SURGICAL FIRST ASSISTANT   *(continued)*

before administration of these agents. Risk factors have been identified that may add to the susceptibility of an adverse reaction. One factor is the route of administration. The risk of reaction from intravascular administration of contrast media occurs more than from extravascular administration (through the gastrointestinal tract). Reactions occurring through intravascular administration are usually mild and self-limiting, and those from extravascular administration are rare. However, either route can produce serious, and at times life-threatening reactions. Other risk factors include advanced age and class IV congestive heart failure as these can increase the likelihood of renal failure following administration of the contrast media. Patients who have had a previous reaction to contrast materials are understandably at higher risk, although reactions do no re-occur in all patients. Patients with chronic renal insufficiency, asthma, and diabetes mellitus must have these diseases addressed and treated before the administration of any contrast media.

ADVERSE REACTIONS

As previously mentioned in the chapter, the identification of allergies is essential before administering any radiographic contrast agents. Symptoms for reactions are categorized according to their severity (Table A). It should be noted that reactions can occur 20 to 30 minutes after injection of the agent and up to 7 days after the procedure. In addition to allergic reactions, an adverse effect of special importance is nephrotoxicity resulting in **acute renal failure (ARF).** Renal insufficiency is caused by a dosage-related toxic injury to the renal tubules. Patients should be assessed for risk factors that may contribute to ARF (Table B). The assessment should also include renal function studies before contrast is administered by obtaining a blood, urea, nitrogen (BUN) and creatinine laboratory tests. These are the best indicators of renal function and the results must be available before the procedure. Current treatment to reduce **nephrotoxicity** is **hydration** to keep the kidneys flushing during the procedure and to minimize the volume of contrast media administered.

Table **A**   Symptoms of Adverse Reactions for Contrast Media

Mild	*Moderate*	*Severe*
Scattered **urticaria**	Persistent vomiting	Cardiac arrhythmia
Nausea	Headache	Hypotension
Vomiting	Facial edema	Severe bronchospasm
Diaphoresis	Mild bronchospasm	Laryngeal edema
Coughing	Dyspnea	Seizures
Dizziness	Palpitations	Pulmonary edema

(continued on following page)

ADVANCED PRACTICES FOR THE SURGICAL FIRST ASSISTANT   *(continued)*

Table **B**   Risk Factors for Contrast-Induced Nephropathy

Patient Factors	*Procedural Factors*
Pre-existing renal conditions	High volume of contrast administered
Diabetes	Failure to verify renal lab function tests
Dehydration	Failure to obtain medical history
Advanced age	Failure to aggressively hydrate
Nephrotoxic medications	Space procedures at least 5 days apart
Congestive heart failure	
Liver disease	

MEDICATIONS

Current studies suggest the administration of acetylcysteine, an antioxidant, may reduce the incidence of contrast-induced ARF. Patients may be given acetylcysteine the day before, the day of, and two days after the procedure. Other medications used to reduce the incidence of adverse reactions to contrast media include methylprednisolone (Medrol) and prednisolone (Prednisolone), which are corticosteroids; diphenhydramine (Benadryl), which is an antihistamine used to treat allergic symptoms; hydroxyzine (Vistaril) to relieve itching, nausea, and vomiting caused by allergies; and histamine H_2 receptor blockers such as cimetidine (Tagamet).

Many factors must be considered before any medications are given to the patient receiving contrast media for radiologic imaging. The surgical first assistant must assist the physician in providing the best patient care by identifying patient risk factors, minimizing adverse effects, and managing reactions of contrast agents.

NEW DIAGNOSTIC IMAGING PROCEDURES

New diagnostic approaches for whole body imaging are using quantum dots, or nanocrystals, as fluorescent and bioluminescent reporters (or tags) that are genetically encoded. These "glowing" tags can provide information for better understanding of human biology as well as help develop treatments for diseases such as cancer, infection, and cardiovascular disease.

One example of this new imaging technology used to diagnose cardiovascular disease and malfunction is an ultrasound contrast agent that consists of millions of tiny bubbles. These bubbles scatter light and allow the physician to see which part of the heart muscle is not functioning properly. The ultrasound component of this technology is highly sensitive and produces a characteristic transient effect for better diagnosis. Other applications include imaging systems to obtain and process information on the molecular and cellular levels of our bodies, models to track neurological damage and repair the central nervous system, and radiodiagnostic agents to label white blood cells without the need to remove and reinject blood into patients. Research is ongoing for these and many more applications using molecular imaging.

KEY CONCEPTS

- Different agents, such as contrast media, dyes, and staining agents are used in surgery to facilitate diagnosis of various pathologic conditions.
- Contrast media are used to demonstrate anatomic structures or abnormalities under radiographic examination.
- Dyes are used to mark (color) tissue or structures for direct visualization.
- Staining agents are used to provide visual contrast between normal and abnormal tissue.

DIURETICS

Medications Covered in Chapter 7

Generic Name	Brand Name	Category
bumetanide	Bumex	Loop diuretic
ethacrynic acid	Edecrin	Loop diuretic
furosemide	Lasix	Loop diuretic
bendroflumethiazide	Naturetin	Thiazide diuretic
chlorothiazide	Diuril, SK-Chlorothiazide	Thiazide diuretic
hydrochlorothiazide	Esidrix, HydroDIURIL, Oretic	Thiazide diuretic
amiloride	Midamor	Potassium-sparing diuretic
spironolactone	Aldactone	Potassium-sparing diuretic
triamterene	Dyrenium	Potassium-sparing diuretic
acetazolamide	Diamox	Carbonic anhydrase inhibitor
mannitol	Osmitrol	Osmotic diuretic

OBJECTIVES

After completing this chapter, you should be able to:

1. State the general purpose of a diuretic.
2. Describe the physiology of the kidney.
3. Identify anatomic structures of the nephron.
4. List diseases that use diuretics for management.
5. Describe the impact of long-term diuretic therapy on the patient about to undergo a surgical procedure.
6. Discuss the type of patient who may come to surgery on long-term diuretic therapy.
7. Differentiate between the purposes for long-term and short-term use of diuretics.
8. List the two most common diuretics administered intraoperatively and their purpose.

KEY TERMS

congestive heart failure (CHF)
creatinine
diuresis
diuretic
dysrhythmia
electrolyte

glaucoma
homeostasis
hyperkalemia
hypertension
hypokalemia
nephron

Diuretics are medications administered to prevent reabsorption of sodium and water by the kidneys. As a result, the patient excretes large amounts of dilute urine. Diuretics are used in the management of several chronic medical conditions such as **hypertension, congestive heart failure (CHF),** and **glaucoma.** A simple statement about the physiology of fluid and **electrolyte** balance is the principle: where the fluid goes, so go the electrolytes.

Most diuretics also cause excretion of electrolytes other than sodium, including potassium and calcium. Potassium (K^+) may be seriously depleted in patients taking certain diuretics, a condition known as **hypokalemia.** If patients on long-term diuretic therapy require surgery, blood chemistry tests are performed to determine serum potassium levels (normal 3.5 to 5.0 mEq/L). Potassium levels that are either too low or too high may cause cardiac **dysrhythmias** under anesthesia (Insight 7–1). Patients with hypokalemia may require administration of intravenous potassium prior to nonemergency surgery. The necessity of preoperative potassium treatment may cause a delay in procedure start time or scheduled date, so operating room staff should be mindful of such possibilities. Long-term diuretic therapy is most frequently seen in elderly patients with systemic fluid management conditions.

Short-term use of diuretics is indicated when a condition requires a rapid but temporary reduction in fluid. An example of short-term use of diuretics is intravenous administration by the anesthesia provider during some surgical procedures. Diuretics may be used during surgery to reduce intraocular pressure, intracranial pressure, or to protect kidney function. During intraocular surgery such as retinal detachment, a diuretic may be given to prevent the accumulation of fluid due to the inflammatory response to tissue manipulation. Diuretics may be administered during craniotomy to prevent brain swelling, especially

---

Insight 7–1   **Physiology Insight: The Importance of Potassium in Cardiac Function**

Potassium (K^+), a mineral element, is the primary intracellular electrolyte in the body. It plays a vital role in many body functions, such as nerve impulse conduction, acid–base balance, and promotion of carbohydrate and protein metabolism. Every body cell, especially muscle tissue, requires a high potassium content to function. It facilitates contraction of both skeletal and smooth muscles—including myocardial (heart muscle) contraction. Potassium levels in the body have a very narrow normal range (3.5 to 5.0 mEq/L) and even a slight deviation in either direction can cause problems. An excess of potassium (*hyper*kalemia) alters the normal polarized state of cardiac muscle fibers. This results in a decrease in the rate and force of the heart's contractions. Very high potassium levels can block conduction of cardiac impulses. This results in rapid heart rate (tachycardia) initially and, later, slow heart rate (bradycardia). If potassium levels are too low (*hypo*kalemia), the heart can develop an abnormal rhythm (arrhythmia). Both hyperkalemia and hypokalemia can lead to muscle weakness and flaccid paralysis. Abnormal potassium levels can diminish excitability and conduction rate of the heart muscle and lead to cardiac arrest. The cause of abnormal levels is usually not dietary deficiency. Many foods contain potassium, including meats, milk, peanut butter, potatoes, bananas, apples, carrots, tomatoes, and dark-green leafy vegetables. Rather, hypokalemia can result from excessive vomiting and diarrhea, severe trauma such as burns, chronic renal disease, excessive doses of cortisone, or long-term diuretic therapy for chronic conditions such as hypertension (high blood pressure). Hyperkalemia results from renal dysfunction, such as the kidneys' inability to excrete excess amounts of potassium, or when there is decreased urine output or renal failure.

---

when the tissue has been damaged by traumatic injury. During vascular procedures on the aorta (especially those near the kidney) diuretics may be given to keep fluid flowing through the kidneys, thus providing a measure of continued kidney function. Note that the risk of hypokalemia is significantly reduced when diuretics are used for short-term treatment of such specific temporary conditions.

Although diuretics are not administered from the sterile back table, it is important that surgical technologists understand how the use of diuretics affects the surgical patient. There are two primary issues that the surgical team must consider.

1. Long-term diuretic therapy may cause the delay or rescheduling of a surgery, so the patient's potassium levels must be verified prior to opening the sterile field.
2. Short-term intraoperative use of diuretics requires the insertion of an indwelling urinary catheter in the patient before surgery. A urinary drainage bag with an accurate measuring device is often used to record urinary output at regular intervals.

To understand the action of diuretics, it is necessary to briefly review renal physiology. Consult your physiology textbook for additional information.

REVIEW OF RENAL PHYSIOLOGY

The primary function of the renal (urinary) system is to maintain **homeostasis** by filtering blood and removing excess water and dissolved substances, or *solutes*, such as sodium and potassium. The **nephron** (Fig. 7–1) is a microscopic filtering unit that removes

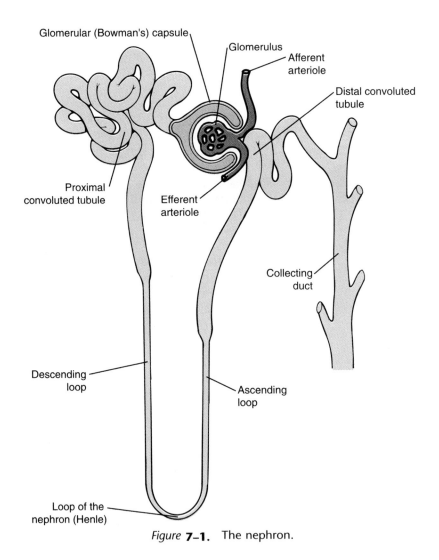

Figure **7–1.**   The nephron.

water and waste solutes. Millions of nephrons are present within the kidneys. Blood is brought to the nephron through the afferent arteriole into Bowman's capsule, where filtration occurs. Filtration is the process of forcing fluids and solutes through a membrane by pressure. Filtered blood then returns to the circulatory system via the efferent arteriole. The remaining fluid, or *filtrate*—which contains all the substances present in blood, except formed elements and most proteins—then undergoes tubular reabsorption. Only specific amounts of needed substances, including water, are reabsorbed. Tubular reabsorption takes place in the proximal convoluted tubule and the ascending and descending limbs of the loop of the nephron (loop of Henle).

The filtrate next receives such materials as potassium, **creatinine**, and hydrogen ions from blood surrounding the tubule; this process is called tubular secretion. Tubular secretion, which takes place in the distal convoluted tubule, eliminates waste products and controls blood pH. Additional water is reabsorbed when filtrate proceeds to the collecting ducts. Filtrate is emptied from collecting ducts into the renal pelvis to the ureter and bladder and is excreted as urine.

DIURETICS

Most diuretics exert effects at different locations along the nephron. Diuretics cause elimination of excess fluid by preventing reabsorption of sodium and water, increasing urine output. Diuretics are classified by site of action and the mechanism by which the solute is altered (Table 7–1).

LOOP DIURETICS

Loop diuretics are highly potent diuretics used to remove fluid arising from renal, hepatic, or cardiac dysfunction and to treat acute pulmonary edema. Hepatic dysfunction may be due to cirrhosis or liver failure. The most common cardiac dysfunction requiring treatment with diuretics is CHF (Insight 7–2). The oral form of high-ceiling diuretics may be used in treatment of hypertension. Loop diuretics work by decreasing the reabsorption of sodium (Na^+) and chloride (Cl^-) ions along the whole renal tubule, especially in the ascending loop of Henle. These diuretics exert a potent effect, because the site of action is so broad. Examples of loop diuretics are bumetanide (Bumex), ethacrynic acid (Edecrin), and furosemide (Lasix). Furosemide is the most commonly used agent in this category. In surgery, furosemide is particularly useful

Table **7–1**   Diuretics by Classification

Class	Generic Name	Trade Name
Loop diuretics	bumetanide	Bumex
	ethacrynic acid	Edecrin
	furosemide	Lasix
Thiazide diuretics	bendroflumethiazide	Naturin
	chlorothiazide	Diuril, SK-Chlorothiazide
	hydrochlorothiazide	Esidrix, HydroDIURIL, Oretic
Potassium-sparing diuretics	amiloride	Midamor
	spironolactone	Aldactone
	triamterene	Dyrenium
Carbonic anhydrase inhibitors	acetazolamide	Diamox
Osmotic diuretics	mannitol	Osmitrol

in intracranial procedures. Furosemide decreases intracranial pressure by quickly removing fluid that accumulates in response to the trauma of intracranial procedures or injuries. When furosemide is administered intravenously, onset of **diuresis** can be expected within 5 to 15 minutes and will continue for approximately 2 hours. The initial dose of furosemide is 20 to 40 mg intravenously, to be given over a period of 1 to 2 minutes. A second dose may be administered 2 hours later.

THIAZIDE DIURETICS

Thiazide diuretics are low potency diuretics used to treat essential hypertension and mild chronic edema. Thiazides work by inhibiting the reabsorption of sodium (Na^+) and chloride (Cl^-) ions in the end of the ascending loop of the nephron and the beginning of the distal convoluted tubule. Examples of thiazide diuretics include bendroflumethiazide (Naturetin), chlorothiazide (Diuril,

---

Insight 7–2   **Pathology Insight: Congestive Heart Failure**

Congestive heart failure, or pump failure, is the inability of the heart to pump sufficient blood to meet the body's demands. Back-pressure from stagnant blood slows down the venous blood return to the heart. When the right ventricle fails, congestion of organs and extremities results. The patient's legs become swollen, especially at the end of the day, and the liver becomes enlarged due to fluid retention. The enlarged liver presses on nerves, which causes pain and nausea. Pressure in the abdominal veins can lead to an accumulation of fluid in the abdominal cavity (ascites). Left ventricular failure leads to pulmonary congestion and edema as fluid builds up in the alveoli. This accumulation of fluids in the lungs causes shortness of breath (dyspnea). As there is less blood flowing to the major organs, their ability to function is impaired. The brain receives less blood, and this means less oxygen (hypoxia). The patient experiences confusion, loss of concentration, and mental fatigue. This also leads to changes in mental status. The kidneys cannot function properly, and this results in less urine formation (oliguria). Renal failure leads to abnormal retention of water and sodium, which leads to generalized edema. Patients with progressive congestive heart failure face life-threatening fluid overload and total heart failure. To compensate for decreased cardiac output, the body has adaptive mechanisms to try to meet the body's needs. As the failing heart tries to maintain a normal output of blood, it enlarges the pumping chambers to hold a greater blood volume. This increases the amount of blood pumped with each chamber's contraction. The heart also begins to increase its muscle mass. This allows for more force with each contraction. Along with this, the sympathetic nervous system helps out by activating adaptive processes to increase the heart rate, redistribute peripheral blood flow, and retain urine. These adaptive measures achieve almost normal cardiac output, but only for a short period of time. They eventually harm the pump because they require an increase in myocardial oxygen consumption. As the mechanism continues, myocardial reserve is exhausted. This leads to heart failure.

SK-Chlorothiazide), and hydrochlorothiazide (Esidrix, Hydro DIURIL, Oretic).

POTASSIUM-SPARING DIURETICS

Potassium-sparing diuretics are low potency diuretics commonly used to treat edema and hypertension and to help restore potassium levels in hypokalemic patients. Potassium-sparing diuretics are usually administered in combination with other diuretics such as thiazides and loop diuretics to minimize potassium loss. Potassium-sparing diuretics prevent the reabsorption of sodium in the distal convoluted tubules by altering membrane permeability. This change in membrane permeability also prevents potassium loss. Potassium-sparing diuretics exert a mild diuretic effect because only a small amount of the glomerular filtrate ever reaches the distal convoluted tubule. Common agents in this category include amiloride (Midamor), spironolactone (Aldactone), and triamterene (Dyrenium). Adverse effects can include **hyperkalemia.**

CARBONIC ANHYDRASE INHIBITORS

Carbonic anhydrase inhibitors are low potency diuretics used to treat mild acute closed-angle glaucoma and chronic open-angle glaucoma (see Chapter 10). These diuretics act on the proximal convoluted tubule, so urine output is not significantly impacted. Carbonic anhydrase is active in formation of aqueous humor in the eye. By inhibiting carbonic anhydrase, these drugs decrease production of aqueous humor, thus lowering intraocular pressure. The most common carbonic anhydrase inhibitor is acetazolamide (Diamox). Acetazolamide may be given orally to cataract patients after surgery because pressure may build up in the eye as a response to manipulation of tissues.

OSMOTIC DIURETICS

Osmotic diuretics are highly potent diuretics. The mechanism of action of osmotic diuretics is unlike that of any diuretics previously described. Osmotic diuretics actually increase blood pressure and volume by drawing fluid out of tissues and into the circulatory system rapidly (Fig. 7–2). Thus, osmotic diuretics are contraindicated in patients with hypertension and edema. Osmotic diuretics are *not* used for management of chronic conditions such as CHF. Osmotic diuretics are used to prevent acute renal failure after cardiac surgery, to treat increased intracranial pressure, and to reduce intraocular pressure in open-globe procedures of the eye such as retinal detachment.

As the name implies, these drugs exert their effects through the process of osmosis. Remember, osmosis is the process of water moving through a semipermeable membrane from an area of lesser concentration of solute (e.g., sodium) to an area of greater concentration of solute. Water moves toward the diuretic agent present in the glomerulus, thus preventing the water from being reabsorbed. Water is then excreted with the diuretic agent in the urine. There is no significant change in sodium reabsorption, so electrolyte balance should remain relatively unaffected.

The most commonly used osmotic diuretic is mannitol (Osmitrol). Mannitol may be used to provide a rapid reduction in

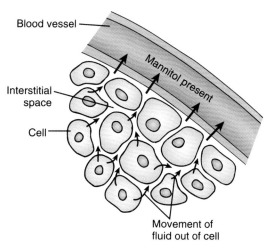

Blood vessel

Interstitial space

Cell

Mannitol present

Movement of fluid out of cell

Figure **7**-**2.**   Mannitol causes a change in the osmolarity of blood, drawing interstitial and intracellular fluid into the bloodstream. This action eventually increases the amount of fluid excreted by the kidneys.

intraocular pressure in patients experiencing acute angle–closure glaucoma. It is administered intravenously, warmed, through a filter to prevent crystallization. Mannitol may also be given during some neurosurgical procedures to reduce intracranial pressure. In vascular procedures, particularly on the aorta, mannitol may be used to protect kidney function by increasing the volume of fluid entering the kidneys.

ADVANCED PRACTICES FOR THE SURGICAL FIRST ASSISTANT
Chapter 7—Diuretics

KEY TERMS

diuresis   **hypokalemia**

As discussed in the chapter, diuretics are administered for the management of several medical conditions: to decrease hypertension, to decrease edema (peripheral and pulmonary) in CHF, to decrease edema in renal or liver disorders, and to treat glaucoma. Diuretics achieve their treatment goals by bringing about a negative fluid balance, mobilizing excessive extracellular

(continued on following page)

ADVANCED PRACTICES FOR THE SURGICAL FIRST ASSISTANT   *(continued)*

fluid, and reducing excess fluid volume. When the patient on diuretics is scheduled for surgery, preoperative evaluations are required. The surgical first assistant must understand the physiological effects on the body and any possible surgical complications that may arise from these medications. **Hypokalemia,** depletion of potassium in the blood serum, is often caused by the affects of diuretics on the kidneys. Thiazide and loop diuretics cause the highest rate of potassium loss. Diuretics increase the body's flow of urine **(diuresis).** Although water and sodium are excreted from the body by the kidneys, other electrolytes such as potassium are also excreted. Potassium is one of the essential minerals needed by the body to maintain homeostasis. It helps regulate normal heart rhythm, blood pressure, and nerve connections. Potassium is also needed to convert blood sugar into glycogen for energy that can be stored in the muscles. Next to calcium and phosphorus, potassium is the most abundant mineral found in the body. Potassium cannot be produced by the body and must be replaced through diet or supplements. See Table A for a list of foods rich in potassium. Nearly 98% of the total potassium is found inside the cells, with the remaining 2% in the blood serum. Small fluctuations in the blood serum potassium may have adverse affects in the functions of the heart, nerves, and muscles. All patients on diuretic therapy are routinely tested preoperatively for blood serum potassium levels. Abnormal levels should be corrected prior to any elective surgical procedure.

POTASSIUM LEVELS

Potassium levels in the blood serum are identified through analysis of a blood sample. In most cases the test is part of a routine chemical analysis that also includes other minerals. A normal level of potassium is 3.5 to 5.0 mEq/L (milliequivalent per liter). A level of 3.0 mEq/L with symptoms or 2.5 mEq/L with or without symptoms is considered severe hypokalemia and requires aggressive inpatient treatment. Patients with levels between 3.0 and 3.5 are considered mildly hypokalemic and are usually treated on an outpatient basis with diet or oral supplements.

Table **A**   Foods High in Potassium Content

apricots	meats	spinach
bananas	milk	sunflower seeds
beans	oranges and juice	sweet potatoes
cantaloupe	peaches	tomatoes
chocolate	potatoes	vegetable juice
fish	poultry	whole grains
honeydew	prunes	winter squash
kiwi fruit	pumpkin	yogurt
lima beans	raisins	

ADVANCED PRACTICES FOR THE SURGICAL FIRST ASSISTANT *(continued)*

TREATMENT OF HYPOKALEMIA

Treatment of hypokalemia involves replacing the potassium with diet or a supplement to obtain and maintain a normal serum potassium level. Treatment by oral intake or a supplement is adequate for minor depletion of potassium and can be performed at home over a period of time. Because of the slow release of potassium into the system, oral replacement treatment is by far the best method for replacement without any serious side effects. Acute hypokalemia (level >2.5 mEq/L) is a serious life-threatening condition and needs to be replaced by intravenous administration of potassium, such as potassium chloride, as an inpatient. Cardiac monitoring is necessary due to possible arrhythmia caused by the fluctuations of potassium levels. Dosage required for correction is based on the accepted formula that 10 mEq/L of potassium chloride will increase the blood serum level by 0.1 mEq/L. Intravenous administration of 10 or 20 mEq/hour not exceeding 200 mEq/L is usually recommended for severe hypokalemia.

KEY CONCEPTS

- Diuretics are agents administered to reduce the amount of fluid accumulating in patients with renal, hepatic, or cardiac dysfunction, as well as to relieve excessive intracranial or intraocular pressure. Excess fluid is removed through excretion of urine.
- Patients receiving long-term diuretic therapy have an increased risk of hypokalemia. If a surgical patient is hypokalemic, potential exists for cardiac dysrhythmias when under general anesthesia. To detect hypokalemia, blood chemistry analysis is performed preoperatively for all surgical patients taking diuretics. The sterile field should not be opened until the potassium levels are verified.
- Some surgical procedures require short-term intraoperative administration of diuretics. Diuretics are given intravenously in surgery during some ophthalmic, intracranial, and vascular procedures. An indwelling urinary catheter must be inserted on all surgical patients who may receive diuretics intraoperatively.
- The most common diuretics administered during surgery are mannitol (Osmitrol) and furosemide (Lasix).

8

HORMONES

OBJECTIVES

After completing this chapter, you should be able to:

1. Define terminology related to the endocrine system.
2. List endocrine glands and hormones secreted by each.
3. State the purpose for administration of each hormone.
4. Describe medical and surgical uses for hormones.
6. List hormones that may be administered from the sterile field.
7. List procedures that may require administration of hormones from the sterile field.

KEY TERMS

amenorrhea
androgen
dysmenorrhea
endometriosis
fibrocystic disease of the breast
fight-or-flight response
hyperparathyroidism
hyperthyroidism

hypoglycemic drugs
hypogonadism
hypoparathyroidism
hypothyroidism
menopause
osteoporosis
palliatives
recombinant DNA technology

H ormones are chemicals released by endocrine glands into the bloodstream (Fig. 8–1). These diverse substances maintain homeostasis (relatively constant conditions in the body) by altering the activities of specific target cells. Functions regulated by hormones include reproduction, growth and development, and metabolism. Hormones have a wide range of actions and effects, and each hormone has a specific function at a specific location in the body. In addition to naturally occurring hormones, several synthetic hormones have been developed. Most hormones are administered as replacement therapy in the medical rather than the surgical setting. But some hormones are used in surgery and may be administered from the sterile back table during the course of a procedure.

ENDOCRINE SYSTEM REVIEW

The endocrine system works with the nervous system to relay messages to maintain homeostasis. The endocrine system communicates by sending chemical messengers (hormones) to target cells located all over the body. Hormones are produced by endocrine glands and secreted into the extracellular space. They enter capil-

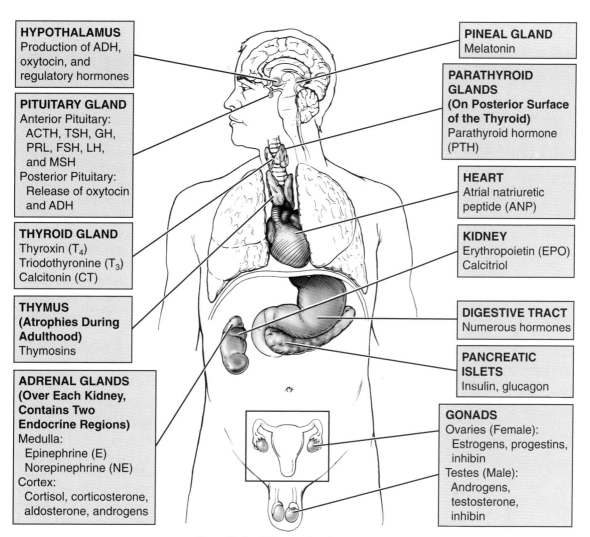

HYPOTHALAMUS
Production of ADH, oxytocin, and regulatory hormones

PITUITARY GLAND
Anterior Pituitary:
  ACTH, TSH, GH,
  PRL, FSH, LH,
  and MSH
Posterior Pituitary:
  Release of oxytocin
  and ADH

THYROID GLAND
Thyroxin (T_4)
Triodothyronine (T_3)
Calcitonin (CT)

THYMUS
(Atrophies During
Adulthood)
Thymosins

ADRENAL GLANDS
(Over Each Kidney,
Contains Two
Endocrine Regions)
Medulla:
  Epinephrine (E)
  Norepinephrine (NE)
Cortex:
  Cortisol, corticosterone,
  aldosterone, androgens

PINEAL GLAND
Melatonin

PARATHYROID
GLANDS
(On Posterior Surface
of the Thyroid)
Parathyroid hormone
(PTH)

HEART
Atrial natriuretic
peptide (ANP)

KIDNEY
Erythropoietin (EPO)
Calcitriol

DIGESTIVE TRACT
Numerous hormones

PANCREATIC
ISLETS
Insulin, glucagon

GONADS
Ovaries (Female):
  Estrogens, progestins,
  inhibin
Testes (Male):
  Androgens,
  testosterone,
  inhibin

Figure **8–1.**   **The endocrine system.**

laries and are carried by the bloodstream to target cells. Hormones bind to receptor sites on cells and cause a change in cell physiology. Chemical messages take longer to work than those relayed by the nervous system, but effects generally last longer. Hormonal effects are many and varied, but actions on the body may be categorized into four main groups:
  • Regulation of internal chemical balance and volume
  • Response to environmental changes, including stress, trauma, and temperature changes

- Growth and development
- Reproduction

Hormones can be classified as steroid and nonsteroid. Steroid hormones are derived from lipids structurally similar to cholesterol and include aldosterone, cortisol, estrogen, progesterone, and testosterone. Nonsteroid hormones are synthesized from amino acids. The simplest hormones are amines, derived from a single amino acid. Amine hormones include epinephrine, norepinephrine, thyroxine, and triiodothyronine. Hormones made of short chains of amino acids are called peptide hormones. Antidiuretic hormone (ADH) and oxytocin are examples of peptide hormones. Protein hormones are longer, folded chains of amino acids. Examples of protein hormones are growth hormone (GH), parathyroid hormone (PTH), insulin, and glucagon (see Table 8–1).

The vast majority of endocrine disorders are due either to hyposecretion or hypersecretion of hormones. Treatment for hyposecretion may include administration of hormones for supplement or for replacement. Hypersecretion may be treated medically with drugs to reduce secretion or surgically by gland removal, depending on indications.

ENDOCRINE GLANDS

PITUITARY GLAND

The pituitary gland, known as the "master gland," has a vital role in reproduction and growth, and it regulates the function of the renal system and thyroid gland. The pituitary gland is divided into two lobes—the anterior or adenohypophysis and the posterior or neurohypophysis. Hormones secreted by the adenohypophysis include growth hormone (GH), thyroid-stimulating hormone (TSH), adrenocorticotropic hormone (ACTH), prolactin (PRL) and gonadotropic hormones, which include follicle-stimulating hormone (FSH) and luteinizing hormone (LH). The neurohypophysis secretes oxytocin and antidiuretic hormone (ADH) (see Insight 8–1).

A pituitary hormone of particular importance to the surgical technologist is oxytocin. Oxytocin stimulates the uterine contractions necessary for normal labor and delivery. If a patient is unable to produce sufficient oxytocin naturally, it may be administered intravenously to induce labor. After delivery of the infant, the uterus must continue to contract in order to expel the placenta and to stop postpartum bleeding from the placental attachment site. After a cesarean section, the uterus is examined for sufficient contractions to naturally stop postpartum bleeding. If

Table **8–1** Hormone Classifications	
Steroid	*Nonsteroid*
aldosterone	epinephrine
cortisol	norepinephrine
estrogen	thyroxine
progesterone	triiodothyronine
testosterone	antidiuretic hormone (ADH)
	oxytocin
	growth hormone (GH)
	parathyroid hormone (PTH)
	insulin
	glucagons

natural contractions are not firm enough, oxytocin may be injected directly into the uterine muscle. The scrubbed surgical technologist uses a syringe to draw up the desired dose of oxytocin from a vial held by the circulator, changes needles, and then passes the medication to the surgeon. Oxytocin is available as Oxytocin, Pitocin, and Syntocinon.

⚠ CAUTION

It is critical to avoid confusion of Pitocin with Pitressin. Pitocin is oxytocin, but Pitressin is vasopressin, which contains antidiuretic hormone (ADH) and oxytocin in a ratio of 20 : 1. It is used subcutaneously or intramuscularly to stabilize fluid balance in patients with diabetes insipidus. The surgical technologist must be alert to drug names that sound similar. When in doubt, always clarify the order.

THYROID GLAND

The thyroid gland is a vascular structure consisting of two lobes joined by an isthmus. The largest of the endocrine glands, the thyroid is located below the larynx, on both sides of the trachea in the anterior neck. It sets the rate of body metabolism. In children an underfunctioning thyroid (**hypothyroidism**) can stunt growth and retard mental development. Lack of thyroid hormones slows metabolism. An adult with hypothyroidism is sleepy, tires easily, is less mentally alert, has reduced endurance, and has a slow heart rate (bradycardia). Overfunctioning of the thyroid, called Graves' disease or **hyperthyroidism**, causes restlessness, nervousness, sweating, and tachycardia (rapid heart rate). The thyroid secretes three important hormones: thyroxine, triiodothyronine, and calcitonin. Thyroxine (T_4) and triiodothyronine (T_3) are regulated by thyroid-stimulating hormone (TSH), which is produced in the pituitary gland. These hormones are essential for normal growth and development; they also help regulate metabolism of carbohydrates, lipids, and proteins. Both T_3 and T_4 require iodine salts for production. Iodine salts are obtained from foods after absorption through the intestines. After absorption, iodine salts are transported by the bloodstream to the thyroid for use in hormone production. Calcitonin helps to control calcium and phosphate concentrations in the blood, and it is regulated by blood levels of these ions. Calcitonin can affect calcium and phosphate levels by inhibiting the rate of release from bone, increasing the rate of incorporation of these ions into bone, and increasing excretion of these ions by the kidneys.

Thyroid hormones are administered to treat hypothyroidism caused by disease or surgical removal of the thyroid gland. Naturally occurring thyroid hormone has been extracted from the thyroid gland of pigs (porcine) and is labeled as desiccated thyroid (Thyroid USP) and thyroglobulin (Proloid). Many types of synthetic thyroid hormone are available, including levothyroxine (Levothroid, Synthroid), liothyronine (Cytomel), and liotrix (Euthroid, Thyrolar).

Antithyroid medications may be used to treat hyperthyroidism. A common antithyroid agent is methimazole (Tapazole), which may be used before surgery to reduce the size of a thyroid tumor or to inactivate thyroid tissue.

PARATHYROID GLANDS

The parathyroid glands are small, yellowish-brown ovals, approximately 6 mm in length, and frequently covered with adipose tissue. The glands are usually found embedded in the posterior surface of the thyroid gland. The number of parathyroid glands may vary from 2 to 6, with 90% of the patients having four: two on each side of the thyroid gland. They produce parathyroid hormone (PTH), or parathormone, which monitors circulating concentrations of calcium ions in the blood. Parathyroid hormone has four major functions: to stimulate osteoclasts, accelerating mineral turnover and the release of calcium from bone; to inhibit osteoblasts, reducing the rate of calcium deposition in bone; to enhance the reabsorption of calcium at the kidneys, reducing its loss via urine; and to stimulate the formation and secretion of calcitriol at the kidneys for the enhancement of calcium and phosphate absorption by the digestive tract. Inadequate amounts of PTH result in low calcium concentrations and **hypoparathyroidism.** This can cause a condition called tetany, characterized by prolonged muscle spasms involving the face and extremities. If calcium concentrations become too high, **hyperparathyroidism** results. In this condition, bones can grow thin and brittle, skeletal muscles weaken, and the central nervous system is depressed. An example of a parathyroid hormone is teriparatide (Forteo), which is a synthetic version produced by recombinant DNA technology.

Insight 8–1   **Recombinant DNA Technology**

Human growth hormone is used for long-term treatment of children with growth failure caused by hyposecretion of GH. Growth hormone obtained from domestic mammals such as cows and pigs does not work for humans. For many years the only source for growth hormone therapy was that extracted from the glands of human cadavers; however, this practice was terminated when several patients died from a rare neurological disease attributed to contaminated glands. So, another source had to be found. That source is **recombinant DNA technology.** This is defined as several techniques for cutting apart and splicing together different pieces of DNA. Segments of foreign DNA are transferred to another cell or organism, and the substances the DNA carries the code for are produced. Thus, these cells or organisms become factories for the production of the substances coded for by the inserted DNA.

For example, this process is carried out to make *Humulin* (insulin). Although bovine and porcine insulin is similar to human insulin, the composition is slightly different. This difference can cause problems for a number of diabetic patients' immune systems, which produce antibodies against it. So researchers inserted the insulin gene into a suitable vector (*E. coli* bacterial cell) to produce an insulin that is chemically identical to what is produced in humans.

Another hormone that is produced using recombinant DNA technology is parathyroid hormone (PTH). This medication has a special side effect: when given in daily injections it promotes strong bones. Thus, it has also been approved as a treatment for osteoporosis.

ADRENAL GLANDS

The adrenal glands are pyramid-shaped glands positioned on top of each kidney. The adrenals are highly vascular and consist of a central portion, the medulla, and an outer portion, the cortex. The adrenal medulla produces, stores, and secretes the hormones epinephrine (adrenaline) and norepinephrine (noradrenaline), collectively called catecholamines. The catecholamines are *sympathomimetic,* meaning they mimic effects of the sympathetic portion of the autonomic nervous system. Epinephrine and norepinephrine work with the sympathetic nervous system to prepare the body for the **fight-or-flight response** to stress. Effects of these hormones include increased heart rate, increased force of cardiac muscle contraction, vasoconstriction, elevated blood pressure, increased respiratory rate, and decreased digestive system activity.

Epinephrine is of particular interest to the surgical technologist because it is used frequently in surgery. Epinephrine is often used in combination with local anesthetics to prolong anesthesia. When injected in dilute amounts (1:100,000 or 1:200,000), epinephrine causes local vasoconstriction; this means it reduces blood flow so it reduces the absorption rate of the anesthetic. Epinephrine may also be used topically for hemostasis. In middle ear procedures, for example, tiny pledgets of Gelfoam are typically dipped in more concentrated epinephrine (1:1000) and applied to areas of capillary bleeding.

⚠ CAUTION

In ear surgery, epinephrine 1:1000 is ONLY used for topical application—*never* injection. If epinephrine 1:1000 is mistakenly injected, deadly tachycardia and hypertension may result. The surgical technologist must exercise particular caution when labeling and handling medications for ear surgery, because two significantly different strengths of epinephrine are present on the sterile back table. As an example, in tympanoplasty, epinephrine 1:1000 is used for topical hemostasis in the middle ear while a local anesthetic with dilute epinephrine (1% lidocaine with epinephrine 1:100,000 or 1:200,000) is injected for hemostasis. Both solutions are clear. To pass the correct medication at the correct time, the surgical technologist *must* know the route of administration for both strengths of epinephrine. The scrubbed surgical technologist must observe the delivery of these medications to the sterile field, and immediately label each drug—its identity *and* its strength—as it is accepted into the sterile field to avoid errors. In addition, topical strength epinephrine (1:1000) must *never* be kept in a syringe on the back table. Rather, a shallow container (such as a sterile Petri dish) should be used for topical epinephrine, to prevent the drug from being mistakenly drawn up into a syringe for injection.

TECH TIP   Local anesthesia containing epinephrine will have a red label or red printing noting its concentration.

Adrenal cortex hormones are classified in two major groups—glucocorticoids and mineralocorticoids—collectively known as steroids. The most important mineralocorticoid is aldosterone, which maintains homeostatic levels of sodium in the blood. Most significant to the surgical technologist are the glucocorticoids, which are used to reduce or inhibit the inflammatory response after surgical procedures such as shoulder arthroscopy or cataract extraction. Steroids are used medically to help prevent rejection of donated organs (Insight 8–2), to reduce the inflammatory response in patients with arthritis, and as replacement therapy for Addison's disease (Insight 8–3). Steroids administered for diseases such as arthritis are used as **palliatives.** Palliative drugs relieve symptoms, but they do not cure the condition or disease.

Steroids may be administered orally, topically, intramuscularly, or rarely, intravenously. Hormones may be long- or short-acting, depending on the agent used. Naturally occurring steroids include cortisone, hydrocortisone, aldosterone, and deoxycorticosterone. Many synthetic steroids have been produced. A partial list of synthetic steroids includes synthetic cortisone (Cortisone, Cortone),

---

Insight 8–2   **Immunosuppressant Agents**

Medical advancements now allow defective body organs to be replaced with healthy donor tissue. This introduces foreign tissue into the recipient's system and will trigger the immune response that can result in the destruction of the transplanted tissue. Thus, tissue must be matched between donor and recipient to avoid rejection. However, even with careful tissue matching, some incompatibilities will exist (except in cases of identical twins or autotransplantation). Glucocorticoids are used to prevent or alleviate the effects of the immune response when the response is detrimental. They are used for the treatment of autoimmune disorders, to prevent rejection of transplants, to suppress hypersensitivity reactions, and to alleviate cerebral edema. For transplant patients, the medication therapy will be lifelong or as long as the transplanted tissue is in place.

Glucocorticoids act by inhibiting synthesis of chemical mediators, such as histamines, and so reduce swelling, redness, warmth, and pain. They also suppress the infiltration of phagocytes to decrease lysosomal enzyme damage and suppress the proliferation of lymphocytes to reduce the immune component of inflammation.

When the immune system is suppressed with glucocorticoids, infectious organisms have the opportunity to multiply. Minor infections may become clinically significant after such therapy, so use in some patients, such as those with fungal or herpes infections, must be avoided. Glucocorticoids should be used cautiously in patients with diabetes mellitus, peptic ulcers, inflammatory bowel disorders, hypertension, congestive heart failure, or renal problems.

Insight 8–3   **Pathology Insight: Addison's Disease**

Addison's disease, also known as adrenocortical hypofunction, occurs when the adrenal cortex does not secrete adequate amounts of steroid hormone. The disorder was first described by Thomas Addison in 1855, when the primary cause was tuberculosis. Today, however, autoimmune disease is the most common cause. Why? Because the body's circulating antibodies react specifically against adrenal tissue to destroy it. Tumors or hemorrhage of the adrenal glands can also cause the disorder, as can hypopituitarism—decreasing adrenocorticotropic hormone (ACTH) secretion—or abrupt withdrawal of long-term corticosteroid treatment. The disorder can occur at any age, even infancy, and is found in both males and females. Medical treatment involves replacement hormones such as prednisone or hydrocortisone drugs and fludrocortisone. John F. Kennedy suffered from Addison's disease. He had almost no adrenal tissue; but by taking replacement hormones he was able to function in one of the world's most demanding jobs—the presidency of the United States (1960–1963).

synthetic hydrocortisone (Hydrocortone, Cortef, Solu-cortef), prednisone (Deltasone, Deltra), prednisolone (Delta-cortef, Hydeltra TBA), methylprednisolone (Medrol, Depo-medrol, Solu-medrol), triamcinolone acetonide (Aristocort, Kenacort, Kenalog 40), dexamethasone (Decadron), and betamethasone (Celestone).

PANCREAS

The pancreas, which is posterior to the stomach and behind the parietal peritoneum, is divided into three anatomic areas: the head, which lies within the loop of the duodenum; the body; and the tail. A unique feature of the pancreas is that it functions as an exocrine gland for digestion and as an endocrine gland for release of hormones. The exocrine pancreas is the primary source for the vital digestive enzymes amylase, lipase, and proteinase. A duct from the gland—the pancreatic duct—transports these digestive enzymes to the duodenum.

The endocrine portion of the pancreas is closely associated with blood vessels, which facilitate the transport of pancreatic hormones to the body. Pancreatic hormones are produced by clusters of cells called the islets of Langerhans. Two pancreatic hormones, insulin and glucagon, regulate metabolism of glucose, a simple sugar used as an energy source. Glucagon is a protein; it stimulates the liver to break down glycogen into glucose, thus increasing blood sugar levels. Insulin, also a protein, stimulates the liver to form glycogen from glucose, thus lowering blood sugar levels. In patients with type I diabetes, the body fails to produce insulin, so an outside source must be provided. Insulin was first obtained from animals, but human insulin (Humulin) is now produced via recombinant DNA technology.

In type II diabetes, the body fails to respond to the action of insulin on target cells. Type II diabetes may be effectively managed with diet and exercise or administration of oral **hypoglycemic drugs**, which include glyburide (Diabeta), chlorpropamide (Diabinese), and tolazamide (Tolinase).

OVARIES

The ovaries, located in the pelvic area, are paired glands that produce estrogen and progesterone. Estrogen and progesterone are critical to the development and maintenance of female sex characteristics, including the menstrual cycle, pregnancy, and lactation. These hormones are available in several forms—tablets, capsules, and oil (intramuscular use only)—and are administered to treat **amenorrhea**, **dysmenorrhea**, and the side effects of **menopause.** Estrogen and progesterone are used as replacement therapy after menopause or oophorectomy to prevent osteoporosis (Insight 8–4) and as oral contraceptives. Estrogens are also used for palliative treatment of advanced androgen-dependent prostate cancer and metastatic breast cancer. Common estrogens available are chlorotrianisene (TACE), conjugated estrogens (Premarin), and estradiol (Estrace).

Insight 8–4   **Pathology Insight: The Role of Estrogen in Osteoporosis**

Osteoporosis is a disorder in which the skeletal system loses too much mineralized bone volume. Normal bones are remodeled throughout life. Until about age 30, bone formation exceeds bone resorption. Later, however, bone resorption outpaces formation; the result is a net bone loss of about 0.5% per year after age 30. After menopause, bone resorption is accelerated in women because estrogen production decreases. Bone tissue needs estrogen in order to absorb calcium. Estrogen also increases vitamin D metabolism—a process necessary for calcium absorption from the intestines. Without proper levels of estrogen in the body, the amount of calcium stored in bones is diminished and bones become more porous—that is, osteoporotic. The skeleton weakens, so it is less able to support body weight. Osteoporotic bone can be seen on routine spine x-rays. The shape of the bone is the same, but the image is less distinct; this suggests porous, or weaker, bone.

A more sensitive test is a bone-density scan known as dual x-ray absorptiometry, or DEXA. Many times, however, the first indication of osteoporosis is a fracture—in the femur at the hip, in the radius near the wrist, or as compression fractures of the vertebrae. Over time, osteoporotic symptoms include loss of height, stooped posture, and back pain. Estrogen replacement plays an important role in the treatment plan for osteoporosis. In addition, patients receive dietary calcium or calcium supplements together with a regular, reasonable exercise regimen.

Estrogen, which is also available in cream form, is occasionally used on vaginal packing placed after vaginal hysterectomy. One type of progesterone available is medroxy-progesterone (Provera).

TESTES

The testes are paired glands located in the scrotum. Endocrine cells are distributed throughout the testes and produce male sex hormones called **androgens.** Androgens, primarily testosterone, are critical for the development of male sex organs and maintenance of secondary sex characteristics. Androgens, especially testosterone (Depo-Testosterone, Delatest), are administered if replacement therapy is indicated, as seen in **hypogonadism.** Testosterone may also be used to treat some types of advanced breast cancer in females. The androgen danazol (Danocrine) is used to treat diseases in females such as **endometriosis** and **fibrocystic disease of the breast.** Patients scheduled for an endometrial ablation may be placed on Danocrine therapy a few weeks prior to surgery to reduce the volume of the endometrial layer.

ADVANCED PRACTICES FOR THE SURGICAL FIRST ASSISTANT
Chapter 8—Hormones

KEY TERMS

euthyroid	hypercalcemia	hypocalcemia

TREATMENT OPTIONS

The thyroid and parathyroid glands are among the most common glands of the endocrine system to be affected by a disorder or a disease. Treatment usually requires both drug therapy and surgery. The hormones secreted by these glands are essential for homeostasis; therefore any abnormal secretion must be corrected. Medical therapy is usually directed by an endocrinologist, whereas surgical removal requires an endocrine surgeon (general or head and neck surgeon). The advanced practitioner acting as a surgical first assistant may only be exposed to the surgical aspect but should also have knowledge of the medical component. It is important to understand how each affects the other.

THYROID GLAND

As previously described in the chapter, the thyroid consists of two lobes connected by the isthmus and secretes hormones. Ideally, it is important for the surgical patient to be **euthy-**

ADVANCED PRACTICES FOR THE SURGICAL FIRST ASSISTANT   *(continued)*

roid prior to any procedure. If the patient is hyperthyroid (an overfunctioning of the gland and thus overproduction of thyroid hormones), medical management with antithyroid agents or radioactive iodine ablation is indicated. If the patient's condition is not managed, a condition called thyroid storm, or hyperthyroid crisis, could occur. This is a failure of the body to tolerate increased thyroid hormones in response to a stressor (such as surgery). Thyroid storm is defined as an acute, life-threatening, thyroid-hormone–induced hypermetabolic state. Symptoms include hyperpyrexia, cardiac arrhythmias, mental status changes, congestive heart failure, and hemodynamic instability. In the past thyroid storm occurred intraoperatively and postoperatively from thyroid surgery, in patients with Graves' disease and in some cases with toxic nodular goiter. Presently, thyroid storm is rare due to prompt recognition, appropriate medical workup and preoperative treatment (Table A). If the patient is

Table **A**   Medical Treatment of Thyroid Disease

Medicine	Treatment of	Action	Therapeutic Dosage	Side Effects
methimazole (Trapazole)	Hyperthyroidism	Inhibits thyroid hormone synthesis	Initially 15–60 mg/d in three doses PO; maintenance 5–15 mg q8h	Rash, urticaria, headache, gastrointestinal tract symptoms
propylthiouracil (PTU)	Hyperthyroidism	Inhibits conversion of T_3 and T_4 hormones	Initially 300–450 mg/d, maintenance 150–300 mg/d, PO	Rash, hair loss, gastrointestinal symptoms, loss of taste, drowsiness, decreased white blood cells, decreased platelets
iodine (Lugol's solution, potassium iodide solution)	Hyperthyroidism	Reduces size and vascularity of gland	0.1–0.3 mL tid PO, one dose	Drink solution through straw to prevent teeth discoloration
levothyroxine sodium	Hypothyroidism	Increases metabolic rate, replaces thyroid hormones	Initially 0.05 mg qd; maintenance 0.075–0.125 mg qd, PO	Nausea, vomiting, diarrhea, cramps, tremors, nervousness, insomnia, headache, weight loss

PO, Per os.

(continued on following page)

ADVANCED PRACTICES FOR THE SURGICAL FIRST ASSISTANT   *(continued)*

hypothyroid (underfunctioning of the gland), medical management with thyroid hormone replacement therapy is indicated before surgery. This condition, in its advanced stage known as myxedema, is characterized by hypothermia, CO_2 retention, and bradycardia. There may be emergency situations in which the patient must have surgery and is not euthyroid. When this occurs, the surgeon and anesthesia personnel will decide the best medications and treatment plan preoperatively and intraoperatively.

PARATHYROID GLANDS

Parathyroid glands are located in the neck, usually posterior to the thyroid gland. The glands may be found within the thyroid gland, in adipose tissue under the thyroid gland, or in the mediastinum. As stated in the chapter, they secrete parathyroid hormone (PTH), which is responsible for regulating calcium levels in the body. Overfunctioning of the parathyroid glands causes the secretion of too much PTH. Hyperparathyroidism is the most common disorder causing the patient's blood calcium level to be elevated. Hypoparathyroidism is responsible for low levels of calcium. Both conditions may be treated with medication therapy (Table B); however, most cases of hyperparathyroidism are treated surgically.

BLOOD SERUM CALCIUM LEVELS

Calcium is the most abundant and important mineral in the body. It is responsible for building and repairing bones and teeth as well as helping nerve function. It is necessary for the

Table B   Medical Treatment of Parathyroid Disease

Medicine	Condition	Action	Therapeutic Dosage	Side Effects
calcitriol (Rocaltrol)	Hypoparathyroidism, hypocalcemia	Enhancement of calcium deposits in bones	Initially 0.57–2.5 mg daily; maintenance 0.2–1 mg daily, PO	Weakness, headache, nausea, vomiting, dry mouth, constipation
calcium	Hypoparathyroidism	Replaces calcium	500 mg bid, PO after meals	
calcitonin	Hyperparathyroidism	Decreases serum calcium	Initially 0.5 mg/d; maintenance 0.25 mg/d, 0.5 bid, SQ	Fatigue, anorexia, nausea, vomiting, constipation, abdominal pain

PO, Per os.

ADVANCED PRACTICES FOR THE SURGICAL FIRST ASSISTANT   *(continued)*

contracting of muscles, the clotting of blood, and proper function of the heart. Maintaining a normal level of calcium is essential for homeostasis and must be replaced continuously by diet or supplemental agents. Of the body's calcium, 99% is stored in the bones, with the remaining 1% found in the blood. The normal laboratory value of calcium is 9.0 to 10.5 mg/dL but may vary somewhat by laboratory. A patient with a laboratory value lower than the normal is considered to have **hypocalcemia**, whereas patients with values higher than normal have **hypercalcemia.** Hypocalcemia may be caused by radical surgery in the central neck, including total thyroidectomy and radical neck dissection. Patients undergoing any central neck procedure need to have calcium levels tested immediately postoperatively. A drop in the serum calcium level below 7.0 mg/dL may be treated with calcium gluconate administrated intravenously. An initial dose of 100 to 200 mg is administered over a 10- to 20-minute period followed by a slow calcium infusion of 0.1 to 1.5 mg/kg/h. Faster infusions may result in cardiac dysfunction or cardiac arrest. Hypercalcemia may be caused by over-functioning of one or more parathyroid glands. This is usually treated with surgical intervention as described later.

HYPERPARATHYROIDISM

Hyperparathyroidism is described as an oversecretion of PTH causing high calcium levels (hypercalcemia) in patients. There are two basic types of hyperparathyroidism: primary and secondary. Primary hyperparathyroidism, the most common disorder, is often caused by at least one diseased gland (usually adenoma) that overstimulates the secretion of PTH. Surgical removal of the affected gland is usually required. The most common procedure today is minimal invasive excision of the affected gland with rapid PTH study. The gland is localized with the use of a sestamibi scan performed preoperatively in the nuclear medicine department. At the beginning of the procedure a blood sample is drawn and processed to identify the amount of serum PTH. A small incision is made over the location of the affected gland, and the gland is surgically removed. The half-life of PTH is about 10 minutes: therefore after this time, a second blood sample is drawn and processed in the same manner as the first. If the results reveal that the serum PTH level has dropped by at least 50%, it is accepted that only one gland was affected and the surgical procedure is concluded. Postoperative calcium levels are closely monitored for 24 hours.

  Secondary hyperparathyroidism is a result of renal failure, which stimulates the parathyroid glands to secrete more PTH. This condition, when treated with hypocalcemic or vitamin D analog medicine, produces limited results. Surgical management is still the most effective treatment. The surgical procedure requires that all but half of the parathyroid glands be removed. With only half the gland functioning, the PTH level is reduced dramatically. Some surgeons transplant the remaining half gland in the sternocleidomastoid muscle for easy access if more gland needs to be removed at a later date.

(continued on following page)

ADVANCED PRACTICES FOR THE SURGICAL FIRST ASSISTANT   *(continued)*

HYPOPARATHYROIDISM

Hypoparathyroidism is a condition in which the parathyroid glands do not secrete an adequate amount of PTH rendering the patient hypocalcemic. This condition is caused by inadvertent excision of all parathyroid tissue during a total thyroidectomy, and is referred to as true hypoparathyroidism, found in 3% to 5% of total thyroidectomy. Postoperative calcium levels are monitored after total thyroidectomy to determine any functioning parathyroid tissue. If levels are low, replacement parathyroid hormone is prescribed. Another type of hypoparathyroidism, termed pseudohypoparathyroidism, is a rare, inherited familiar disorder. Females are twice as likely to inherit the condition as males. Both disorders are treated with a hypercalcemic medicine to regulate the calcium levels. There is no surgical procedure to correct this disorder.

KEY CONCEPTS

- The endocrine system works with the nervous system to relay chemical messages called hormones.
- Hormones maintain homeostasis by altering activities of specific target cells.
- Hormones' activities include: regulation of internal chemical balance and volume; response to environmental changes; growth and development; and reproduction.
- Most endocrine disorders are due to hyposecretion or hypersecretion of hormones and are treated with medications administered from the medical setting.
- Some hormones are synthesized by recombinant DNA technology.
- Hormones most commonly administered in surgery are oxytocin, epinephrine, and steroids.

MEDICATIONS THAT AFFECT COAGULATION

Medications Covered in Chapter 9

Generic Name	Trade Name	Category
absorbable gelatin	Gelfoam, Gelfilm	Hemostatic
microfibrillar collagen hemostat	Avitene, Instat MCH	Hemostatic
oxidized cellulose	Oxycel, Surgicel, Surgicel NuKnit	Hemostatic
absorbable collagen sponge	Collastat, Helistat, Hemopad, Instat	Hemostatic
thrombin	Thrombogen	Hemostatic
bone wax	N/A	Hemostatic
tannic acid	N/A	Chemical hemostatic
silver nitrate	N/A	Chemical hemostatic
Monsel's solution	N/A	Chemical hemostatic
calcium salts	Calcium chloride	Systemic coagulant
vitamin K phytonadione	Konakion, Mephyton, AquaMephyton	Systemic coagulant
antihemophilic factor (VIII)	Hemofil-M, Koate-HT, Monociate	Blood coagulation factor
factor IX complex	KonyneHT, Profiline Heat-treated, Proplex	Blood coagulation factor
aspirin	N/A	Oral anticoagulant
warfarin	Coumadin	Oral anticoagulant
heparin	N/A	Parenteral anticoagulant
enoxaprin	Lovenox	Parenteral anticoagulant
streptokinase	Streptase	Thrombolytic
urokinase	Abbokinase	Thrombolytic
antistreplase	Eminase	Thrombolytic
alteplase	Activase	Thrombolytic

OBJECTIVES

After completing this chapter, you should be able to:

1. Define terms related to blood coagulation and medications that affect coagulation.
2. Describe the physiology of blood clot formation.
3. List agents that affect coagulation by category.
4. Identify the category of various agents that affect coagulation.
5. State the purpose of each category of medications that affect coagulation.
6. Describe the action of medications that affect coagulation.
7. List uses, routes of administration, side effects, and contraindications for agents that affect coagulation.
8. Describe the impact of preoperative oral anticoagulant therapy on the surgical patient.
9. List examples of surgical procedures in which agents that affect coagulation may be administered.
10. Compare and contrast administration route, onset of action, antagonist, and purpose of parenteral and oral anticoagulants.
11. List the administration route for each medication that affects coagulation.

KEY TERMS

anticoagulants
coagulants
coagulation (clotting) factors
hemostatics
parenteral

platelet aggregation
systemic
thrombolytics (fibrinolytics)
thrombosis

Blood naturally contains both **coagulants**, which promote clotting, and **anticoagulants**, which inhibit clotting. Normally, anticoagulants are dominant; they keep blood in liquid form. But when damage occurs to blood vessels, the body's coagulation mechanism begins clot formation to prevent excessive blood loss. At times, it becomes necessary to enhance or assist natural coagulation. During surgical intervention, the blood supply to an area may be disrupted, causing blood loss. Intraoperatively, damaged blood vessels are controlled with the use of thermal hemostasis (electrosurgical unit) or mechanical hemostasis (such as ligatures or hemostatic clips). The natural coagulation process usually works effectively on damaged capillaries, arterioles, and venules. But this process may be assisted. Topical **hemostatics** are coagulants used on areas of capillary bleeding as an adjunct to natural hemostasis. And when natural **coagulation**

factors are absent or insufficient, **systemic** coagulants are used to restore or enhance the coagulation process. Although systemic coagulants are usually administered in the medical setting, they may be given immediately preoperatively or intraoperatively.

Conversely, blood coagulation may also be undesirable. Systemic anticoagulants are used to prevent or delay the onset of the coagulation sequence during surgical procedures performed on blood vessels, for example. Heparin is one such systemic anticoagulant. It is routinely administered during peripheral and cardiovascular surgical procedures to prevent adverse clotting. Most other systemic anticoagulants are administered in the medical setting to prevent conditions such as deep vein **thrombosis** (DVT) or pulmonary embolism (PE). Patients on long-term anticoagulation require special consideration when undergoing an invasive surgical procedure, because of their delayed coagulation time.

When a blood clot, or thrombus, forms within an intact blood vessel, a mechanism in the blood acts to dissolve the clot naturally. If the natural anticoagulation process is inadequate, **thrombolytics** may be administered to speed clot breakdown. Thrombolytics are used to treat existing blood clots as seen in conditions such as DVT, PE, coronary artery thrombosis, and myocardial infarction.

PHYSIOLOGY OF CLOT FORMATION

The body's coagulation mechanism prevents blood loss due to trauma or damage to small blood vessels. (Trauma to large blood vessels, however, requires surgical intervention—thermal or mechanical hemostasis—to control blood loss.) Damage to a small blood vessel causes spasm, which causes a platelet plug to form, which leads to coagulation. In fact, blood clot formation is a cascade of events occurring in three basic stages (Fig. 9–1).

Stage 1: Thromboplastin (also known as prothrombin activator) is formed.

Stage 2: Thromboplastin converts prothrombin (known as factor II) into thrombin.

Stage 3: Thrombin converts fibrinogen (known as factor I) to fibrin.

Fibrin is a mesh of protein threads—a net that traps blood cells to form a clot.

Stage 1 involves two different mechanisms for the formation of thromboplastin—the extrinsic pathway and the intrinsic pathway. The *extrinsic* pathway is initiated by factors outside the blood. It is triggered by a clotting factor released from damaged

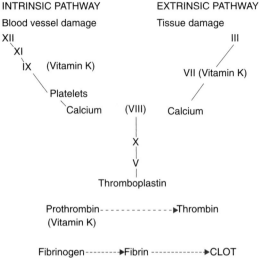

INTRINSIC PATHWAY   EXTRINSIC PATHWAY

Blood vessel damage   Tissue damage

XII   III

  XI

    IX (Vitamin K)

               VII (Vitamin K)

     Platelets

       Calcium   (VIII)   Calcium

                 X

                 V

          Thromboplastin

Prothrombin - - - - - - - - - - - - - ▶Thrombin
(Vitamin K)

Fibrinogen - - - - - - - - ▶Fibrin - - - - - - - - - - - - - ▶CLOT

Figure **9–1.** Blood coagulation pathways.

tissue, that is, tissue thromboplastin, or factor III. The extrinsic pathway can produce a clot in seconds. Tissue thromboplastin (factor III) combines with antihemophilic factor VIII (AHF) and calcium to activate the Stuart-Prower factor X. When activated, factor X reacts with proaccelerin (factor V) and calcium to form thromboplastin.

The *intrinsic* pathway is initiated by substances contained in the blood. This pathway is more complex and takes several minutes. When a blood vessel is damaged, the Hageman factor (factor XII) is activated. Factor XII then activates plasma thromboplastin antecedent (PTA; factor XI), which activates plasma thromboplastin component (PTC; factor IX). Then, as in the extrinsic pathway, activated factor IX combines with antihemophilic factor and calcium to activate factor X and factor X reacts with proaccelerin (factor V) and calcium to form thromboplastin.

The clotting cascade requires calcium at all stages—that is, calcium enables many of the steps. Vitamin K also plays a vital role in coagulation. It is required, for example, to synthesize prothrombin (factor II), proconvertin (factor VII), plasma thromboplastin component (factor IX), and the Stuart-Prower factor (X). See Table 9–1 for a summary of blood coagulation factors.

Occasionally, clotting may take place within an unbroken blood vessel; this abnormal clotting is called thrombosis. If it

Factor	Name	Function
I	Fibrinogen	Converted to fibrin
II	Prothrombin	Converted to thrombin
III	Tissue thromboplastin	Triggers extrinsic pathway
IV	Calcium	Essential in all three stages of clotting
V	Proaccelerin	Accelerates conversion of prothrombin to thrombin
VI		Factor VI is no longer believed to be involved in blood coagulation.
VII	Proconvertin	Essential for extrinsic pathway
VIII	Antihemophilic factor	Accelerates activation of factor X
IX	Plasma thromboplastin component (Christmas factor)	Essential for intrinsic pathway; accelerates activation of factor X
X	Stuart-Prower factor	Essential for intrinsic and extrinsic pathways
XI	Plasma thromboplastin antecedent	Essential for intrinsic pathway; accelerates activation of factor IX
XII	Hageman factor	Essential for intrinsic pathway
XIII	Fibrin-stabilizing factor	Strengthens fibrin clot

*Table **9–1*** Blood Coagulation Factors

forms in an artery, such a clot (thrombus) may cut off blood supply to an area. If a thrombus forms in a vein, it may inhibit return of blood to systemic circulation. Or a venous clot may break off and become an embolus—traveling to the heart, brain, or lungs—causing severe complications, even death. Blood clots may dissolve naturally; this is because blood normally contains a clot-dissolving enzyme, fibrinolysin. But if the body's natural declotting mechanism is inadequate, medical or surgical intervention may be required. For example, arterial embolectomy may be necessary when blood clots form in the femoral, popliteal or tibial artery. If a blood clot forms in a vein, medical treatment may be sufficient. With bed rest and administration of a thrombolytic agent, such a clot may dissolve.

COAGULANTS

Coagulants are drugs that promote, accelerate, or make possible blood coagulation. There are two major categories of coagulants: hemostatics and systemic coagulants. Hemostatics are topical agents used almost exclusively in the surgical setting. Systemic coagulants are generally used in the medical setting.

HEMOSTATICS

Hemostatics are agents that enhance or accelerate blood clotting at a surgical site. These agents serve as adjuncts to natural coagulation, which controls minor capillary bleeding. Thus, hemostatics are not effective against arterial or major venous bleeding. Hemostatics used in surgery are applied topically in the form of films, powders, sponges, or solutions. Several different types of hemostatic agents are available (Table 9–2), and each is supplied in sterile packaging for delivery to the sterile field.

Table 9–2   Topical Hemostatics by Category

Absorbable Gelatin

Gelfilm
Gelfoam powder
Gelfoam sponge

Microfibrillar Collagen Hemostat

Avitene
Instat MCH

Oxidized Cellulose

Oxycel
Surgicel
Surgicel NuKnit

Absorbable Collagen Sponge

Collastat
Helistat
Hemopad
Instat
Superstat

Thrombin

Thrombogen

Bone Wax

Chemical Hemostatics

tannic acid
silver nitrate
Monsel's solution

Absorbable Gelatin

Absorbable gelatin hemostatics are animal in origin, made from purified pork skin gelatin USP. Applied topically, with pressure, to bleeding sites, these agents are thought to be mechanical, rather than chemical, in their mode of action. Gelatin hemostatics are absorbed completely in four to six weeks, depending on such factors as the amount used and the surgical site. Gelatin hemostatics may be used dry or moistened with saline; however, they should not be used in the presence of infection. Examples of gelatin hemostatics include Gelfilm as well as Gelfoam powder and sponges (Fig. 9–2). Dry Gelfilm has the consistency of stiff cellophane; moistened, it becomes pliable. As a film, it can be cut into desired shapes and sizes. Gelfoam powder can be made into a paste by mixing with saline. The powder form promotes granulation tissue, so it may be used on areas of skin ulceration. Gelfoam sponges are also available. They come in many sizes (Table 9–3) for various applications, and may be torn or cut to desired shapes. Gelfoam is commonly used in orthopedic, general, and neurosurgical procedures. Gelfoam is also used in otologic surgery such as tympanoplasty. It is cut into

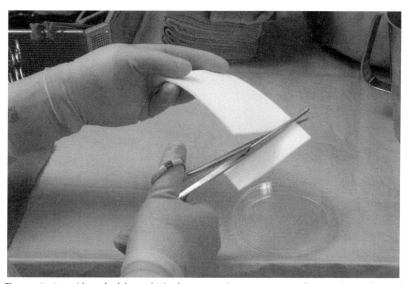

Figure **9–2.**   Absorbable gelatin hemostatic agents may be cut into desired shapes and sizes.

Table **9–3** Gelfoam Sponge Sizes	
Manufacturer's Code	**Actual Size**
12–3	20 mm × 60 mm (12 sq cm) × 3 mm thick
12–7	20 mm × 60 mm (12 sq cm) × 7 mm thick
50	80 mm × 62.5 mm (50 sq cm) × 10 mm thick
100	80 mm × 125 mm (100 sq cm) × 100 mm thick
200	80 mm × 250 mm (200 sq cm) × 10 mm thick

tiny pieces called pledgets, which may be used to pack the area around a tympanic graft or to apply a very small amount of epinephrine (topically) on bleeding surfaces inside the middle ear.

Microfibrillar Collagen Hemostat

Avitene is a dry, fibrous preparation of purified bovine corium collagen (Fig. 9–3). Direct application to bleeding surfaces attracts platelets to the substance, thus triggering further **platelet aggregation** into thrombi. Avitene should be applied with dry instruments only, as it will adhere to wet surfaces. Wetting also decreases its hemostatic efficiency. In addition contact with nonbleeding surfaces must be avoided as adhesions may result. Excess Avitene should be removed by irrigation within a few minutes. Avitene is available in powder form (in amounts of 0.5 g, 1 g, and 5 g), in sheets of various sizes, and packaged in delivery devices for endoscopic and specialty applications.

Instat MCH is derived from bovine deep flexor tendon, a source of pure collagen. The microfibrillar form allows the surgeon to grasp only the amount needed with a forceps. Onset of action is 2 to 4 minutes. Instat MCH is absorbable, but removal is recommended. It is available in 0.5- and 1-g containers.

Oxidized Cellulose

The hemostatic action of oxidized cellulose is not yet clearly understood. When applied to bleeding surfaces, oxidized cellulose swells, becoming a gelatinous mass that serves as a nucleus for clotting. Oxidized cellulose is absorbable, but removal is recommended after hemostasis is achieved. Oxidized cellulose comes in gauze or cotton form and is best applied when dry. The cotton form should be separated into strands or small pieces prior to use.

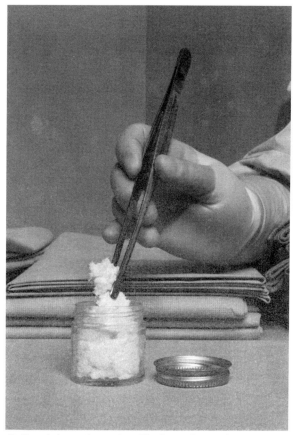

Figure **9–3.**   Avitene is a microfibrillar collagen hemostatic agent.

The gauze form may be cut to desired shape and size. Oxidized cellulose is commonly used in neurosurgery and otorhinolaryngology. Examples of oxidized cellulose include Oxycel (gauze and cotton), Surgicel gauze, and Surgicel NuKnit (a knitted fabric), all available in multiple sizes (Table 9–4).

Absorbable Collagen Sponge

Absorbable collagen sponges are made from purified bovine collagen. The sponge is cut to desired shape and applied with pressure to a bleeding site. When applied to bleeding surfaces, the sponge promotes platelet aggregation. Collagen may reduce the bonding strength of methyl methacrylate (bone cement), so it should not be applied to bone prior to placement of a prosthesis

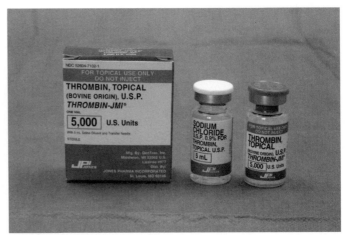

Figure **9–4.**   Thrombin must be reconstituted with sterile water or saline.

Table **9–4** Surgicel and Surgicel NuKnit Sizes	
Surgicel	**Surgicel NuKnit**
$^1/_2 \times 2$ inches	1×1 inches
2×3 inches	1×3.5 inches
2×14 inches	3×4 inches
4×8 inches	6×9 inches

requiring cement fixation. Examples of absorbable collagen sponges are Collastat, Helistat, Hemopad, and Instat. One brand of collagen sponge, Superstat, contains calcium chloride. When applied, the sponge activates the body's coagulation mechanism to achieve hemostasis in 2 to 3 minutes. Superstat should be applied dry and covered with a laparotomy or gauze sponge. It is contraindicated in neurosurgical applications. Superstat is available in two sizes, with calcium chloride concentrations of 1.5% and 3%.

Thrombin

Thrombin is a topical hemostatic agent of bovine origin. It may come prepared in a spray bottle kit or in a powder form that must be reconstituted with sterile water or saline (Fig. 9–4). Thrombin should be used immediately after preparation, or it should be refrigerated and used immediately after reconstituting. Thrombin works by catalyzing the conversion of fibrinogen to fibrin, thus increasing the speed of the natural clotting mechanism. Thrombin may be applied topically in solution or as a powder.

 CAUTION

Thrombin must *never* be introduced into large blood vessels because significant intravascular clotting and death may result. In addition, to avoid inadvertent injection, thrombin should never be kept on the sterile back table in a syringe.

Thrombin is measured in units rather than milligrams and comes in strengths from 1,000 to 20,000 units for different applications. The speed of thrombin's clotting action depends on the concentration used—typically 100 units/mL (1,000 units of thrombin with 10 mL of diluent). Concentrations as high as 2,000 units per milliliter may be used if needed. Areas of profuse bleeding, as in liver trauma, may require the highest concentration of thrombin.

Bone Wax

Bone wax is a topical hemostatic agent made from beeswax. It comes packaged for sterile delivery in a foil-type wrapper inside a peelable package (Fig. 9–5). Bone wax is used primarily in orthopedics and neurosurgery to control bleeding on bone surfaces. It acts as a mechanical barrier rather than as a matrix for clotting.

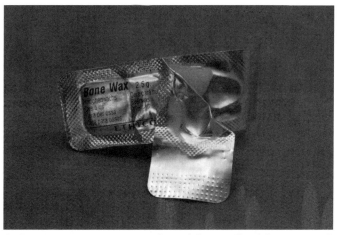

Figure **9–5.**   Bone wax comes packaged for sterile delivery in a foil-type wrapper inside a peelable package.

Bone wax is a pliable, opaque, waxy substance that is sparingly applied directly onto bone. It may harden when kept outside of the foil package for extended periods of time.

Chemical Hemostatics

Some hemostatic agents, such as tannic acid and silver nitrate, chemically cauterize bleeding surfaces. Tannic acid is a powder made from an astringent plant. Applied topically to mucous membranes, it helps stop capillary bleeding. Tannic acid may be used after tonsillectomy in combination with other agents. One such agent is 1% Neosynephrine (a vasoconstrictor). Another example is mixing the tannic acid with a combination of agents (which include glycerine, propylene glycol, zephiran chloride, ephedrine sulfate, and phenylephrine solution) to form Simiele's solution. A tonsil sponge is saturated with the tannic acid and Neosynephrine mixture or the Simiele's solution and applied to the tonsillar fossa to control minor bleeding.

Silver nitrate is another cauterizing agent, especially when mixed with potassium nitrate. This combination is molded onto applicator sticks (which come in 6- and 12-inch lengths) and is used to cauterize wounds. It can also remove granulation tissue or warts. Silver nitrate sticks also come in 18-inch lengths for use with a sigmoidoscope. The applicator tips are moistened with water and applied to the desired area for treatment. Silver nitrate has a caustic effect on mucous membranes and should not be used around eyes. It may also discolor the treatment site with repeated application.

Another chemical hemostatic agent is Monsel's solution, a deep brown solution of ferrous sulfate, sulfuric acid, and nitric acid diluted with water. Monsel's solution may be applied to the bleeding surface remaining after a cervical cone biopsy.

⚠ CAUTION

Monsel's solution may be easily confused with another brown-colored solution on the back table for cervical cone biopsy, Lugol's solution (see Chapter 6). Lugol's solution is a mild iodine solution used to stain the cervix to reveal the area of dysplasia for biopsy. If Monsel's solution is applied to the cervix instead of Lugol's solution, the biopsy area may be damaged by the cauterization effects of the acids. The scrub and circulator must verify both solutions during delivery to the back table and the containers must be labeled immediately.

*Table **9–5*** Systemic Coagulants	
Calcium Salts	**Blood Coagulation Factors**
Calcium chloride	*Antihemophilic factor (VIII)*
Vitamin K	Hemofil-M
	Koate-HT
Konakion	Monociate
Mephyton	
AquaMephyton	*Factor IX complex*
	KonyneHT
	Profiline Heat-treated
	Proplex

SYSTEMIC COAGULANTS

Systemic coagulants are agents that replace deficiencies in the natural clotting mechanism. If needed, systemic coagulants are usually administered preoperatively. Occasionally, the anesthesia provider may administer a systemic coagulant intraoperatively. Systemic coagulants may be used to replace calcium, vitamin K, or some of the coagulation factors in the blood. Such deficiencies in coagulation substances may be due to heredity, as in hemophilia, or they may be acquired, as a vitamin K deficiency. Systemic coagulants may be administered intravenously, intramuscularly, orally, or subcutaneously, depending on the medication used. See Table 9–5 for a summary of systemic coagulants.

Calcium Salts

Calcium, which is the body's most common mineral, is critical for numerous body functions, including blood coagulation. If calcium levels fall during surgery, natural coagulation becomes less efficient, so calcium salts may be administered intravenously to assist the mechanism. During transfusions, for example, anesthesia providers must monitor blood calcium levels very closely, because the processing of donated blood tends to strip it of calcium. Typically, an injection of a 10% solution of calcium chloride ($CaCl_2$) is used to restore calcium levels intraoperatively. Calcium may also be given preoperatively. In the medical setting, calcium may be given by mouth (in tablet form) or injected intramuscularly.

CAUTION

Calcium salts are not given to patients with a history of malignant hyperthermia (MH). Why? Because one aspect of MH is increased calcium release from muscle cells. (See Chapter 16.)

Vitamin K

Vitamin K is a fat-soluble vitamin; it promotes blood clotting by increasing synthesis of prothrombin in the liver. In the surgical patient, a deficiency in vitamin K can lead to excessive bleeding. Decreased vitamin K levels are seen in patients on oral anticoagulants, such as coumarin derivatives. Some antibacterial therapies also cause vitamin K deficiency. If needed, vitamin K may be administered by subcutaneous injection 6 to 24 hours preoperatively, because it takes several hours to produce an acceptable effect. When emergency surgery is necessary and cannot be delayed for vitamin K, fresh frozen plasma may be administered for immediate hemostasis. Vitamin K is also used in the medical setting to counteract anticoagulant-induced prothrombin deficiency. It does not directly counteract oral anticoagulants, but stimulates prothrombin formation by the liver. Vitamin K will not counteract the action of heparin. Administration of vitamin K intravenously has resulted in severe anaphylactic reactions; therefore, it is given intravenously only when other routes are not feasible and when the risks have been recognized and considered. Vitamin K is available as phytonadione (Konakion, Mephyton, or AquaMephyton).

Blood Coagulation Factors

Deficiency of any clotting factor interferes with effective coagulation. Two blood factors administered intravenously in the medical setting are antihemophilic factor (AHF), known as factor VIII, and factor IX complex. Factor VIII, a plasma protein essential for conversion of prothrombin to thrombin, is prepared from human blood plasma. This factor is absent in patients with hemophilia A and must be administered intravenously as needed prior to an operative procedure. Antihemophilic factor is available as Hemofil-M, Koate-HS, and Monociate. Factor IX complex is a concentrate of dried plasma fractions—mainly coagulation factors II, VII, IX, and X. Factor IX complex may be administered preoperatively as needed in patients with hemophilia B. It is also used in the medical setting to reverse coumarin-induced hemorrhage.

Factor IX complex is available as Konyne-HT, Profiline Heat-treated, and Proplex.

ANTICOAGULANTS

Anticoagulants are drugs that prevent or interfere with blood coagulation. Anticoagulants are administered in the medical setting to prevent venous thrombosis, pulmonary embolism, acute coronary occlusions after myocardial infarction (MI), and strokes caused by an embolus or cerebral blood clot. Anticoagulants do not dissolve existing clots; rather, they prevent new clots from forming. A surgical patient with a history of arterial stasis, or who must be immobilized for a prolonged period of time after surgery, may be placed on prophylactic anticoagulant therapy. Anticoagulants are used in surgery to prevent clot formation as a response to trauma or manipulation of blood vessels. Patients receiving anticoagulants are carefully monitored for signs of hemorrhage, a common side effect. Minor hemorrhage may be evident as bruising, nosebleed (epistaxis), blood in urine (hematuria), or bloody stools (melena).

PARENTERAL ANTICOAGULANTS

Parenteral anticoagulants (Table 9–6) are drugs administered intravenously, subcutaneously, or topically that interfere with blood clotting. Heparin sodium is the most commonly used parenteral anticoagulant. It is derived from porcine intestinal mucosa and is available in solution for injection. Heparin is measured in units rather than milligrams and is available in doses of 1,000 to 20,000 units/mL. Heparin works at several points in the clotting cascade by inhibiting factor X, interfering with the conversion of prothrombin to thrombin, and by inactivating thrombin, thus preventing conversion of fibrinogen to fibrin. Heparin also interferes with platelet aggregation. Onset of action is rapid, usually within 5 minutes, with duration of 2 to 4 hours. Adverse reactions include increased risk of hemorrhage and thrombocytopenia (decrease in platelets), so heparin is contraindicated in patients

Table **9–6**   Parenteral Anticoagulants and Antidote

Anticoagulant	Antidote
heparin sodium	protamine sulfate
enoxaprin sodium	protamine sulfate

Insight 9–1   **Blood Coagulation Studies**

Two laboratory tests are routinely used to assess blood coagulation. Prothrombin time (PT, pro-time) is an evaluation of the extrinsic and common coagulation system. PT is used to monitor anticoagulant therapy by vitamin K antagonists such as warfarin. PT screens for adequate amounts of factors I, II, VII, and X. Partial thromboplastin time (PTT) and activated partial thromboplastin time (APTT) evaluate the intrinsic and common coagulation pathways. PTT is used to monitor heparin therapy. PTT screens for deficiencies of all coagulation factors except VII and XIII. Previously, results of PT varied by the method used and so were reported with the appropriate reference range. The reporting of PT results has been standardized with the use of the International Normalized Ratio (INR). The INR is the PT ratio obtained using the World Health Organization's reference preparation as the source of thromboplastin.

with existing severe thrombocytopenia. Coagulation studies (Insight 9–1) are used to monitor heparin's therapeutic action.

If a high risk of pulmonary embolism exists, heparin may be administered preoperatively by subcutaneous injection at least 1 hour prior to a surgical procedure. Heparin is the primary anticoagulant used intraoperatively. It is administered intravenously 3 minutes prior to placement of an arterial occluding clamp. Three minutes is usually sufficient to allow systemic distribution of heparin, preventing the formation of blood clots caused by arterial stasis. Some older types of vascular graft materials must be preclotted prior to insertion to minimize blood loss. Preclotting a graft requires saturation with blood, which must be withdrawn prior to systemic heparinization to be effective.

Heparin is frequently used from the sterile back table during peripheral vascular procedures. A dilute solution, such as 5000 units of heparin in 1000 mL of normal saline, is used as a topical arterial irrigant.

⚠ CAUTION

Careful attention must be paid to identifying the correct strength of heparin administered, because 1 mL of heparin can contain 1000 units, 5000 units, 10,000 units, or 20,000 units (Table 9–7). Remember that the dose of drug administered is the strength *times* the volume. It is possible to administer the same volume of heparin, yet give a dose 20 times more than ordered. The circulator and scrub must always read aloud and verify the number of *units* of heparin placed in solution for irrigation, as well as the volume. The container must be carefully labeled and the scrub must repeat the solution strength to the surgeon when passing it.

Table **9–7** Heparin Strengths	
Strength	*Volume*
Vials	
1000 units/mL	10 mL, 30 mL
5000 units/mL	1 mL, 10 mL
10,000 units/mL	1 mL, 4 mL
Heparin in Tubex Cartridges	
1000 units/mL	1 mL
2500 units/mL	1 mL
5000 units/mL	1 mL
7500 units/mL	1 mL
10,000 units/mL	0.5 mL, 1 mL
20,000 units/mL	1 mL
Heparin Lock Flush (Vials)	
10 units/mL	10 mL, 30 mL
100 units/mL	10 mL, 30 mL
Heparin Lock Flush (Tubex Cartridge)	
10 units/mL	1 mL, 2.5 mL
100 units/mL	1 mL, 2.5 mL

Heparin may be used intraoperatively in many types of vascular procedures. During a femoral embolectomy, for example, heparin is administered through an arterial irrigating catheter to clear the artery of remaining clot or embolic debris. In cardiovascular procedures requiring extracorporeal circulation, heparin is administered to prevent coagulation of blood in the pump tubing. Heparin, in various strengths, is also used during placement of a venous access port or catheter. Again, proper identification—and careful labeling—of different strengths of heparin on the back table is mandatory (Fig. 9–6). For instance, a port or catheter may be flushed prior to insertion with a mild heparin solution, such as 10 units/mL; then when it is in position, it may be flushed with a solution of 100 units/mL. The scrubbed surgical technologist is responsible for passing the correct heparin solution at the correct time.

The antidote for heparin is protamine sulfate, a parenteral anticoagulant that binds with and inactivates heparin. Protamine may be used to treat a heparin overdose, or to reverse heparin-induced

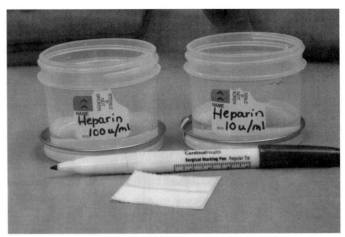

Figure **9–6.** Heparin solutions on the sterile back table must be labeled.

anticoagulation. Protamine is administered by slow intravenous injection. In surgery, protamine may be administered by the anesthesia provider prior to wound closure if anticoagulation is still evident.

Enoxaparin sodium (Lovenox) is a parenteral anticoagulant used to prevent postoperative deep vein thrombosis following hip or knee replacement. A sterile, low-molecular-weight heparin derived from porcine intestinal mucosa, Lovenox is administered by subcutaneous injection. A preparation of the drug can be sent home with the patient, avoiding prolonged hospitalization for anticoagulant therapy. Enoxaprin is contraindicated in patients with active major bleeding or those with hypersensitivity to heparin or pork products. It should not be given in combination with other anticoagulants, including aspirin. Side effects include local irritation, pain at the injection site, fever, and nausea. Rare adverse effects include hemorrhagic complications and thrombocytopenia. Levels of enoxaprin are monitored with a complete blood count (CBC) and platelet counts. Protamine sulfate may be administered by slow intravenous injection as an antidote to excessive enoxaprin anticoagulation.

ORAL ANTICOAGULANTS

Oral anticoagulants are used for long-term management of thromboembolic disease such as deep vein thrombosis or pulmonary embolism. Oral anticoagulant therapy is also used to prevent blood clots associated with cerebrovascular thromboembolic disease. Warfarin sodium (Coumadin), a coumarin derivative, is a widely prescribed oral anticoagulant. Coumarin derivatives act by inhibiting vitamin K activity in the liver, thereby preventing formation of coagulation factors II, VII, IX, and X. Warfarin, which is highly bound to plasma proteins (see Chapter 1), is metabolized in the liver and excreted in the urine. The onset of action of warfarin is prolonged, usually 12 to 72 hours; and its duration is 5 to 7 days. The effectiveness of warfarin therapy is assessed by measuring prothrombin time (PT), which should be approximately twice normal. As drug interactions are common with warfarin, all other medications must be closely monitored. Some common side effects include hemorrhagic episodes such as epistaxis, hematuria, and bleeding gums. The antidote for excessive warfarin anticoagulation is vitamin K.

Oral anticoagulant therapy poses a particular problem when a patient requires surgical intervention. In select cases, warfarin may be temporarily discontinued approximately one week prior to an elective surgical procedure. However, patients on oral anticoagulants who require emergency surgery exhibit prolonged bleeding times. When indicated, fresh frozen plasma may be administered for hemostasis in emergency situations. Meticulous hemostasis is also necessary to minimize blood loss in patients on oral anticoagulant therapy.

Aspirin (acetylsalicylic acid, or ASA) is also considered an oral anticoagulant; it prevents clot formation by inhibiting platelet aggregation. Aspirin may be given after myocardial infarction or recurrent transient ischemic attacks (TIAs) to reduce risk of further incidence. The administration of just 300 mg of aspirin can double normal bleeding time for up to seven days. Thus, if possible, patients on aspirin therapy should discontinue use at least one week prior to elective surgery.

THROMBOLYTICS

Thrombolytics (Table 9–8) are agents given intravenously in the medical setting to help dissolve blood clots. These drugs activate

Table **9–8** Thrombolytics	
Generic Name	*Trade Name*
streptokinase	Streptase
urokinase	Abbokinase
antistreplase	Eminase
alteplase	Activase

plasminogen to form plasmin, which digests fibrin. And when fibrin breaks down, the clot dissolves. Thrombolytics are used to treat acute myocardial infarction when coronary artery thrombosis is present. Anticoagulant therapy may be used in conjunction with thrombolytic agents, because clot formation is an ongoing process. The major side effect of thrombolytics is hemorrhage, so patients are closely monitored. Mild side effects include skin rash, itching, nausea, and headache. Streptokinase (Streptase), an enzyme produced by a strain of streptococci, and urokinase (Abbokinase), derived from human tissue, are examples of thrombolytic agents. Antistreplase (Eminase) is a combination of streptokinase and human plasminogen.

Alteplase (Activase) is a thrombolytic agent produced by recombinant DNA technology. It is a biosynthetic form of a naturally occurring enzyme, human tissue-type plasminogen activator (t-PA). Alteplase is used concurrently with heparin in treatment of acute myocardial infarction. In specific cases, alteplase may also play a role in the treatment of strokes, pulmonary emboli, and peripheral vascular occlusions. Because it is a human enzyme, fewer allergic and hypersensitivity reactions occur with alteplase than with other thrombolytic agents. Another advantage of alteplase is its ability to act specifically—targeting clots rather than exerting systemic effects.

ADVANCED PRACTICES FOR THE SURGICAL FIRST ASSISTANT
Chapter 9—Medications That Affect Coagulation

KEY TERMS

anticoagulation therapy
international normalized ratio (INR)
prothrombin time (PT)

ANTICOAGULATION THERAPY

A common medication protocol that affects the vascular system is **anticoagulation therapy.** It is crucial that the surgical first assistant be familiar with medications and how this therapy is used in the preoperative, intraoperative, and postoperative settings. In anticoagulation therapy the blood-clotting action is diminished or eliminated. It can be implemented as short-term or long-term therapy. A higher degree of anticoagulation carries a higher risk of

ADVANCED PRACTICES FOR THE SURGICAL FIRST ASSISTANT   *(continued)*

bleeding. These patients must be thoroughly educated on the effects of anticoagulation medications, and they are closely monitored while the therapy is in progress. There are various medications used for anticoagulation depending upon the conditions being treated and the length of time the treatment is required (Table A).

Table **A**   Anticoagulant and Antiplatelet Medications

Drug	Route	Uses	Dosage	Time	Side Effects
Anticoagulants					
heparin sodium	SC, intravenous bolus, intravenous drip	Treat thromboembolism, deep vein thrombosis, pulmonary embolism; prevent blood clotting	80–100 u/kg intravenous bolus, 20,000–40,000 qd IV	1–2 hrs	Bleeding, itching, burning
warfarin sodium (Coumadin)	PO	Long-term prophylaxis for thromboembolism	Initial 200–300 mg/day; maintenance 25–200 mg/day	3–5 days	Rash, fever, nausea, abdominal cramps, anorexia, diarrhea
Antiplatelets					
aspirin	PO	Prophylaxis for myocardial infarction, stroke, transient ischemic attack	81–325 mg/day	10–12 hrs	Bleeding, bruising, gastrointestinal symptoms
clopidogrel (Plavix)	PO	Prophylaxis for myocardial infarction, stroke, transient ischemic attack, thromboembolism	75 mg/day	8 hrs	Heartburn, dizziness, aching muscles, gastrointestinal discomfort, headache
dipyridamole (Persantine)	PO	Prophylaxis for thromboembolism; reduce damage from myocardial infarction; prevent recurrence; prevent complications during heart bypass surgery	75–100 mg qid	10 hrs	Abdominal distress, headache, dizziness, itching

PO, Per os; *SC,* subcutaneous.

(continued on following page)

ADVANCED PRACTICES FOR THE SURGICAL FIRST ASSISTANT   *(continued)*

SHORT-TERM THERAPY

Short-term anticoagulation therapy is used intraoperatively on vascular procedures and for the postoperative prevention of deep vein thrombosis (DVT) or pulmonary embolus (PE) in the surgical patient. The most common medication used for short-term therapy is heparin sodium. It is the medicine of choice for intraoperative anticoagulation because of its relatively short half-life (one hour). For example, in cardiac surgery using cardiopulmonary bypass, the usual dosage with heparin sodium administered intravenously is not less than 150 and up to 400 u/kg (units per kilogram of patient weight). This will obtain total anticoagulation of the patient's blood. The surgeon should be notified after one hour has lapsed since the last dosage. Additional doses may be required to maintain anticoagulation for the remainder of the procedure. Protamine sulfate is administered to reverse the affects of heparin sodium. Protamine sulfate should be administered very slowly to prevent hypotension. As stated, heparin sodium is used as the first line of treatment for DVT and pulmonary embolus. In addition, it is used for acute intravascular thrombosis. Therapy is started with an intravenous bolus of 80 u/kg, then followed by a continuous heparin drip throughout the acute phase. For complete anticoagulation, an intravenous drip of heparin sodium is administered at a rate of 20,000 to 40,000 units per day.

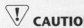 **CAUTION**

Heparin sodium comes in many strengths (as seen in Table 9–7). Always check the strength before mixing or allowing administration of this medication.

LONG-TERM THERAPY

Long-term anticoagulation therapy is usually necessary for patients with vascular disease or vascular implants such as stents or heart valves. It carries the high risk of bleeding, which can be a major or life-threatening complication. The risk of thrombus or embolus formation must outweigh the risk of bleeding. Warfarin sodium (Coumadin) is the most common medication for long-term anticoagulation to treat any thromboembolic condition such as deep vein thrombosis and pulmonary embolus. It is also used to prevent thrombus formation for patients with atrial fibrillation. Warfarin is an oral anticoagulant that suppresses the amount of vitamin K produced in the liver. When the amount of vitamin K is reduced, clotting factors II, VII, IX, and X are suppressed.

Warfarin sodium prolongs the clotting time, which is assessed by the **prothrombin time (PT)** laboratory test and must be closely monitored. Laboratory values of PT may be different between specific laboratories depending on the type of reagent used. To control this variability, the **international normalized ratio (INR)** laboratory test was introduced. This has been widely accepted as the test of choice to monitor and adjust the effects of warfarin sodium to maintain the appropriate level of anticoagulant in the patient. The effects of war-

ADVANCED PRACTICES FOR THE SURGICAL FIRST ASSISTANT *(continued)*

farin sodium can differ among the patient population making dosage difficult to control, especially at the beginning of the therapy. Initial and maintenance dosages of warfarin sodium are individualized according to the INR results. The INR is mathematically calculated from a PT (clotting time). Therapeutic ranges of anticoagulants are controversial within the medical community. It is commonly accepted that an INR range of 2.0 to 3.0 is sufficient to maintain a level of anticoagulation that is beneficial for the treatment of most thromboembolus conditions.

Other oral medications that affect the clotting factor of blood are antiplatelet medicines. The most common is aspirin, which is often discounted by healthcare workers as a drug therapy. Aspirin is used mainly for prophylactic coverage to prevent the formation of a thrombus in arteries. Patients at risk for myocardial infarction (MI), stroke, or transient ischemic attack (TIA) will benefit from aspirin therapy. Recommended dosage is 81, 162, or 325 mg/day orally. Due to aspirin's long-acting effects, patients requiring surgery of any kind should discontinue the use of aspirin at least seven days prior to their procedures. Adverse effects include heartburn, gastrointestinal symptoms, and nausea.

Other antiplatelet medications include clopidogrel (Plavix) and dipyridamole (Persantine). These medicines may be prescribed individually or be used in combination with an anticoagulation medication. Indications for use as a stand-alone therapy are usually in patients with high risk for, or history of a thromboembolic event. These include prevention of MI, stroke, and TIA. These medications have relatively long half-lives and should be discontinued several days in advance of any surgical procedures.

Clopidogrel (Plavix) is prescribed to prevent formation of thrombus in arteries. Like aspirin, clopidogrel is used as a prophylactic therapy for patients with history or high risk for arterial thromboembolic event, MI, stroke, or TIA. Recommended dosage is 75 mg/day orally. Common side effects may include gastrointestinal discomfort, headache, dizziness, aching muscles, and heartburn. Excessive bruising may also occur while taking this medication.

Dipyridamole (Persantine) is used to prevent thrombus in patients who have had heart valve surgery. As stated, it may also be used in combination with other medications (such as aspirin) to reduce the damage from MI, to prevent a recurrence, and to prevent complications during heart bypass surgery. Usual dosage is 75 to 100 mg orally four times a day. Common side effects may include abdominal distress, dizziness, headache, and itching.

☞ **Note:** Antiplatelet medicines have no benefit for use in venous thrombus conditions.

KEY CONCEPTS

- Blood naturally contains both coagulants and anticoagulants, but anticoagulants are normally dominant because they keep blood in its flowing, liquid form.
- Blood coagulation is a process that minimizes blood loss when small blood vessels are disrupted. The formation of a blood clot is the result of a three-stage cascade of events.
- Clot formation may be initiated via two different pathways—extrinsic or intrinsic.
- Thrombosis is the formation of a blood clot within an unbroken blood vessel. If natural coagulation or anticoagulation is inadequate, medical or surgical intervention may be necessary.
- Drugs that affect blood coagulation fall into two main categories: coagulants and anticoagulants.
- Coagulants assist the body's natural clotting mechanism. Coagulants applied topically during surgery to control minor bleeding and capillary oozing are called hemostatics.
- Anticoagulants work to prevent undesired clotting, slow the normal clotting mechanism, or help break up existing clots.
- Anticoagulants fall into three basic categories: parenteral anticoagulants, oral anticoagulants, and thrombolytics.
- Heparin is the most common parenteral anticoagulant used in surgery, usually during peripheral and cardiovascular procedures.
- Thrombolytics are administered intravenously to break up existing blood clots.

10

OPHTHALMIC AGENTS

(continued on following page)

Medications Covered in Chapter 10   *(continued)*

Generic Name	Brand Name	Category
tropicamide	Mydriacyl Ophthalmic Topicacyl, Opticyl	Cycloplegic
gentamicin	Garamycin, Genoptic	Antibiotic
tobramycin	Tobrex	Antibiotic
neomycin	Neosporin	Antibiotic
bacitracin	A-K Tracin	Antibiotic
erythromycin	Illotycin	Antibiotic
sulfacetamide	Sulamyd	Antibiotic
cocaine solution (4%)	Cocaine solution	Topical anesthetic
tetracaine	Pontocaine	Topical anesthetic
proparacaine	Alcaine, Ophthaine	Topical anesthetic
lidocaine	Xylocaine	Injectable anesthetic
bupivicaine	Marcaine, Sensorcaine	Injectable anesthetic
acetazolamide	Diamox	Carbonic anhydrase inhibitor, diuretic
dichlophenamide	Daranide	Carbonic anhydrase inhibitor, diuretic
dorzolamide	Trusopt	Carbonic anhydrase inhibitor, diuretic
methazolamide	Glauctabs	Carbonic anhydrase inhibitor, diuretic
mannitol	Osmitrol	Osmotic diuretic
glycerine	Glyrol, Osmoglyn	Osmotic diuretic
isorbide	Ismotic	Osmotic diuretic
timolol	Timoptic	Beta-adrenergic blockers
betaxolol	Betoptic	Beta-adrenergic blockers
carteolol	Occupress	Beta-adrenergic blockers
levobunolol	Betagan	Beta-adrenergic blockers
dexamethasone and tobramycin	TobraDex	Steroid and antibiotic
predonisolone and gentamicin	PRED-G	Steroid and antibiotic
dexamethasone, neomycin and polymixin B	Maxitrol	Steroid and antibiotic
betamethasone	Celestone suspension	Steroid
dexamethasone	Maxidex suspension, Decadron Ointment and solution	Steroid
prednislone	PredMild, PredForte suspensions	Steroid
aspirin	N/A	Steroid
ketorolac	Acular	NSAID
diclofenac	Voltaren	NSAID
flurbiprofen	Ocufen	NSAID
suprofen	Profenal	NSAID
fluorescein sodium	Fluor-I-Strip, Flu-Glo, AK-Fluor, Fluorescite	Dye
rose bengal	Rose Bengal	Dye
lissamine green	Lissamine Green	Dye
indocyanine green	IC-Green	Dye

OBJECTIVES

After completing this chapter, you should be able to:

1. Describe the basic anatomy of the eye.
2. Define terminology related to ophthalmic medications.
3. State the purpose of each category of ophthalmic medications.
4. List examples of ophthalmic medications in each category.
5. Describe how ophthalmic agents are used in surgery.

KEY TERMS

constrict	mydriatic
cycloplegic	nonsteroidal anti-inflammatory drugs (NSAIDs)
dilate	ophthalmic viscosurgical device (OVD)
glaucoma	proteolytic
miotic	

Ophthalmic surgical procedures often require the use of several medications from the sterile back table. Initially, the scrubbed surgical technologist must properly identify and label all medications received into the sterile field. In addition, the surgical technologist must understand the purpose of each drug in order to pass it to the surgeon at the appropriate time. This is especially important during procedures where the operative microscope is used. The surgeon must focus attention and vision through the lens and cannot continually refocus away from the operative field. In this chapter we'll discuss definitions, purposes, routes, and agents in each ophthalmic drug category used in surgery. A review of basic anatomy is included for reference.

ANATOMY REVIEW

The eye (Fig. 10–1) is a complex sense organ that receives visual stimuli and transmits signals via the optic nerve (cranial nerve II) to the brain for interpretation. Accessory structures include eyebrows, eyelids, eyelashes, and the lacrimal system. The lacrimal system produces, distributes, and removes tears, which keep eye surfaces moist and clean. A thin, transparent mucous membrane called the conjunctiva lines the inside of the eyelids and the anterior surface of the eyeball (globe). Only about 17% of the globe is

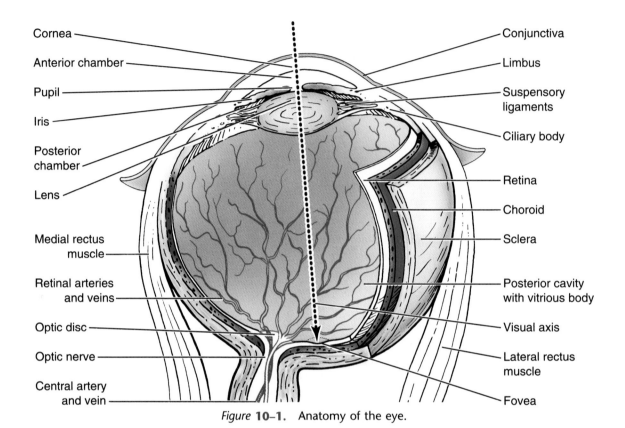

Figure **10-1.** Anatomy of the eye.

visible; the remainder is protected within the bony orbit where it is supported on a cushion of fat and fascia. The globe consists of three layers of tissue; fibrous, vascular, and nervous. The fibrous outer coat of the eye is composed of dense, white connective tissue, called sclera. Sclera gives the globe its shape, provides protection, and can be seen through the conjunctiva as the "white" of the eye. The anterior covering of the eye is made of clear, non-vascular fibrous tissue called the cornea. The cornea does not contain blood vessels to provide its nourishment; rather, it is nourished by being bathed in a solution called aqueous humor and from oxygen in the air. It serves as the "window" of the eye. The area where the cornea and sclera meet is called the limbus. Deep to the limbus is a venous sinus called the canal of Schlemm.

The vascular layer of the eye is called choroid. The anterior, and thickest, portion of choroid is the ciliary body. The ciliary body secretes aqueous humor from structures called ciliary processes.

Ciliary muscle arises in the ciliary body and attaches to the lens, altering its shape to accommodate near or distant vision. The iris is attached to the ciliary process and is positioned between the cornea and lens. The pigmented iris consists of radial and circular muscle fibers whose function is to change the size of its opening, called the pupil. The pupil regulates the amount of light entering the eye by **constricting** or **dilating.** The nervous layer of the eye, called the retina, is present only posteriorly and covers the choroid. Images focused onto the retina trigger sensory receptors characterized as rods and cones. Signals are then transmitted via the optic nerve to the occipital lobe of the brain for recognition.

The lens is positioned just behind the iris and serves to focus images onto the retina. The lens consists of protein fibers arranged in onion-like layers. The lens, which is normally transparent, is covered by a clear fibrous capsule and held in place by suspensory ligaments called zonula.

The interior portion of the globe contains two cavities, anterior and posterior, separated by the lens. The anterior cavity is further separated into anterior and posterior chambers. The anterior chamber is posterior to the cornea and anterior to the iris. The posterior chamber is behind the iris and anterior to the lens. The entire anterior cavity is filled with aqueous humor (fluid) secreted by the ciliary processes. Aqueous humor flows forward in the anterior cavity and drains through the trabecular meshwork into the canal of Schlemm. If a blockage occurs in the trabecular meshwork, intraocular pressure builds, causing **glaucoma.** The posterior cavity, which is between the lens and retina, is filled with a thick substance called vitreous humor. Vitreous humor gives the globe its shape, keeps the retina in position, and contributes to intraocular pressure. Unlike aqueous humor, vitreous humor is not replaced.

The eye contains a barrier similar to the blood–brain barrier. The blood–eye barrier prevents effective absorption of most systemically administered medications. For this reason, the most common administration route for ophthalmic medications is topical application; as drops, suspensions, ointments and on medicated disks or pledgets inserted onto the eye (Insight 10–1). A few agents may be given orally or parenterally. Ophthalmic agents administered topically enter systemic circulation through the conjunctival vessels and the nasolacrimal system. About 80% of eyedrops enter the nasolacrimal system, then drain from nose to mouth and enter the stomach where absorption takes place.

Figure 10–2 illustrates the proper steps for administration of topical ophthalmic solutions. After administration of the

---

Insight 10–1   **Administering Ophthalmic Medications with Pledgets**

Another method for instilling ophthalmic medications is pledgets. The medication-soaked pledgets are placed in the conjunctival cul-de-sac after the eye has been anesthetized with local anesthetic drops. An example of this method is instilling mydriatic or cycloplegic medication preoperatively. Antibiotic and local anesthetic medications can also be added to the pledget mixture (placing all medications into a sterile medicine cup), then inserting the pledget with sterile tissue forceps. An ophthalmic medication that comes prepackaged in this manner is the pilocarpine ocular system (Ocusert). Ocusert is a wafer-thin disc impregnated with pilocarpine, used to produce miosis and decrease intraocular pressure. The disk is placed into the lower conjunctival sac, where it delivers the appropriate amount of medication every hour for 7 days.

☞**Note:** Eye sponges (spears) can be used as pledgets.

---

medications, compression of the lacrimal sac prevents rapid drainage of medication into the lacrimal system where it is carried away from the eye.

☞ **Note:** It is important to follow aseptic technique when applying ophthalmic medications. The tip of the medication applicator should not touch the patient's tissue or the bottle is considered to be contaminated and must be discarded immediately after use. Also, such contact could result in a corneal abrasion. When using ointments for the first time, the first quarter inch should be squeezed from the container and discarded.

CATEGORIES OF OPHTHALMIC AGENTS

ENZYMES

Enzymes are proteins that act as catalysts; that is, they speed up chemical reactions. Two enzymes are used in ophthalmic surgery. Alpha-chymotrypsin (Alpha-Chymar, Zolyse) may be injected during intracapsular cataract extraction to break down the suspensory ligaments (zonula) holding the lens in place. Alpha-chymotrypsin is a **proteolytic** enzyme; specifically, it dissolves the protein structure of fibrous connective tissue in zonula. Current techniques of cataract extraction—phacoemulsification and extracapsular cataract extraction—leave zonula intact, so the use of proteolytic enzymes has become less frequent. Hyaluronidase is a protein enzyme extracted from highly purified bovine or sheep testicular enzyme (hyaluronidase). Mixed with injectable local

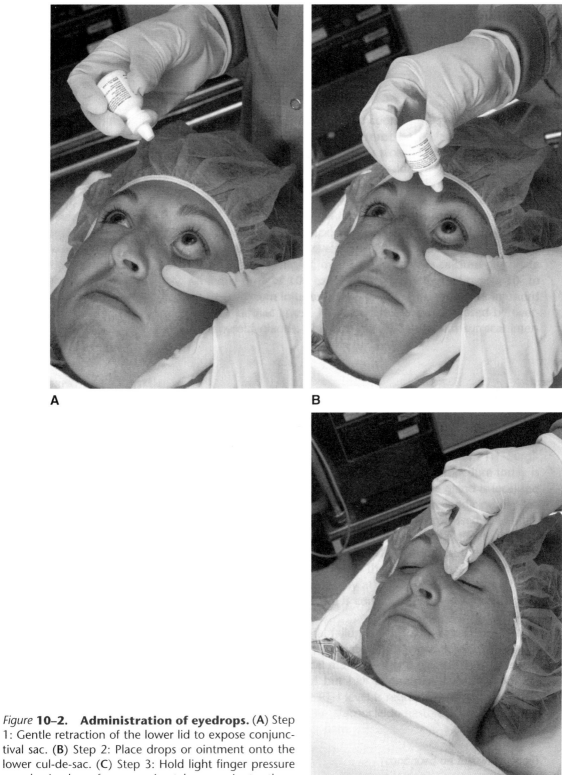

Figure **10–2. Administration of eyedrops. (A)** Step 1: Gentle retraction of the lower lid to expose conjunctival sac. **(B)** Step 2: Place drops or ointment onto the lower cul-de-sac. **(C)** Step 3: Hold light finger pressure over lacrimal sac for approximately one minute; then, with eye closed, remove excess medication from the inner corner of the eyelid with a cotton ball.

anesthetic agents, hyaluronidase increases the rate and extent of anesthetic diffusion through tissue for nerve block.

☞ **Note:** As of January 2001, hyaluronidase marketed as Wydase was no longer being produced by Wyeth-Ayerst Company, because of quality assurance issues. Wydase was the most common form of hyaluronidase used in ophthalmic procedures. At this time, a new hyaluronidase product derived from sheep testicular tissue has been developed by ISTA Pharmaceuticals and marketed as Vitrase. Vitrase is packaged sterile in vials and must be reconstituted with sodium chloride injection, then used immediately after preparation. Edema is the most frequently reported side effect of hyaluronidase.

IRRIGATING SOLUTIONS

Irrigating solutions are used during ophthalmic procedures to cleanse the operative site and keep the cornea moist. The most common ophthalmic irrigating solution is balanced salt solution (BSS). BSS is a sterile, physiologically balanced irrigant. It is packaged in sterile containers of 15 and 30 mL for topical use from the sterile field; it also comes in bottles of 250 and 500 mL for infusion using administration tubing sets. Dextrose 50% can be added to balanced salt solution (Endosol, BSS Plus, Endosol Extra) for the diabetic patient. During most ophthalmic procedures (and any other procedures that involve blood in the eye area) the scrubbed surgical technologist will periodically irrigate the cornea with BSS. Other ophthalmic irrigating solutions (A-K Rinse, Blinx, Irigate, Dacriose) are available for over-the-counter purchase.

VISCOELASTIC AGENTS

Viscoelastic agents are thick, jelly-like substances injected into the eye during certain ophthalmic procedures. These agents are often injected into the anterior chamber during cataract extraction (phacoemulsification) to keep the chamber expanded, prevent injury to surrounding tissue and protection of the cornea. Viscoelastic agents may also be used as a vitreous substitute or tamponade (compression). Examples of viscoelastic agents include sodium hyaluronate (Healon, Healon 5, Amvisc-Plus, Vitrax, Provisc), 2% hydroxypropyl methylcellulose (Ocucoat), and sodium chondroitin sulfate 4%–sodium hyaluronate 3% (Viscoat). Viscoelastic agents are supplied, premeasured, in sterile syringes with blunt-tipped cannulas. Most should be kept refrigerated until use. Side effects include a transient rise in intraocular pressure, iritis, corneal edema, and corneal decompensation. Note that the term **ophthalmic viscosurgical device (OVD)** is being used for viscoelastic agents because they are no longer considered as only medications used to maintain space and coat ocular tissues. Rather, they are an integral part of cataract surgery and are being used in combinations as newer techniques for ophthalmic surgery are being developed. For example, the DuoVisc viscoelastic system combines two viscoelastic materials, Viscoat and Provisc, into a single system to be used during a cataract procedure.

MIOTICS

Miotics are medications that constrict the pupil by stimulating the sphincter muscle of the iris. Because constriction of the pupil (miosis) reduces intraocular pressure, miotics are frequently used in short-term treatment of glaucoma. Miotics may be used intra-operatively when pupillary constriction is indicated, as in laser iridectomy. Occasionally miotics are used to maintain the position of an implanted lens after cataract extraction. Miotics may be administered by injection or topical application. Side effects include eye, eyebrow, or eyelid pain; blurred vision; abdominal cramps; and diarrhea.

Acetylcholine chloride is a miotic agent available in a solution of mannitol marketed as Miochol-E. It may be used for initial treatment of chronic open-angle glaucoma and acute glaucoma; this is because miosis facilitates drainage of aqueous humor. Miochol-E may be injected during surgery to decrease intraocular pressure and to cause miosis if needed. Miosis lasts about 10 minutes. Miochol-E should be reconstituted immediately before use. Carbachol (IsoptoCarbachol) is used topically to reduce intraocular pressure in glaucoma, and by injection (Miostat) into the anterior chamber as needed intraoperatively. Pilocarpine hydrochloride (Pilocar, IsoptoCarpine), in 1% and 4% ophthalmic solution, is another topical miotic. Pilocarpine (as acetylcholine) acts directly on the smooth muscle of the iris to stimulate miosis. Pilocarpine increases flow of aqueous humor through the trabecular meshwork, thus it is most useful in treating open-angle glaucoma.

MYDRIATICS AND CYCLOPLEGICS

Both **mydriatics** and **cycloplegics** are paralytic agents used to dilate the pupil prior to ophthalmoscopy. Both kinds of agents cause *mydriasis*—dilation of the pupil—by paralyzing the sphincter muscle of the iris. Cycloplegics also paralyze the accommodation mechanism. (This means that patients may be unable to see near objects clearly.) After topical instillation of mydriatics or cycloplegics, the lacrimal sac should be compressed for 2 to 3 minutes to avoid rapid systemic absorption of the medication (see Fig. 10–2). Common mydriatic agents are atropine and phenylephrine. Atropine sulfate (Atropisol, IsoptoAtropine), a belladonna alkaloid, is available for ophthalmic use in solutions of 0.25% and 2%, and in ointment of 0.5% and 1% for topical application. Atropine may be used to dilate the pupil for a few weeks after surgery if needed. Atropine's onset is approximately 30 minutes, while peak effect is seen in 30 to 40 minutes; duration is 7 to 10 days. Atropine is also a potent cycloplegic. Homatropine hydrocromide (IsoptoHomatropine) is similar to atropine, but has a faster onset of approximately 10 to 30 minutes, and a shorter duration of up to 3 days. Phenylephrine (Neo-Synephrine, AK-Dilate) is available in solutions of 2.5% and 10% for topical ophthalmic use. Its onset is approximately 30 minutes, with effects lasting 2 to 3 hours. Cycloplegic agents include cyclopentolate HCL (Cyclogyl, AK-Pentolate, Pentolair) available in 0.5% to 2% solutions and tropicamide (Mydriacyl, Ophthalmic, Tropicacyl, Opticyl) available in 0.5% and 1% solutions. Side effects include tachycardia, photophobia, dry mouth, edema, conjunctivitis, and dermatitis.

OINTMENTS AND LUBRICANTS

Several diverse ophthalmic medications are available in ointment form. Antibiotics are frequently used in ophthalmology to treat external ocular infections and as prophylaxis against postoperative infections. Ophthalmic antibiotic preparations include aminoglycosides such as gentamicin, neomycin, and tobramycin. Interestingly, no nephrotoxicity or ototoxicity has been noted with ophthalmic use of aminoglycosides (see Chapter 5). Gentamicin (Garamycin, Genoptic) is available in 0.3% solution or ointment, tobramycin (Tobrex) in 0.3% solution or ointment, and neomycin in a solution of 2.5 mg/mL or ointment 5 mg/g. Neomycin is also available as Neosporin, combined with polymixin and bacitracin. Other common ophthalmic antibiotics include bacitracin ointment (A-K Tracin) in 500 units/g, erythromycin (Ilotycin) 0.5% ointment, and sulfacetamide (Sulamyd) in 10% and 30% solution and 10% ointment.

Lubricants are also available in ointment form. Ophthalmic lubricants are frequently used when a general anesthetic is administered for any surgical procedure. Under general anesthesia, eyelids are relaxed and the corneal reflex is absent. To prevent corneal drying or damage and maintain integrity of the epithelial surface, a lubricant such as Lacri-lube or Duratears is applied to each eye and the eyelids are taped closed. On emergence from anesthesia, patients may exhibit blurred vision; although this blurring is due to the ointment, they should be prevented from rubbing their eyes. Be alert to any patient allergic reactions to preservatives found in these medications.

 CAUTION

It is possible to injure the cornea, even through closed eyelids. Always take precautions to avoid injury of the eye area.

ANESTHETICS

Anesthetics are medications that interfere with normal transmission of pain impulses to the brain. Most ophthalmic surgical procedures require the use of a topical or an injected anesthetic agent. Cocaine solution (1% and 4%) was the initial topical anesthetic agent used in ophthalmology; but it is used rarely now. Two common topical ophthalmic anesthetics are tetracaine hydrochloride (Pontocaine) and proparacaine hydrochloride (Alcaine, Ophthaine). Both medications are available in a 0.5% ophthalmic solution. Their onset is under 1 minute, and duration is 10 to 20 minutes. Many ophthalmic procedures are scheduled with an anesthesia provider on "standby" to administer sedation and monitor the patient. This is called MAC—monitored anesthesia care (see Chapter 14).

Ophthalmic procedures requiring an extensive area of anesthesia are performed under a regional, retrobulbar (see Chapter 14) or peribulbar block. This type of anesthesia, which provides both sensory and motor (movement) block, is done with a local anesthetic, such as lidocaine or bupivicaine. In retrobulbar block, the agents are injected near the optic nerve (Fig. 10–3). In peribulbar block, the injections are made in the soft tissue superior (above) and inferior (below) to the eyeball. Other agents may be added to the anesthetic, such as hyaluronidase (Vitrase). Hyaluronidase, as discussed previously, is an enzyme mixed with anesthetics (50 to 300 units per mL appropriate to purpose) to increase diffusion of the anesthetic through the tissue, and to improve the effectiveness of the block. This is contraindicated if malignancy is present. Another agent added to an anesthetic is epinephrine. Epinephrine

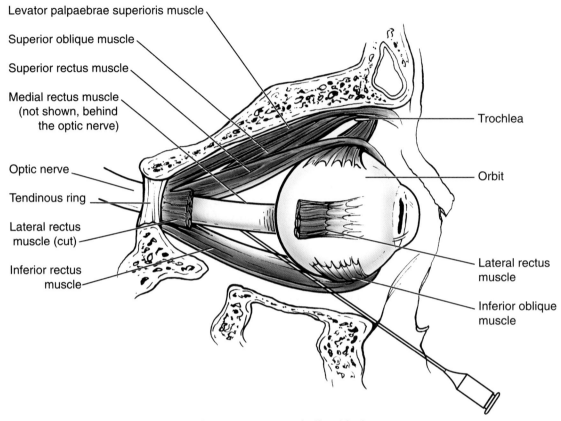

Levator palpaebrae superioris muscle

Superior oblique muscle

Superior rectus muscle

Medial rectus muscle
(not shown, behind
the optic nerve)

Optic nerve

Tendinous ring

Lateral rectus
muscle (cut)

Inferior rectus
muscle

Trochlea

Orbit

Lateral rectus
muscle

Inferior oblique
muscle

Figure **10–3.** Retrobulbar block.

is a powerful vasoconstrictor; it is used to prevent rapid absorption of the anesthetic, thereby prolonging the block.

ANTIGLAUCOMA AGENTS

The word **glaucoma** is a general term that refers to a group of conditions characterized by increased intraocular pressure. This pressure damages the optic nerve and may cause blindness. There are two main causes for this condition: either aqueous humor is overproduced, or the drainage mechanism is blocked. Although glaucoma is easily treated in the medical setting, untreated it can lead to blindness. The most common form of glaucoma is chronic open-angle glaucoma. In open-angle glaucoma, the trabecular meshwork cannot drain aqueous fluid effectively. A far rarer form is narrow-angle glaucoma (also called angle-closure glaucoma) which may be acute or chronic and is found in only about 5% of all glaucoma patients. Angle-closure glaucoma is caused by an abnormally narrow junction between the cornea and iris, blocking the flow of aqueous humor into the trabecular meshwork.

Because pupillary constriction may open the trabecular meshwork and facilitate drainage of excess fluid, short-term treatment often involves miotics. However, long-term management of increased intraocular pressure may be accomplished with several different types of agents including miotics, beta-adrenergic blockers, and diuretics (see Chapter 7), particularly carbonic anhydrase inhibitors. Carbonic anhydrase is an enzyme present in the ciliary body; it catalyzes secretion of aqueous humor. A carbonic anhydrase inhibitor such as acetazolamide (Diamox) interferes with production of carbonic anhydrase; thus it reduces production of aqueous humor and decreases intraocular pressure. Acetazolamide, which reduces aqueous humor production by 50% to 60%, is administered orally to manage chronic open-angle glaucoma, or given intravenously to treat acute angle-closure glaucoma. With oral administration, ocular effects are seen in 1 to 2 hours, with a duration of 3 to 5 hours. Other carbonic anhydrase inhibitors include dichlophenamide (Daranide), dorzolamide (Trusopt), and methazolamide (Glauctabs). Side effects include lethargy, anorexia, drowsiness, nausea, vomiting, and hypokalemia.

Osmotic diuretics may also be used for short-term treatment of glaucoma. By raising the osmotic pressure of blood, osmotic diuretics cause fluid to be drawn out of the eye, lowering intraocular pressure. Ocular effects of osmotic diuretics last about 4 hours. Osmotic diuretics may be used immediately before surgery to reduce intraocular pressure, or they may be given during procedures to treat retinal detachment to aid in scleral closure. Osmotic diuretics are also used in cases of acute angle-closure glaucoma to facilitate the response of the iris muscle to miotics. The most common osmotic diuretic used in ophthalmic surgery is mannitol (Osmitrol). Mannitol in a 5% to 20% solution is given intravenously in a dose of 1 to 2 g/kg of patient weight. For example, 500 mL of a 20% mannitol solution may be administered over a period of 30 to 60 minutes. When mannitol is administered preoperatively, an indwelling urinary catheter is usually inserted into the patient's bladder to accommodate resulting diuresis (increased excretion of urine). Maximum effect is noted approximately an hour after administration. Other osmotic diuretics used in ophthalmology include glycerine 50% solution (Glyrol, Osmoglyn) and isorbide 45% solution (Ismotic), both administered orally. Side effects from osmotics are commonly headache, nausea, vomiting, and diarrhea.

A group of medications known as beta-adrenergic blockers are also used to treat glaucoma. By blocking beta-adrenergic receptor sites, these drugs reduce aqueous fluid production. Systemic side effects of beta-adrenergic blockers include decreased heart rate and blood pressure. Timolol (Timoptic) is used to treat chronic open-angle glaucoma. Although its exact mechanism not yet known, it has been reported to decrease production of aqueous humor and increase outflow. Timolol, in 0.25% or 0.5% ophthalmic solution, is administered in a dosage of one drop in the affected eye twice a day. One dose of timolol may reduce intraocular pressure for up to 24 hours. Unlike miotics, no accommodation problems are noted with use. Other beta-adrenergic blockers include betaxolol (Betoptic) 0.5% solution, carteolol (Occupress) 1% solution, and levobunolol (Betagan) 0.25% and 0.5% solution. Side effects include mild ocular irritation, eye pain, headache, decreased corneal sensitivity, transient dry eye syndrome, and blurring of central vision.

ANTI-INFLAMMATORY AGENTS

Two categories of anti-inflammatory agents are used in ophthalmology: steroids and **nonsteroidal anti-inflammatory drugs (NSAIDs)**. Steroids are hormones (see Chapter 8) with a wide range of effects; they are used in ophthalmology to decrease ocular inflammatory response to trauma, decrease corneal inflammation, protect the eye from scarring, and postoperatively to decrease swelling. They are contraindicated in the presence of infection because steroids are not bactericidal and tend to hide the symptoms of infection. However, steroid preparations are available in combination with antimicrobial agents. Examples are TobraDex, which combines the anti-inflammatory action of dexamethasone 0.1% with the antibiotic tobramycin 0.3%; PRED-G, which is prednisolone in combination with the antibiotic gentamicin; and Maxitrol ointment, which combines the antibiotics neomycin and polymixin B with dexamethasone. Steroids may be administered via four routes: topical, systemic, periocular, or intravitreal. Common steroids used are betamethasone (Celestone suspension), dexamethasone (Maxidex suspension, Decadron ointment and solution), and prednisolone (PredMild, PredForte suspensions).

Ocular NSAIDs are used to prevent or treat cystoid macular edema, iritis, and conjunctivitis. They are also used to reduce postoperative inflammation following cataract surgery. Ophthalmic solutions of ketorolac 0.5% (Acular) and diclofenac 0.1% (Voltaren) are available. Nonsteroidal anti-inflammatory drugs may also be used to inhibit intraoperative miosis, particularly flurbiprofen 0.03% (Ocufen) and suprofen 0.1% (Profenal). Side effects include burning and stinging when administered.

DIAGNOSTIC AGENTS

Several agents are available for diagnostic purposes. Most of these used in surgery are dyes, which color or mark tissue. Ophthalmic dyes are instilled topically to diagnose abnormalities of the cornea and conjunctival epithelium or to locate foreign bodies. Dyes may also be used to observe the flow of aqueous humor or to demonstrate lacrimal system function. Examples of dyes used in ophthalmology are fluorescein sodium, rose bengal, and lissamine green. These dyes are available as individually wrapped sterile paper strips, which are moistened with a sterile solution and applied to the anterior surface of the eye. Fluorescein sodium (Fluor-I-Strip, Ful-Glo, AK-Fluor, Fluorescite) is a nontoxic, water-soluble dye that is applied to the cornea or conjunctiva to identify denuded areas of epithelium or foreign bodies. It diagnoses corneal abrasions by staining damaged or diseased corneal tissue bright green. A foreign body will be surrounded by a green ring. Fluorescein sodium should not be used with soft contact lenses, because they may absorb the dye. Rose bengal and lissamine green in 1% solutions stain devitalized cells better than fluorescein sodium. These dyes are primarily used for demarcation of devitalized conjunctival epithelium seen in "dry eye" syndrome (keratoconjunctivitis sicca).

Indocyanine green (IC-Green) is a diagnostic dye used for ophthalmic angiography. It is given intravenously outside the surgical setting in order to visualize the choroidal vascular network. The dye leaks slowly from these choroidal capillaries, which allows vessels in the deeper tissues to be seen (because they are not masked by the dye). As these deeper layers are visualized, tumors and other problems that may not be detectable with regular angiography at this point can be located and treated. Indocyanine green is a fluorescent, sterile, water-soluble dye that comes in powder form and must be reconstituted with sterile water. Once prepared, it must be used within 10 hours. It contains sodium iodide, so caution must be used for patients with iodide allergies.

ADVANCED PRACTICES FOR THE SURGICAL FIRST ASSISTANT
Chapter 10—Ophthalmic Agents

KEY TERMS

extracapsular   phacoemulsification
intracapsular

CATARACT EXTRACTION

The surgical technologist practicing in ophthalmology must combine the science of patho-physiology and anatomy of the eyes with a current knowledge of the pharmaceutical agents used in the treatment of eye disorders and surgical procedures. One of the most common eye disorders is cataracts. Cataracts are the leading cause of decreased vision in the United States. Of Americans between the age of 65 and 73 years, 50% have some degree of cataract formation. This increases to 70% after the age of 75 years. With surgical removal being the only treatment, cataract surgery is the most common and successful of all surgical proce-dures today. More than 1 million cataracts are removed each year. A cataract is defined as an opacity or clouding of the crystalline lens of the eye. Although most cataracts are age related (senile cataract), they may be associated with other factors. These include trauma, metabolic diseases, congenital factors, prolonged corticosteroid usage, and exposure to radi-ation or ultraviolet (UV) light. Cataracts may develop in one or both eyes. Each cataract tends to mature or develop at a different rate. Therefore the patient's vision may be affected in one eye more than the other. Because of this differential, only one cataract is removed at a time. Cataract extraction is an intraocular procedure. Cataracts can be extracted by one of two methods: **intracapsular** or **extracapsular.** The most commonly performed surgical interven-tion for cataracts in the United States is extracapsular extraction with **phacoemulsification** and intraocular lens implant.

Today's patient undergoing an ophthalmic procedure, such as cataract extraction, is most likely to be done on an ambulatory (same-day surgery) basis. This means the perioperative team must coordinate patient preparations in a very short period of time. The success of sur-gical intervention depends on the skills and knowledge of the team.

CAUTION

Medications that are intended for usage in the eyes are potent, and one medication error can result in permanent blindness. Therefore all medications and irrigating solutions should be confirmed and labeled immediately.

PREOPERATIVE MEDICATIONS

Preoperative medications are extremely important to the outcome of the procedure and to the patient's safety. Conventionally, preoperative preparation for cataract extraction involved

ADVANCED PRACTICES FOR THE SURGICAL FIRST ASSISTANT   *(continued)*

the installation of multiple drops. Today the growing trend is to use the pledgets for administration of all preoperative medications as discussed earlier in the chapter. This is considered an economical, time-saving, effective, and safe method to deliver the drops. These may include, but are not limited to, a mydriatic for maximum pupil dilation, which is essential for lens extraction. A short-acting mydriatic such as phenylephrine hydrochloride (Neo-Synephrine) 2.5% or 10% is preferred. This can be used alone or in combination with a cycloplegic. Tropicamide (Mydriacyl) 1% is the most commonly used agent that causes cycloplegia (paralysis of accommodation, inhibits focusing) and it also has a mydriatic effect. A non-steroidal anti-inflammatory agent such as ketorolac (Acular) 0.5% may be used to decrease the inflammatory process and to help maintain pupil dilation. A topical, broad-spectrum anti-infective agent such as ofloxacin (Floxin) 0.3% ophthalmic solution may be used to sterilize the eye to prevent the intraocular introduction of bacteria.

ASSISTANT ADVICE

When administering topical mydriatic or cycloplegics for pupil dilation preoperatively, a patient with dark irises may need a larger dose because more pigment requires more of the medication to achieve the desired effect.

TOPICAL METHOD OF LOCAL ANESTHESIA

The topical method of local anesthesia for cataract extraction has increased in popularity. A combination of anesthetic eyedrops such as tetracaine hydrochloride (Pontocaine) 0.5% is instilled into the eye and is enhanced with infiltration anesthetic such as methylparaben-free (MPF) lidocaine (Xylocaine) 1% or 2%, which is placed into the anterior chamber through the incision.

INTRAOPERATIVE MEDICATIONS

As discussed in the chapter, intraoperative medications may include balanced salt solution (BSS) used for intraocular irrigation and to moisten the cornea. A viscoelastic agent is injected into the anterior chamber to deepen the chamber and widen the pupil to facilitate the use of the phacoemulsification. Following the placement of the intraocular lens implant, timolol (Timoptic) 0.5% drops may be used to decrease intraocular pressure. Note that ofloxacin

(continued on following page)

ADVANCED PRACTICES FOR THE SURGICAL FIRST ASSISTANT *(continued)*

(Floxin) and ketorolac (Acular) 0.5%, mentioned in Preoperative Medications, may be used again. An alternative to this is a subconjunctival injection of the corticosteroid and antibiotic. Some commonly injected corticosteroids (anti-inflammatory agents) may include betamethasone (Celestone) or dexamethasone (Decadron). Cefazolin (Ancef, Kefzol) or gentamicin (Garamycin) are commonly used antibiotics for these injections. Some surgeons prefer to patch and shield the eye following the procedure.

ASSISTANT ADVICE Irrigation of the eye is commonly performed during ophthalmic procedures to prevent drying of the cornea and to remove blood and debris from the eye. This should be done from the inner canthus to the outer canthus of the eye to prevent the irrigation and debris from pooling.

POSTOPERATIVE MEDICATIONS

The patient is usually released within a few hours postoperatively (unless there are any postoperative complications). Postoperative medications sent home with the patient will usually include the same topical anti-inflammatory and antibiotic agents used during the surgical procedure. The patient may also be sent home with the same topical agent used during the procedure to decrease intraocular pressure and is instructed to avoid activities that could increase this pressure. Normally the patient is seen by the ophthalmologist the next day for postoperative evaluation.

KEY CONCEPTS

- The eye is a complex sense organ comprised of many anatomical structures.
- The blood–eye barrier prevents effective absorption of most systemically administered medications, thus the most common method of administration for ophthalmic medications is topical.
- Enzymes are used to increase anesthetic diffusion through tissue for nerve blocks, and to dissolve zonula.
- Irrigating solutions cleanse the operative site and keep the cornea moist.

- Viscoelastic agents are used to keep the anterior chamber expanded and to prevent injury to surrounding tissue.
- Miotics constrict the pupil and can be used for short term treatment of glaucoma, and to maintain position of the lens after cataract surgery.
- Mydriatics and cycloplegics dilate the pupil by paralyzing the sphincter muscle of the iris.
- Many ophthalmic medications are available in ointment form including antibiotics and lubricants.
- Ophthalmic anesthesia is achieved with topical agents, and when a more extensive area is involved, a retrobulbar or peribulbar block can be administered.
- *Glaucoma* is a general term referring to increased intraocular pressure.
- There are several categories of medications that are used to treat glaucoma: miotics, beta-adrenergic blockers, and osmotic diuretics.
- Steroids and NSAIDs are used as anti-inflammatory agents in ophthalmics.
- Steroid preparations are available in combination with antimicrobials.
- Diagnostic agents used in ophthalmics are dyes.

FLUIDS AND IRRIGATION SOLUTIONS

Medications Covered in Chapter 11

Generic Name	Brand Name	Concentrations	Category
sodium chloride, normal saline		0.9%	Intravenous solution, irrigant
sodium chloride		5%, 3%, 0.33%, 0.45%, 0.225%	Intravenous solution
dextrose in water		2.5%, 5%, 10%, 20%, 25%, 30%, 40%, 50%, 60%, 70%	Intravenous solution
dextrose in normal saline		5%, 10%	Intravenous solution
lactated Ringer's solution, Hartmann's solution			Intravenous solution
plasmalyte			Intravenous solution
isolyte E	Ionosol, Normosol		Intravenous solution

(continued on following page)

Medications Covered in Chapter 11   *(continued)*

Generic Name	Brand Name	Concentrations	Category
RhoD immune globulin	RhoGam		Blood compatibility medication
albumin		5%, 25%	Volume expander, intravenous solution
plasma protein fraction		5%	Volume expander
dextran	Macrodex, Rheomacrodex	40, 70, 75	Volume expander
hetastarch	Hespan		Volume expander
	Hemopure*		Blood substitute
	PolyHeme*		Blood substitute
	Oxyglobin*		Blood substitute
hyaluronan	Viscoseal	0.5%	Synovial fluid replacement
sterile water			Irrigant
sorbitol		3%	Irrigant
glycine		1.5%	Irrigant
	Hyskon		Irrigant
	Physiosol		Irrigant
	Interceed, Seprafilm		Adhesion barrier
	Spraygel*		Adhesion barrier

*Currently undergoing clinical trials for full FDA approval.

OBJECTIVES

After completing this chapter, you should be able to:

1. Briefly describe the physiology of fluid loss in the surgical patient.
2. List fluid electrolytes and their functions crucial to homeostasis.
3. Define terms and abbreviations related to fluid replacement.
4. State objectives of parenteral fluid therapy in surgery.
5. List common intravenous solutions and their purposes in surgery.
6. List supplies needed to start an intravenous line.
7. List basic functions and types of blood.
8. State average adult circulating volume of blood, hemoglobin, and hematocrit values.
9. List the formed elements present in blood.
10. Define terms and abbreviations related to blood.
11. Briefly describe antigen–antibody interactions in blood types.
12. List and describe indications for blood replacement in the surgical patient.
13. List available options for blood replacement.

14. Describe components of whole blood used for replacement.
15. Define autologous and homologous blood donation.
16. Describe the process of intraoperative autotransfusion.
17. List volume expander solutions used in surgery.
18. List blood substitutes used in clinical trials.
19. Describe the procedure for blood replacement in surgery using donor blood from the blood bank.
20. List and describe fluids used as irrigation solutions in surgery.
21. List and describe supplies and equipment used for irrigation.

KEY TERMS

antibody	hemoglobin	hypokalemia
antigen	hemolysis	hyponatremia
arrhythmia	homologous	hypovolemia
autologous	hypercalcemia	intravenous
autotransfusion	hyperkalemia	isotonic
electrolyte	hypernatremia	metabolic acidosis
hematocrit	hypocalcemia	

One of the primary goals of surgical patient care is to maintain the patient in as stable a physiologic state as possible. As fluids are essential to survival, blood and fluid replacement are two of the most common means used in surgery to assist in maintaining homeostasis. Blood loss may be due to trauma or to the surgical procedure itself. The volume of blood lost must be carefully assessed and replaced if significant. The surgical patient's fluid and electrolyte balance must also be assessed and monitored. Most surgical patients have preoperative fluid and food restrictions prior to surgery, so fluid replacement is usually indicated. This is accomplished by administering **intravenous** (IV) fluids and medications. Intravenous means administration through a vein. Such fluids may be ordered for replacement of lost fluids, to maintain fluid and electrolyte balance, or to administer IV medications. *Replacement fluids* are often ordered to replenish losses caused by hemorrhage (in surgery), vomiting, and diarrhea (in the medical setting). *Maintenance fluids* sustain normal fluid and electrolyte balance. In addition, fluids are used to irrigate body tissues during surgical procedures. These irrigation solutions must be physiologically acceptable to tissues while providing visualization, removing blood and debris, and adding medications to the surgical site. The surgical technologist observes blood or fluid replacement and assists with irrigation procedures in the surgical suite daily.

FLUID AND ELECTROLYTE MANAGEMENT

PHYSIOLOGY REVIEW

In a healthy adult approximately 60% of the total body weight is made up of fluids, **electrolytes,** and nonelectrolytes. Fluids are distributed into two distinct compartments: intracellular fluid (ICF) and extracellular fluid (ECF).

The major electrolytes break down into sodium (Na^+), chloride (Cl^-), potassium (K^+), calcium (Ca^{2+}), phosphate (HPO_4^{2-}), and magnesium (Mg^{2+}) ions. Other electrolytes are bicarbonate (HCO_3^-), sulfate (SO_4^{2-}), and carbonic acid (H_2CO_3). The nonelectrolytes present in normal body fluid are glucose, urea, and creatinine. Electrolytes have three main purposes in homeostasis: controlling the volume of body water by osmotic pressure, maintaining the acid–base balance, and serving as essential minerals. See Table 11–1 for a list of major electrolytes and functions. Altering of normal concentrations of these elements can result in serious, and possibly life-threatening, complications.

Chloride is the most abundant anion in extracellular fluid and helps regulate osmotic pressure between intracellular and extracellular spaces. Magnesium plays an important part in the sodium–potassium pump and also activates enzymes required to break down adenosine triphosphate (ATP). Phosphate is stored in teeth and bone and is released when needed. Phosphate is a necessary element in the formation of DNA and RNA, in synthesis of ATP, and in buffering of acid–base reactions.

Two electrolytes with particular importance to surgery are calcium and potassium. Calcium is the most abundant mineral in the body and is necessary for the formation and function of bones and teeth. Calcium is also involved in the blood-clotting process, neurotransmitter release, muscle contraction, and cardiac function. Too much calcium, **hypercalcemia,** or too little, **hypocalcemia,** can cause cardiac **arrhythmias,** muscle spasms, and weak heartbeats. Normal calcium levels are 4.5 to 5.5 mEq/L. Potassium serves several critical functions in homeostasis. Potassium helps maintain fluid volume in cells, controls pH, and is vital in the transmission of nerve impulses. Either too much potassium, **hyperkalemia,** or too little, **hypokalemia,** causes serious metabolic problems. Because potassium is critical to neuromuscular function, cardiac arrhythmias are often seen in patients with potassium imbalances. Many elderly patients may be taking diuretics (see Chapter 7) and can easily become hypokalemic, so a potassium level must be determined on all surgical patients

Table **11–1** Major Electrolytes and Functions		
Electrolyte	*Chemical Symbol*	*Function*
sodium	Na^+	Osmotic pressure, nerve impulse transmission
chloride	Cl^-	Osmotic pressure, aids digestion
potassium	K^+	Osmotic pressure, acid–base balance, nerve impulse transmission
calcium	Ca^{2+}	Bone growth and development, blood coagulation, enzyme activity, neuromuscular function
magnesium	Mg^{2+}	Enzyme action in synthesis of adenosine triphosphate, muscle contraction, protein synthesis
phosphate	HPO_4^{2-}, $H_2PO_4^-$	Acid–base balance
bicarbonate	HCO_3^-	Acid–base balance
sulfate	SO_4^{2-}	Acid–base balance
carbonic acid	$H_2CO_3^-$	Acid–base balance

taking diuretics. Normal potassium levels are 3.5 to 5 mEq/L. A potassium or calcium imbalance is of special concern in surgical patients because of increased risk of cardiac arrhythmias or arrest when a general anesthetic is administered. Elective surgery may be postponed until potassium and calcium levels have been restored to a safe range.

 Note: Potassium is an electrolyte that can be added at higher concentrations in premixed IV solutions or added to the IV solution before infusion preoperatively.

⚠️ **CAUTION**

IV potassium can cause severe and potentially fatal cardiac rhythm disturbances. Thus, patients should be carefully monitored and when possible, oral potassium is preferable.

Sodium controls distribution of water in the body and maintains fluid and electrolyte balance. Sodium is the principle cation of extracellular fluid and is vital to neuromuscular function. If there is too much sodium in the body, the condition is called **hypernatremia**. This condition frequently results from a relative water loss and the cells become dehydrated. If there is too little, it is called **hyponatremia**. This results from excessive water ingestion or retention, or inadequate sodium intake.

INTRAVENOUS FLUIDS

Appropriate fluid and electrolyte management are integral components of surgical patient care, both for maintaining homeostasis and also for positive surgical outcomes. Nearly every surgical patient receives intravenous fluids. An IV drip is started on the patient for two purposes: to establish a direct access to the circulatory system for medication administration and to administer parenteral fluids. Parenteral fluid therapy has three objectives: to maintain daily fluid requirements, to restore previous losses, and to replace current losses. To accomplish these objectives, several fluids are available and are used for specific purposes. The IV fluids most commonly used in the surgical setting are called *crystalloids*. These are solutions composed mainly of water with dissolved electrolytes, dextrose solutions, and multiple-electrolyte solutions.

Common Intravenous Fluids Administered in Surgery

Sodium chloride (NaCl) in a 0.9% solution (**isotonic**) is the agent of choice for fluid replacement and simple hydration and is the most common IV fluid used in surgery. Sodium chloride is packaged in 1000-, 500-, 250-, and 100-mL bags for IV administration. It comes in a variety of concentrations (the amount of sodium chloride in solution), which include 5%, 3%, 0.9%, 0.45%, 0.33%, 0.225%. Sodium chloride is used when chloride loss is greater than or equal to sodium loss, for treatment of **metabolic acidosis** in the presence of fluid loss and to replenish lost sodium. Sodium chloride is the IV fluid used when transfusing blood products because it does not **hemolyze** (fill with fluid and rupture) blood cells.

Normal saline and physiological saline are common terms for 0.9% sodium chloride. The concentration of sodium chloride in normal saline is 0.9 g per 100 mL of solution. Another common IV saline concentration is 0.45% sodium chloride. Notice that 0.45% is half the strength of 0.9% NaCl, and it is sometimes written as $^1/_2$ NS (for half normal saline). Other saline concentrations are 0.33% NaCl or $^1/_3$ NS, and 0.225% NaCl or $^1/_4$ NS.

Dextrose is used in patients who require an easily metabolized source of calories: it is the best available carbohydrate and provides energy for cellular activity. Dextrose is available in various concentrations in water and in normal saline. Dextrose in water is used to hydrate the surgical patient, spare body protein, and enhance liver function. Because the trauma and stress of surgery causes some water and sodium retention, intraoperative intravenous therapy often involves administration of limited amounts of dextrose 5% in water (D_5W). Dextrose in water is also prepared in 2.5%, 10%, 20%, 25%, 30%, 40%, 50%, 60%, and 70% solution.

The percentage of solution determines the clinical use of dextrose. Lower concentrations (less than 10%) are used for peripheral hydrations, providing calories, and assessing kidney function (if patients do not need electrolyte replacement). In higher concentrations, dextrose is used for reversing hypoglycemia, providing calories when less fluid is indicated, and, with amino acids, for total parenteral nutrition.

Dextrose is frequently used in saline solutions—for example, 5% in normal saline (D_5NS). It is packaged in bags of 1000-, 500-, 250-, and 150-mL. This fluid is used for temporary treatment of circulatory insufficiency and shock from hypovolemia, in the absence of a plasma extender, and for early treatment with plasma for loss of fluid due to burns. Dextrose 10% in normal saline ($D_{10}NS$) is supplied in 1000- and 500-mL bags and is used to replenish nutrients and electrolytes.

It should be noted that dextrose solutions given intravenously increase insulin and oral hypoglycemic requirements for the diabetic patient. Dextrose is not used in conjunction with transfusion of blood products because it causes hemolysis of blood cells.

Ionosol B (MB and T) and 5% dextrose injection are maintenance and replacement electrolyte solutions. They provide a source of water, electrolytes, and carbohydrates to cover hydration, insensible water loss, and urinary excretion. Ionosol comes packaged in 500- and 1000-mL plastic bags; Ionosol MB and T also come in 250-mL size.

Normosol (M and R) and 5% dextrose injection is a solution of balanced electrolytes in water used intravenously for parenteral replacement of acute losses of extracellular fluid with minimal carbohydrate calories. Normosol M comes in 500- and 100-mL containers. Normosol R comes in a 1000-mL size only.

Lactated Ringer's (LR), or Hartmann's solution, is a physiologic salt solution used to replenish the patient's electrolytes and for rehydration to stimulate renal activity. Lactated Ringer's solution, which is used to replace fluid lost from burns or severe diarrhea, closely resembles the composition of extracellular fluid. It should not be used in patients with the inability to metabolize lactate (found in the solution). Patients at high risk are those with liver disease, Addison's disease, severe pH imbalances, shock, or cardiac failure.

Plasma-lyte and Isolyte E are electrolyte-balanced solutions compatible with the pH of blood. They are used to treat the massive loss of water and electrolytes seen in uncontrolled vomiting or diarrhea. The composition of these solutions is similar to the plasma portion of blood.

Intravenous Equipment and Supplies

An intravenous line is established in nearly all surgical patients prior to surgery. A flexible catheter, or angiocath (Fig. 11–1), is inserted via a needle into a vein, usually in the patient's hand or forearm. The needle is removed, leaving the catheter in the vein where it is taped securely in place. The *primary* IV tubing connects to the hub of the IV catheter, and the other end is connected to a container of IV solution. This tubing contains a drip chamber, injection port, and roller clamp (Fig. 11–2). Fluids and most of the medications needed during surgery are administered through the intravenous line. A *secondary* IV tubing may be used with the primary tubing when giving medications via "piggyback." The secondary tubing is shorter and also contains a drip chamber and roller clamp. In this setup, the secondary tubing is hung higher

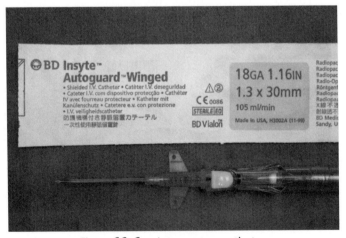

Figure **11–1.** Intravenous catheter.

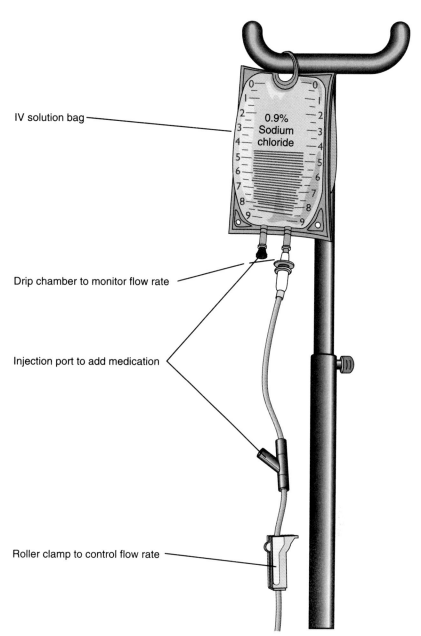

IV solution bag

0.9%
Sodium
chloride

Drip chamber to monitor flow rate

Injection port to add medication

Roller clamp to control flow rate

Figure **11–2.**   Intravenous tubing.

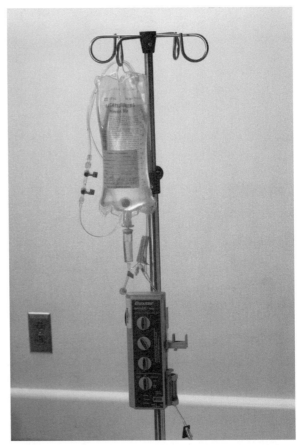

Figure **11–3.**   Electronic intravenous infusion pump and controller.

on the IV pole than the primary IV tubing so that the secondary medication infuses first. Secondary lines are used with antibiotics. At times, the IV tubing may be placed in an electronic infusion pump system (Fig. 11–3).

BLOOD REPLACEMENT

PHYSIOLOGY REVIEW

Blood performs several critical functions in maintaining homeostasis. It is used to transport oxygen, nutrients, wastes, hormones and enzymes throughout the body. Blood also maintains the body's acid–base balance (pH), its temperature, and its water content. The immune response is carried through the circulatory system as well. Blood is so crucial to maintaining life processes that it has a self-protection mechanism—clotting—to prevent harmful loss.

In an average adult, the circulating blood volume is approximately 70 mL/kg of body mass. To keep the body functioning normally, this blood volume should be maintained. Some surgical patients are at high risk for substantial blood loss during surgery; these include patients needing cardiac and peripheral vascular procedures, or those with trauma. The goal of blood replacement in scheduled surgical procedures is to maintain the circulating volume of blood as well as its oxygen-carrying capacity.

Blood consists of two main components: formed elements and plasma (fluid). The formed elements include erythrocytes (red blood cells or RBCs), leukocytes (white blood cells or WBCs), and platelets. Erythrocytes contain **hemoglobin**, a protein responsible for transport of oxygen and carbon dioxide between the lungs and the cells. Leukocytes provide protection against foreign microbes by phagocytosis and antibody production. Platelets mediate the clotting process.

Most surgical patients undergo laboratory tests to determine the amount of hemoglobin (Hgb) present in their blood. A normal hemoglobin level is 12 to 16 g/100 mL of blood in adult females and 14 to 18 g/100 mL in adult males. A low hemoglobin level indicates reduced oxygen-carrying capacity. Because oxygen levels must be optimum during general anesthesia, elective surgery may be canceled if the hemoglobin dips below normal levels. Another important measure of the oxygen-carrying capacity of the blood is **hematocrit**. Hematocrit is the volume of erythrocytes in a given volume of blood and is expressed as a percentage. Normal hematocrit levels range from 35 to 52%, varying by age and gender (Table 11–2).

Table **11–2**   Blood Values

	Females	*Males*
Circulating blood volume	4–5 L (4.2–5.3 qts)	5–6 L (5.3–6.4 qts)
Hemoglobin	12–16 g/100 mL	14–18 g/100 mL
Hematocrit	35–46%	40–52%
Red blood cells	4.2–5.4 million/mm^3	4.7–6.1 million/mm^3
Platelets	150,000–4,000,000/mm^3	Same

In cases of known or anticipated blood loss, the patient's blood must be typed and cross-matched to administer compatible donor blood. The blood type is determined by proteins called **antigens** present on the surface of RBCs. Blood type is inherited, and there are many types and groupings based on the antigens present on the RBCs. The major groupings of concern in surgery are ABO and Rh. Patients may be type A, B, AB, or O. Type A blood contains the A antigen, type B has the B antigen, type AB contains both, and type O blood has neither. Blood is also designated as Rh-positive (Rh antigen present) or Rh-negative (no Rh antigen present). Each person also has the corresponding **antibody** present in his or her plasma; that is, type A has anti-B, type B has anti-A, type O has both anti-A and anti-B, and type AB has neither (Fig. 11–4). If type A blood is administered to a type B patient, the recipient's antibodies will attack the donor RBCs, causing a potentially fatal transfusion reaction. A blood cross-match is performed to determine compatibility between the donor and the recipient. A sample of donor RBCs is mixed with the recipient's serum and the results are examined to determine compatibility. See Table 11–3 for more information on blood types.

RhoD immune globulin (RhoGam) is a medication used to treat possible blood compatibility reactions. It is an injectable blood product manufactured from human plasma that contains antiD to suppress the immune response of an Rh-negative mother to an Rh-positive fetus. If the anti-Rh antibody is given right after delivery, it blocks the sensitization of the mother and prevents Rh disease from occurring in the woman's next Rh-positive preg-

Table 11–3 Blood Types

Your Blood Type	Percentage of Population with Your Blood Type	Patients Who Can Receive Your Red Blood Cells	Patients Who Can Receive Your Plasma
O^+	38%	O^+, A^+, B^+, AB^+	O^+, O^-
O^-	7%	All blood types	O^+, O^-
A^+	34%	A^+, AB^+	A^+, A^-, O^+, O^-
A^-	6%	A^+, A^-, AB^+, AB^-	A^+, A^-, O^+, O^-
B^+	9%	B^+, AB^+	B^+, B^-, O^+, O^-
B^-	2%	B^+, B^-, AB^+, AB^-	B^+, B^-, O^+, O^-
AB^+	3%	AB^+	All blood types
AB^-	1%	AB^+, AB^-	All blood types

Courtesy of the American Red Cross.

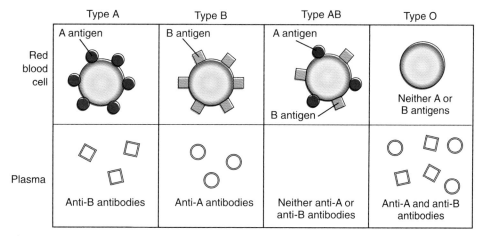

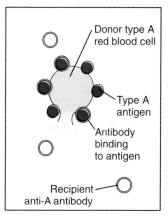

Figure **11–4.**   Antigen and antibody in blood types.   B

nancy. This Rh disease could result in miscarriage in subsequent pregnancies if not treated. RhoD immune globulin is for intramuscular injection only and is routinely given to Rh-negative mothers who deliver Rh-positive babies.

For further explanation of the physiology of blood, labor, and delivery, please refer to your anatomy and physiology textbook.

INDICATIONS FOR BLOOD REPLACEMENT

The first recorded blood transfusion occurred in 1667, when a 15-year-old male was given lamb's blood. This method was popular for a time until transfusion reactions were recognized and reported.

Insight 11–1   **Hemolytic Transfusion Reaction**

If blood is not properly typed and matched before being transfused, a serious and sometimes fatal reaction can occur, called hemolytic transfusion reaction, or hemolytic anemia. This can result from incompatible blood types or Rh factors and must be treated immediately. If the patient is under general anesthesia, the symptoms are a generalized diffuse blood loss and lowered blood oxygen saturation levels (as the red blood cells are not carrying sufficient oxygen). If any suspicious reactions occur during blood transfusion, the following steps should be taken:

1. Stop the transfusion.
2. Report immediately to the surgeon and the blood bank.
3. Send a sample of the patient's blood to the blood bank (to rule out a mismatch).
4. Return any unused portion of the blood unit and blood tubing to the blood bank.
5. Begin appropriate medication therapy, which usually includes steroid therapy as soon as possible.
6. Send urine samples to the lab to check for kidney function.

In some cases the patient may have to undergo renal dialysis to rid the system of mismatched blood.

Since the discovery that even all human blood is not alike, many advances have been made in blood transfusion therapy. Today, blood transfusions are routine because of the knowledge that blood must be compatible in type and Rh factor (Insight 11–1).

The most common indication for blood replacement in surgery is **hypovolemia** or circulatory shock, seen most frequently in trauma and vascular procedures. Other indications include restoration of the oxygen-carrying capacity as seen in anemic patients, and to maintain clotting properties as needed in patients with hemophilia.

Trauma patients may be in critical need of blood in order to sustain vital functions. If immediate replacement is required, and the patient's blood type is known, type-specific-only RBCs (packed cells) may be administered with fluid volume support. If the patient's blood type is unknown, O-negative blood may be administered. In either case, the surgeon must document the need for blood release without compatibility testing.

OPTIONS FOR BLOOD REPLACEMENT

There are several options available to replace blood loss in surgery; these include use of donor blood (**homologous** donation), patient donating own blood prior to surgery (**autologous** donation), patient's own blood collected and used during or after surgery (**autotransfusion**), or use of blood substitutes. Each blood replacement option has indications, advantages, and disadvantages. Some of these options may not be feasible in certain cases, depending on the situation.

Homologous Donation

A common method of blood replacement is the use of donor, or homologous blood. (This is also referred to as allogenous blood.) A blood bank is responsible for collecting, processing and releasing donor blood for use. Donor blood, although carefully tested, does present some risk for transmission of blood-borne pathogens such as hepatitis B and C, and human immunodeficiency virus (HIV). Thus, it is used only when clearly indicated.

Blood is separated during processing into components and then administered to treat specific needs. Component replacement therapy is an effective and efficient use of limited resources because a unit of donor whole blood, separated into components, can be used to treat several patients.

Whole Blood

Whole blood consisting of RBCs, plasma (which contains plasma proteins), stable clotting factors, and anticoagulants is rarely used for transfusion today. Whole, fresh blood is indicated only in cases of acute, massive blood loss that requires the oxygen-carrying properties of RBCs and the volume expansion provided by plasma. It is also a source of proteins and some coagulation factors. A unit of whole blood contains enough hemoglobin to raise an anemic adult's hematocrit approximately 3 percentage points.

Packed Cells (RBCs)

Most transfusions of donor blood in surgery involve the use of packed red blood cells (RBCs). The use of packed RBCs with a synthetic volume expander has proven to be as effective as whole blood, while reducing the risks of whole blood transfusion reactions. Packed cells are obtained by removing approximately 200 mL of plasma and most of the platelets from 1 unit (500 mL) of whole blood. The infusion of RBCs helps restore the oxygen-carrying capacity of the patient's own circulatory system. Intravenous fluids are administered concurrently to restore circulating volume if needed.

Plasma

Plasma may be administered when clotting factors are needed in addition to circulating volume. This need is frequently seen when several units of blood have been replaced, as the clotting factors have been removed from donor blood. Plasma is not used for volume expansion alone, because albumin and synthetic expanders are as effective and eliminate the risk of transmission of blood-borne diseases. Plasma is stored as fresh-frozen plasma (FFP) to preserve clotting factors and thawed in a water bath prior to use. It must be administered type-specific and used within 6 hours of thawing.

Platelets

Platelets are administered in surgery when large amounts of donor blood have been used to replace the patient's volume. Because the platelets have been removed from donor blood, the result of massive transfusions may be an inability of the patient's circulatory system to clot properly. Platelets are infused to restore a more normal clotting process. They may also be administered prophylactically in patients who have low platelet counts, as those receiving chemotherapy or with leukemia. At room temperature, platelets must be continually gently agitated to prevent clumping.

Cryoprecipitate

Cryoprecipitate is a plasma component used in the treatment of bleeding caused by hemophilia A, Von Willebrand's factor, and lack of factor XIII. Cryoprecipitate may be administered in surgery when massive amounts of blood have been replaced, severely impacting the normal coagulation process. See Insight 11–2.

Autologous Donation

Patients scheduled for elective surgical procedures in which blood loss is anticipated, such as a total hip replacement, may be allowed to donate their own blood up to one month prior to surgery. This process is called autologous transfusion and usually involves two units of blood. Most patients can safely donate two units of whole blood over a period of weeks just prior to their scheduled procedure, possibly eliminating the need for donor blood. The patient's blood is collected, processed, stored, and released for surgery by the blood bank. Patients often choose this option, if available, to protect themselves from potential blood-borne disease transmission.

Insight 11–2   **Platelet-Rich Plasma for Wound Healing**

From a small volume of the patient's own blood, surgeons can extract a platelet concentrate suspended in plasma that contains various growth factors (cytokines). When this platelet concentrate is reintroduced into the wound, it has the potential to greatly speed up the body's natural healing response in both soft and hard tissues. One company, Biomet, has developed a GPS® II Platelet Concentrate System with an automated platelet collection process. The patient's blood is placed in the collection device, which is then placed within a centrifuge and spun for 15 minutes. The blood is separated into platelet-poor plasma, platelet-rich plasma, and red blood cells. Then, the platelet-rich plasma is collected and placed into the wound.

Autotransfusion

Another form of autologous donation used intraoperatively and postoperatively is called autotransfusion. Autotransfusion involves the collection, processing, and reinfusing of the patient's own blood during the surgical procedure using cell-saver technology with little damage to the RBCs (Fig. 11–5). Several cell-saver machines are available. Some are designed specifically for emergency procedures when rapid infusion is required. Blood can be collected in a suction-type device or via bloody sponges drained into a sterile basin of saline, then aspirated into the machine. However, blood that has been exposed to collagen hemostatic agents and some medications (such as certain antibiotics) cannot be used because clotting in the machine may occur. Another method of autotransfusion is to use a sterile blood collection–suction canister to collect the patient's blood from the operative field. When the canister is filled, the blood is washed in a red cell washer (usually found in the blood bank) and reinfused. In this method, the blood is sent out of the surgical department to be washed and so time is lost before reinfusion.

Autotransfusion is performed during open-heart surgery, vascular procedures, major orthopedic procedures, and some trauma procedures such as splenectomy. Autotransfusion has several advantages over the use of donor blood, including immediate replacement of blood loss without the potential for transfusion reaction or delay for blood typing and cross-matching and no risk of transmission of blood-borne pathogens. In addition, patients with religious objections to donated blood often do not object to autotransfusion. Autotransfusion is not suitable for all patients, because some trauma patients may have lost so much blood already that little volume is left to salvage. A disadvantage of auto-

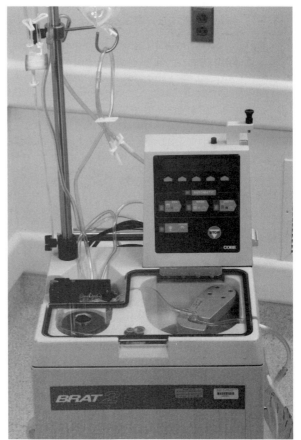

Figure **11–5.**   Cell-saver (autotransfusion) machine.

transfusion is that it cannot be used in the presence of cancer cells, infection, or gross contamination, such as open gastrointestinal tract. Autotransfusion is generally contraindicated during cesarean section because of the presence of amniotic fluid. Autotransfusion is commonplace in most operating rooms today and is an effective option for replacement of blood lost during certain surgical procedures.

Volume Expanders

Volume expanders are used to increase the total volume of body fluid. They are *colloids*, osmotically active, and draw fluid from extracellular fluid (ECF) compartments. Volume expanders can be used when donated blood or autotransfusion is not immediately available for emergency procedures. Several volume expanders are available.

Albumin and plasma protein fraction (PPF) are plasma derivatives used to provide volume expansion when crystalloid solutions, such as saline and dextrose, are not adequate (as for massive hemorrhage). They are also used in the treatment of hypovolemic shock as seen in burn patients who have lost fluid volume but not RBCs. Albumen is available in concentrations of 5%, which is equal to plasma, or as a concentrated 25% in sodium chloride solution. PPF is available as a 5% solution.

Dextran expands plasma volume by drawing fluid from the interstitial space to the intravascular fluid space. It is formed by the action of a bacterium, has osmotic properties, but not oxygen-carrying capacity. Packaged as Dextran 40, it is used prophylactically for thrombosis and embolism. It improves microcirculation independent of basic volume expansion and minimized the changes that occur in the blood viscosity that accompanies shock. Dextran 70 or 75 is used to expand plasma volume in impending hypovolemic shock. It is packaged for IV administration, 6% Dextran 70 in 0.9% sodium chloride (Macrodex) or 10% Dextran 40 in 5% dextrose or 0.9% sodium chloride (Rheomacrodex). The usual dose is 500 mL.

Hetastarch (Hespan) is also a synthetic used for its osmotic properties. It has no oxygen-carrying capacity. Hetastarch is made from hydroxyethyl starch (cornstarch). It acts as albumin in the management of shock. When given intravenously, it expands blood volume by one to two times the amount infused. Hetastarch comes in a 6% solution in 0.9% sodium chloride.

Blood Substitutes

The quest continues for blood alternatives that can transport oxygen to tissues, be given to any blood type, are safe to administer to the patient, and can be stored for long periods of time. A substitute is also needed for people with religious objections to blood transfusion. Three such blood substitutes are undergoing clinical tests to obtain Food and Drug Administration approval.

Hemopure is a product made from highly purified bovine blood and provides a form of hemoglobin to aid in oxygen transport to tissues. It has a shorter circulation time than blood (only 1 to 2 days) but does not require refrigeration. Its manufacturing process claims to rid the product from any risk of infection from viruses, including HIV, hepatitis C, and bovine spongiform encephalopathy (mad cow disease). Hemopure is stable for approximately 2 years at room temperature.

PolyHeme is a solution of chemically modified hemoglobin processed from outdated human red blood cells. Hemoglobin is first extracted from RBCs and then filtered to remove any impurities. Next is a multistep process to create a polymerized hemoglobin form that avoids undesirable effects such as vasoconstriction and kidney or liver dysfunction. PolyHeme's manufacturing process eliminates blood-borne diseases. Its shelf life is approximately 12 months under refrigeration.

Oxyglobin was introduced in the United States in the veterinary market as a treatment for canine anemia. A human version is undergoing clinical trials. Oxyglobin is an ultrapurified bovine hemoglobin formulated in a modified lactated Ringer's solution compatible with all blood types.

PROCEDURE FOR DONOR BLOOD REPLACEMENT IN SURGERY

The process for administration of donated blood products must be carefully monitored at each step to prevent transfusion of incompatible elements. Transfusion of incompatible blood or blood products can cause a fatal transfusion reaction (see Insight 11–1). The patient who needs a transfusion is typed and crossmatched and identified with a special wristband. A requisition slip (Fig. 11–6) with multiple carbon copies is sent to the blood bank with patient name, identification number, amount, and type (which includes blood group and Rh factor) of blood ordered. A copy of the requisition is sent back to surgery with each unit of released blood. The blood (unit) must be checked to verify its unit number and also expiration date. Meticulous records are kept in the blood bank on each unit, and the transporter is required to verify correct information with blood bank personnel and to sign out each unit released.

Once the donor units reach the surgical suite, they are to be placed in an appropriate blood refrigerator, which must have continuous temperature monitoring of 1° to 6° C. Any units needed for immediate transfusion will be taken directly to the operating room. Both circulator and anesthesia provider verify the patient and donor unit information before administration. In addition, the product itself is checked for any clots, discoloration, leaks, or damage to the bag that might result in contamination. If this occurs, the unit should not be used and must be returned to the blood bank.

When multiple units of blood are to be administered over a short period of time, or when cold blood is rapidly administered through a central venous line, the blood must be warmed to

BLOOD BANK REQUISITION				
REGIONAL MEDICAL CENTER ANYTOWN, USA				
☐ PACKED CELLS ☐ FRESH FROZEN PLASMA ☐ PLATELETS SINGLE DONOR ☐ PLATELETS RANDOM OTHER (SPECIFY)		DATE _____		

REGIONAL MEDICAL CENTER
ANYTOWN, USA

☐ PACKED CELLS ☐ FRESH FROZEN PLASMA ☐ PLATELETS SINGLE DONOR ☐ PLATELETS RANDOM OTHER (SPECIFY)

DATE _____

UNIT NO. ABO & Rh	PATIENT NO. ABO & Rh	EXPIRATION DATE

PATIENT _____ BIRTH DATE _____

PHYSCIAN _____

X-MATCHED BY-DATE

HOSPITAL NO. _____

☐ COMPATIBLE

BLOOD BANK RELEASE	TRANSFUSION STARTING RECORD	TRANSFUSION CHECK LIST
DATE BLOOD TAKEN/TECH	TRANSFUSION ORDERED BY	TRANSFUSION STARTED DATE	☐ Order verified from chart ☐ Verbal Order ☐ I have established the identity of the patient.
TIME TAKEN A.M. P.M.	I HAVE CAREFULLY COMPLETED THE CHECK LIST AND ATTACHED PART 1 TO PATIENT'S CHART	TRANSFUSION STARTED TIME A.M. P.M.	☐ The patient's name and hospital number agree with those on the tag. ☐ The blood type and Rh on the tag agree with those on the unit.
TAKEN BY	SIGNED*	MD RN	☐ Blood unit number marked on the tag agrees with the number on the unit. ☐ The blood is not outdated.
	*MUST BE SIGNED BY PERSON STARTING TRANSFUSION		

Figure **11–6.** Blood requisition slip.

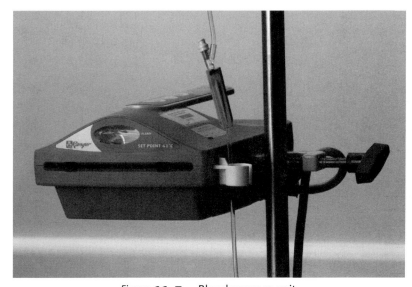

Figure **11–7.** Blood warmer unit.

prevent transfusion complications (Fig. 11–7). If blood must be transfused rapidly, a blood pump will be used. Different types of blood pumps are available, from simple pneumatic pumps to complex electric or battery-operated units that calibrate the infusion rate precisely.

IRRIGATION SOLUTIONS

Irrigation is an essential aspect of most open and endoscopic surgical procedures. These solutions assist in clearing the surgical field of active bleeding and improving visualization during the procedures. Irrigation is gentler on tissues than sponging in preventing desiccation and dryness, which can lead to adhesion formation (Insight 11–3). Endoscopic procedures use irrigation solutions to distend hollow organs, such as the bladder and uterus, and joint spaces such as the knee and shoulder. These solutions also wash out blood, bits of resected tissue, and stone fragments while allowing for specimen collection, as in transurethral resection of the prostate gland. However, it has been demonstrated that irrigation solutions may enter systemic circulation in large volumes, so they must be regarded as systemic medications.

Insight 11–3   Adhesion Barriers

Abdominal and pelvic surgery sometimes results in the formation of adhesions from scar tissue. Scar tissue forms around the incision and can cling to the surface of organs. Adhesions mature into fibrous bands, often with small calcifications and containing blood vessels. They can obstruct or distort organs causing pain, doctor's visits, the need for pain medication, subsequent surgery, and lost work time. An approach to preventing adhesion formation, in addition to excellent surgical technique, has been to use mechanical barriers and fluids. A barrier agent for prevention of adhesions should be nonreactive in tissue, maintain itself as the peritoneum and other structures regenerate (heal), and then be absorbed by the body.

Hyskon, a 32% solution of dextran 70 suspended in glucose, is used as a distention medium and has also been used as a fluid barrier to adhesions. The concept is of a viscous solution that is absorbed in 5 to 7 days and draws fluid equal to $2^1/_2$ to 3 times the original volume into the abdomen or pelvis. This action produces a hydroflotation effect on internal structures to prevent adhesion formation. Spraygel is currently in clinical trials in the United States. It is a synthetic absorbable adhesion barrier that consists of two polyethylene glycol-based liquids that are mixed during spraying. They form an adherent absorbable hydrogel that remains intact for 5 to 7 days during the critical healing period. The agent then degrades into an absorbable, easily excreted byproduct. Spraygel will be available in a laparoscopic spray system as well as an open-surgery applicator.

Mechanical barriers include Interceed and Seprafilm. Interceed is derived from oxidized regenerated cellulose in a mesh form that is positioned over injured tissues. It forms a gelatinous protective layer that is absorbed within two weeks. Complete hemostasis is required before applying Interceed. Seprafilm is a bioabsorbable membrane derived from sodium hyaluronate and carboxymethylcellulose. Once applied, it breaks down into a hydrated gel that is absorbed within seven days.

⚠ CAUTION

Test the temperature of all irrigation solutions, especially those recently taken from the warmer, as too hot of a solution can cause tissue damage. If it feels hot to your gloved hand, it is too hot for the patient and should be mixed with cooler solution.

BASIC IRRIGATION SOLUTIONS

Sodium chloride 0.9% (normal saline) is traditionally the irrigation solution of choice for open surgical procedures. It is a sterile, topical, conductive, electrolyte-containing solution that should never be administered by parenteral injection (there is a separately packaged sodium chloride solution for injection). Sodium chloride is used to rinse indwelling urethral catheters and surgical drainage tubes. It can be used to wash or rinse tissues, or soak surgical dressings and can serve as diluent or vehicle for administering other pharmaceutical preparations (as antibiotics in sodium chloride irrigation). Sodium chloride, if systemically absorbed, can result in alteration of cardiopulmonary and renal function. Excessive volume of the solution or pressure during irrigation, especially in small areas or closed cavities, can result in distention or tissue disruption. If this occurs the irrigation solution should be discontinued immediately. Sodium chloride comes in 150-, 500-, 1000-, 2000- and 3000-mL pour bottles. It also comes in 0.45% concentration in 1500- and 2000-mL sizes.

At the end of the surgical procedure, the surgeon will require a "wet one" and a "dry one," meaning a sponge saturated with clean, sterile sodium chloride irrigation solution and then a dry sponge. These are used to wipe off any blood from the patient's incision site, and any that has splattered or run on the patient's skin. The wet sponge also wipes any residual betadine prep solution from the area. Then the second clean, sterile sponge is used to dry the area and prepare it for the surgical dressings. Also note to check the surgeon's face for any splattered blood, which must be removed before he or she goes out to talk with the patient's family.

⚠ CAUTION

Saline is a conductive solution and so is used with caution in the presence of the electrosurgical unit (ESU). The danger comes from the transfer of heat and current to adjacent tissues. When used in open surgical procedures, most fluid is suctioned from the field and so saline can be used with little risk. However, in endoscopic procedures the ESU is applied within the fluid, in a confined space, and so other irrigation solutions are used that do not have conductive properties.

Sterile water is used more often to rinse instruments to cool them after autoclaving, remove residual disinfectant before coming into contact with patient skin, soak blood from hinges and serrations before terminal cleaning and autoclaving, and cool saw blades or burrs when drilling. It is also used in splash basins to remove powder from surgical gloves immediately pre-operatively and to remove blood from surgical gloves intra-operatively. It is used to dilute prep solutions (betadine scrub solution) and to fill the balloon on Foley catheters. Like saline, sterile water can be used to cleanse indwelling urethral catheters and surgical drainage tubes and soak surgical dressings. Sterile water is nonconductive and can be used for transurethral resection of bladder tumor (TURB) because it is not absorbed through the bladder. It cannot be used for transurethral resection of the prostate (TURP), because it is not isotonic and can result in intravascular **hemolysis** of erythrocytes. Using sterile water for TURP can also result in its absorption in large amounts through vascular openings. Sterile water comes packaged in 250-, 500-, 1000-, 2000-, and 3000-mL containers.

☞ **Note:** There is also a sterile water packaged separately for injection.

 CAUTION

Sterile water is not used for irrigation in procedures using the cell-saver machine, because it would also be suctioned up into the machine. If this occurs, hemolysis of the blood cells may result, thus they cannot be rein-fused. This principle also applies in the presence of cancer cells. Sterile water would not be used to irrigate, as the solution would cause the cells to swell and possibly rupture, spilling their cancerous contents onto other tissues.

Figure 11–8 shows irrigation devices.

Physiosol is a balanced electrolyte solution used as sterile irrigation for wounds and also for washing and rinsing purposes. It can be used as an irrigant for body joints because its pH and electrolyte composition closely resemble that of synovial fluids. In addition, it provides a transparent fluid medium with optical properties for good visualization during arthroscopy. Physiosol

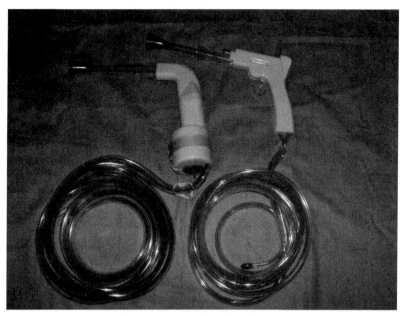

Figure **11–8.** Irrigation devices.

comes in solutions of 6.0 and 7.4 pH, and is packaged in 250-, 500-, and 1000-mL pour bottles and in 1000-mL flexible plastic bags.

IRRIGATION SOLUTIONS USED IN SPECIALTY PROCEDURES

Urologic irrigation solution of 3% Sorbitol is sterile, nonelectrolytic, nonhemolytic, and electrically nonconductive. It is used as an irrigating fluid for the urinary bladder as it provides a high degree of visibility without conducting heat and current from the ESU to tissues. During transurethral procedures, it removes blood and tissue fragments. During this procedure, venous sinuses may be opened and varying amounts of irrigation solutions are absorbed into the bloodstream. Thus, the patient should be monitored for altered cardiopulmonary and renal dynamics and hyperglycemia.

 CAUTION

During all procedures using a distention medium, the rate of flow and total fluid volume of the irrigation solutions must be carefully monitored. Also important is the height at which the IV pole is set as this determines the rate of flow (via gravity) and pressure of the solution.

Insight 11–4   **Transurethral Resection Syndrome**

Transurethral resection syndrome is a condition that results from absorption of fluids during a transurethral resection of the prostate gland (TURP). During a TURP procedure, irrigation fluid is used to visualize the area and wash away (lavage) blood and tissue debris. As the tissue is cut by the electrocautery, bleeding occurs from the open capillaries. The irrigation fluid flow must be at a pressure high enough to clear the surgical site, so this fluid pressure is greater than or equal to the pressure of the blood flow from the tissues. The open capillaries provide an access route for the fluid to enter the bloodstream. This can result in hypervolemia with dilutional hyponatremia and acid–base imbalance (acidosis). When glycine is used as the irrigation solution, its overabsorption can lead to hyperammonemia. Hyperammonemia can lead to cerebral edema, seizures, and death.

See Insight 11–4 on transurethral resection syndrome.

Sorbitol is sometimes used in combination with mannitol as Purisole (2.5% sorbitol, 0.54% mannitol) for transurethral procedures and in hysteroscopy. Mannitol 5% is also used in hysteroscopy when the ESU is used and is indicated to prevent hydrolysis and hemoglobin buildup during TURP.

Glycine 1.5% is a sterile nonconducting fluid used to irrigate body cavities. Its active ingredient is glycine, a naturally occurring amino acid, and like the other irrigants is nonconductive, non-electrolytic, and can be used with ESU. Thus it can be used in TURP and is also used in hysteroscopy. However, over absorption during this procedure can result in water intoxication with hyponatremia and acid–base imbalance (metabolic acidosis). Glycine comes packaged in 1500-mL pour bottles and 3000-mL flexible plastic bags.

Hyskon is a 32% solution of dextran 70 suspended in glucose. A water-soluble glucose polymer, it was originally used as a plasma expander. Hyskon is used to distend the uterus during hysteroscopy and to irrigate blood and tissue debris from the surgical site. It is electrolyte-free and nonconductive, so it can be used with ESU. When large amounts of Hyskon are used, the possibility of systemic effects such as plasma volume expansion can occur.

TECH TIP   Hyskon must be washed off instruments as soon as possible after use because it is difficult to remove when allowed to dry.

SYNOVIAL FLUID REPLACEMENT

Other body fluids are also being replaced, thanks in part to the advancement of arthroscopic surgery. Viscoseal is a 0.5% concentration, isotonic solution of hyaluronan of fermentative origin. Hyaluronan is a vital component of hyaline cartilage and synovial fluid. Viscoseal is used to irrigate joints during arthroscopic surgery, and also as a synovial fluid substitute. During arthroscopic procedures, synovial fluid is washed away by irrigating fluids. Viscoseal, when introduced into the joint, displaces any irrigating solutions left in the space, and leads to the reestablishment of the normal protective hyaluronan coating on the surface of the articular cartilage and synovial membrane.

IRRIGATION EQUIPMENT AND SUPPLIES

Irrigating syringes are bulb-shaped or bulb/barrel syringes (Asepto). They can also be larger standard syringes with special needle attachments for use in vascular surgery. The Asepto syringe is the most commonly used irrigator in open procedures. It is packaged sterile and holds approximately 120 mL. The regular bulb syringe, also called an ear syringe, does not have a barrel and is designed to irrigate smaller areas, such as the ear canal. It is also used to aspirate (remove) fluid from the nose and mouth of an infant, as during cesarean sections.

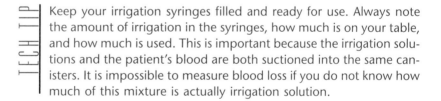

Keep your irrigation syringes filled and ready for use. Always note the amount of irrigation in the syringes, how much is on your table, and how much is used. This is important because the irrigation solutions and the patient's blood are both suctioned into the same canisters. It is impossible to measure blood loss if you do not know how much of this mixture is actually irrigation solution.

Evacuators are syringes used to insert and remove irrigation solutions in closed areas such as the bladder. Examples are an Ellik or a Toomey syringe used for TURP. The Ellik is a double-bowl–shaped glass or plastic container that is filled with irrigation solution and used to flush the prostate area. It aspirates blood clots and resected tissue as the solution is returned back into the evacuator. The Toomey is a large syringe-type container, usually used with a metal adapter inserted onto a catheter for irrigating the bladder/prostate area. It can also be used with an endoscope.

Continuous irrigation, such as for cystoscopy or hysteroscopy procedures, requires a closed, disposable irrigation system. Tubing

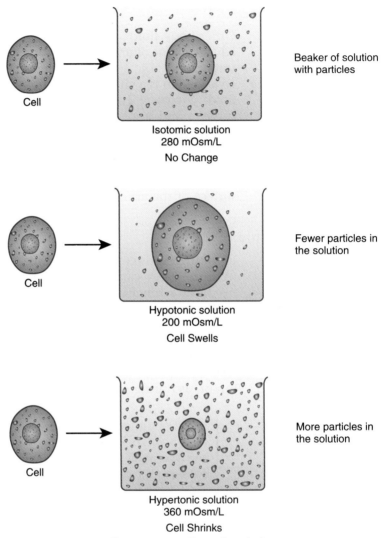

Beaker of solution
with particles

Cell

Isotomic solution
280 mOsm/L

No Change

Fewer particles in
the solution

Cell

Hypotonic solution
200 mOsm/L

Cell Swells

More particles in
the solution

Cell

Hypertonic solution
360 mOsm/L

Cell Shrinks

Figure **11–9.**   Osmotic solutions.

is either straight, as used intravenously, or more commonly Y-shaped to allow attachment of two bags or bottles of irrigation solutions.

Irrigation for endoscopic procedures is accomplished through irrigating channels built into endoscopes, or by irrigating systems inserted into an opening or port. Irrigation solutions can also be manually inserted into endoscopes with a syringe, for small amounts; or a syringe and stop cock attached to irrigation tubing hooked up to bags of solution when larger amounts are required. Pumps are also available that supply more fluid under pressurization. With these systems, the irrigation solutions can be introduced with more force, over a longer period of time, and the pressure is adjustable (see Fig. 11–8).

ADVANCED PRACTICES FOR THE SURGICAL FIRST ASSISTANT
Chapter 11—Fluids and Irrigation Solutions

KEY TERMS

hypertonic	solute
hypotonic	solution
osmolarity	solvent
osmosis	

BODY FLUIDS

When a patient's treatment necessitates intravenous medication and infusion therapy, it is the responsibility of the surgical first assistant to know why such interventions are essential and how they will affect the patient. The surgical first assistant should have an understanding of the pathophysiology of fluids and how they work in the body, and should be able to relate this to the need for intravenous therapy.

As mentioned earlier in the chapter all body fluids are primarily made up of water in which a variety of substances are dissolved. The total volume of water in the body is distributed between two large compartments, the intracellular and extracellular. These two compartments are separated by a semipermeable cell membrane. The extracellular compartment is subdivided into three compartments: the intravascular, interstitial, and transcellular. The compositions of the fluid contained within the two compartments are distinctive in chemical formulation. Intracellular fluid (ICF) is contained within the cell. Fluid found outside of the cell is extracellular (ECF). Even though the two compartments have structural differences and carry out completely different tasks, they are in constant interaction with each other in order to maintain homeostasis. **Osmosis** governs the movement of body fluids between these two compartments. Osmosis is the passage of water through the semipermeable membrane from an area with lower concentration of **solutes** to an area with higher concentration.

☞ **Note:** For the cell membrane to be semipermeable, it must be more permeable to water than to solutes (thus it controls the passage of solutes). In the body, water acts as a **solvent**, able to hold substances as well as acts to dissolve them. Solutes are substances dissolved in water (the solvent), and the combination of the solute and the solvent forms the **solution**.

See Figure 11–9.

(continued on following page)

ADVANCED PRACTICES FOR THE SURGICAL FIRST ASSISTANT *(continued)*

OSMOLARITY OF FLUIDS

In the chapter, the composition and concentration of IV fluids were discussed. The concentration of the solute in the solution determines its **osmolarity** (tonicity). Normal saline (0.9% sodium chloride) is an isotonic solution. This is defined as occurring when fluid that surrounds the cell membrane has the same tonicity and osmotic pull as inside the cell. Therefore the cell goes unchanged. A **hypotonic** solution is when the fluid on the outside of the cell membrane has a lesser tonicity and osmotic pull than the fluid on the inside of the cell membrane. Therefore more fluid flows into the cell, causing it to swell and possibly burst. The opposite of this is a **hypertonic** solution in which fluid on the outside of the cell membrane has a greater tonicity and osmotic pull than on the inside of the cell membrane. Thus more fluid is pushed out of the cell, causing it to shrink and shrivel.

See Table A on osmolarity of sodium chloride solution.

CONTINUOUS AND INTERMITTENT IRRIGATION

As described in the chapter, irrigation and IV fluids are used for a multitude of tasks in the surgical setting. Both IV fluids and irrigation solutions can be administered by two methods: continuous or intermittent. Continuous IV therapy is done to replace and maintain fluids in the body. Continuous irrigation is fluid instilled into an area of the body through a steady flow. An example of this is distending the bladder for transurethral resection of the prostate gland (TURP) or to ensure visualization during an arthroscopy. Intermittent infusions are used for medication administration and secondary fluid replacement. Examples of intermittent administration are IV piggybacks, IV push (bolus), and heparin or saline locks. Intermittent irrigation is also introduced onto an area or into a cavity of the body that is then suctioned or sponged. This is done to remove blood and debris from the site as during a debridement using a pulsed system (see Fig. 11–8), or following a laparotomy by pouring irrigation from the sterile pitcher into the abdomen.

Table **A**   Osmolarity of Sodium Chloride Solution

Solution	Concentration	Indications
Hypertonic	3% and 5%	Cerebral edema and hyponatremia
Isotonic	0.9%	Intravenous fluids
Hypotonic	0.225%, 0.33%, 0.45%	Dehydration and hypernatremia

ADVANCED PRACTICES FOR THE SURGICAL FIRST ASSISTANT   *(continued)*

ASSISTANT ADVICE

The surgical first assistant should constantly monitor the patient's tissue. Irrigation fluid (i.e., normal saline) is applied to prevent drying during the procedure and to prevent overheating of saw blades and burrs, which can cause thermal damage to surrounding tissues.

KEY CONCEPTS

- The human body is made up of fluid electrolytes and nonelectrolytes distributed into intracellular and extracellular fluid compartments.
- Blood and fluid replacement to normal levels are essential for survival.
- Major electrolytes are sodium, chloride, potassium, calcium, phosphate, and magnesium.
- Too much of the electrolyte in the blood is *hyper-*, too little is called *hypo-;* as too much potassium is hyperkalemia, too little is hypokalemia.
- Most surgical patients receive an IV drip to administer and maintain fluids and to establish a direct access to the circulatory system for medication administration.
- Common IV fluids used in surgery are sodium chloride, dextrose in water and sodium chloride, Lactated Ringer's, Ionosol, and Normosol.
- The most common IV fluid used in surgery, 0.9% sodium chloride, is also called normal saline.
- Blood serves many functions in the body, such as transporting oxygen, nutrients, waste, hormones, and enzymes, and maintaining the acid–base balance, temperature, and water content.
- The average adult circulating blood volume is approximately 70 mL/kg of body mass.
- Blood consists of formed elements (RBCs, WBCs, platelets) and plasma.
- Hemoglobin is a protein responsible for carrying oxygen and carbon dioxide between the lungs and the cells.

- Hematocrit is the volume of erythrocytes in a given volume of blood expressed as a percentage.
- The most common indication for blood replacement in surgery is hypovolemia.
- Options for blood replacement include homologous donation, autologous donation, autotransfusion, volume expanders, and—in the future—blood substitutes.
- There is specific hospital protocol to follow when obtaining blood from the blood bank for the surgical patient.
- Irrigation is used to clear the surgical field of blood and tissue debris, distend hollow organs, allow for specimen collection, and act as a diluent or vehicle for the administration of other pharmaceutical preparations.
- The irrigation solution of choice for most surgical procedures is 0.9% sodium chloride (normal saline).
- Normal saline is conductive and not to be used in the presence of the electrosurgical unit (ESU).
- Sterile water is used for a variety of functions, including instrument care and handling, glove cleaning, cooling instruments during surgical cases, and cleaning urethral catheters.
- Special irrigation solutions are used for specific procedures.
- Irrigation equipment includes bulb syringes, Asepto syringes, large standard-sized syringes, irrigating systems, and pump-irrigators.

ANTINEOPLASTIC CHEMOTHERAPY AGENTS

Medications Covered in Chapter 12

Generic Name	Brand Name	Category
nitrogen mustard, mechlorethamine	Mustargen	Alkylating agent
cyclophosphamide	Cytoxan	Alkylating agent
carboplatin	Paraplati	Alkylating agent
methotrexate	MTX, Folex, Mexate	Antimetabolite
5-fluorouracil	5-FU, Adrucil	Antimetabolite
paclitaxel	Taxol	Mitotic inhibitor
docetaxel	Taxotere	Mitotic inhibitor
bleomycin sulfate	Blenoxane	Antibiotic
doxorubicin	Adriamycin	Antibiotic
diethylstilbestrol	Estrobene, DES	Hormone
leuprolide	Lupron	Hormone antagonist
tamoxifen	Nolvadex	Hormone antagonist
erythropoietin	Epogen, Procrit	Biologic response modifier
filgrastim	Neupogen	Biologic response modifier

OBJECTIVES

After completing this chapter, you should be able to:

1. Define terms related to cancer.
2. Discuss different types of abnormal cell growth.
3. List the classifications of antineoplastic agents.
4. Define biologic response modifiers.
5. List the most prevalent carcinogen in the United States.
6. Discuss nanotechnology and its applications in medicine.

KEY TERMS

antineoplastic
benign
cancer
carcinogen
cytotoxic
epidemiology
etiology

malignant
metastasis
neoplasm
remission

The term **cancer** (also called carcinoma or CA) is a common one in the surgical setting. In the United States, cancer is the second leading cause of death, with heart disease being first. Nearly one third of all Americans are affected by some type of cancer during their lives. It may be found in any age group, but is often seen in older people. As the years of human life expectancy continue to increase, there is more evidence of cancer. The rate of occurrence for certain types of neoplastic disease, including breast, lung, and skin cancers, continues to increase, and cases are seen frequently, along with colon cancers, for surgical intervention.

The exact cause of cancer remains unknown. It is understood that before cancer can start, a disruption (possibly in the cell's genetic material) must occur that transforms normal cells into **malignant** ones. Normal body cells divide and multiply, replacing dying ones. When this rate of cell division is disrupted and not controlled, an abnormal growth of cells is formed. This abnormal growth is called a tumor, or **neoplasm**. Neoplasms may be **benign**, which means they resemble normal tissue, grow slowly, are highly organized cells, and do not normally spread into surrounding tissue. These tumors may be surgically removed if they disrupt normal body functions or cause pain. Neoplasms may also be malignant, or cancerous. These cells are unorganized and immature, multiply rapidly, and invade surrounding tissues. They can travel through the circulatory or lymphatic systems and spread to other areas of the body where they form another tumor called a **metastasis**. Many times, surgery is performed to diagnose or remove cancerous tumors. However, surgery may not be the only treatment available to cure the patient of the disease.

CHEMOTHERAPY AGENTS

Pharmaceutical agents play an important role in the treatment of cancer outside the surgical setting. **Antineoplastic** agents can be used as systemic treatment in the primary or main tumor, and in its metastases. This is often in addition to surgical treatment. These agents are **cytotoxic** and thus affect normal cells as well as malignant ones. They are often given intravenously in high doses on an established schedule. This regimen allows normal cells to recover in between chemotherapy medication doses. Antineoplastic agents are used for **remission** or palliative effects. Remission is the abatement (stopping) of symptoms and possible cure of the disease. Palliation (as already discussed in the text) means the relief of symptoms without cure. Antineoplastic agents are classified according to their mechanism of actions: alkylating agents, antimetabolites, mitotic inhibitors, antineoplastic antibiotics, hormones, and hormone antagonists. Steroids and antiemetics are also used along with antineoplastics to help prevent nausea and vomiting—a common side effect of chemotherapy. Other chemotherapy side effects include diarrhea, bone marrow depression, rashes, alopecia (hair loss), and scaling or dryness of the skin. Antineoplastic agents are contraindicated in pregnancy and in patients with renal or hepatic disorders.

Alkylating medications are the largest group of anticancer agents and are toxic to tissues that grow rapidly. They include the first antineoplastic drug, nitrogen mustard, which was introduced for this purpose in the 1940s (mustard gas was used in chemical warfare in World War I). Alkylating agents kill cells by forming cross-links on the DNA strands and affect all phases of the cell cycle. Thus, they are effective against many types of cancers such as acute and chronic leukemias, lymphomas, multiple myeloma, and solid tumors of the breast, ovaries, uterus, lungs, bladder, and stomach. Examples of alkylating agents include cyclophosphamide (Cytoxan) and carboplatin (Paraplatin).

Antimetabolites are the oldest group of anticancer agents (except for the original nitrogen mustard). They disrupt the metabolic processes and some inhibit enzyme synthesis. Thus, the neoplastic cell is unable to divide—resulting in cell death. Antimetabolites are used in the treatment of many cancers such as epidermoid cancers of the head and neck, lung cancer, bladder and brain cancers and breast cancer. Examples include the more commonly known agents methotrexate (MTX, Folex, Mexate) and 5-fluorouracil (5-FU, Adrucil).

☞ **Note:** Methotrexate is also used in confirmed ectopic pregnancy when the embryo is still small. It is injected into the muscle and reaches the embryo via the bloodstream, killing the cells that are developing in the placenta. The embryo is reabsorbed into the body, and the fallopian tube is not damaged.

Mitotic inhibitors are derivatives of plant extracts. They block cell division at a specific phase (M phase or the metaphase stage) of the cell cycle. These agents can be used as single medications or in combination drug therapy. Uses of mitotic inhibitors include treatment of advanced breast and ovarian, colon, and lung cancers, and squamous cell cancers of the head and neck. Examples include the medications paclitaxel (Taxol) and docetaxel (Taxotere), which are derived from the bark and needles of yew trees.

Antineoplastic antibiotics are different from those used for treating infections. These antibiotics target specific types of cancers by inhibiting protein and RNA synthesis and binding DNA, which causes fragmentation of the cell. They, like most antineoplastic agents, have toxic effects. The first antibiotic used in this manner, dactinomycin, was in the treatment of animal tumors in the 1940s. The antibiotics differ and are used to treat a variety of cancers such as squamous cell cancers of the head and neck, testicular cancer, Wilm's tumor, and ovarian, lung, and bladder cancers. Examples include bleomycin sulfate (Blenoxane) and doxorubicin (Adriamycin).

Hormones and hormone antagonists are used in combination therapy for treating various cancers. They include androgens and antiandrogens, estrogens and antiestrogens, and progestins. These agents act as antagonists that inhibit tumor cell growth and compete with endogenous hormones. One example is the use of androgens, which promote regression of breast tumors. Hormone antagonists exert beneficial effects by altering the hormonal environment that promotes cancer growth, for example, as when sex hormones such as estrogen are used to treat prostate cancers. Estrogens suppress androgen production by acting in the pituitary to decrease interstitial cell-stimulating hormone. This results in the decreased production of androgens by the testes, which helps to decrease the progression of prostatic cancer. Hormones (corti-costeroids) also act as anti-inflammatory agents to suppress the tissue's inflammatory process. They are primarily used for treating cancers of the breast, endometrium, and prostate. Examples include diethylstilbestrol (Estrobene, DES), leuprolide (Lupron), and tamoxifen (Nolvadex).

BIOLOGIC RESPONSE MODIFIERS

Biologic response modifiers (BRMs) are agents that have been developed through biochemical technology to boost, or enhance, the body's immune system. They can be used in conjunction with chemotherapy agents. As previously discussed, chemotherapy agents destroy not only cancer cells but also normal cells such as white blood cells (WBCs), which are essential in protecting the body from infections. BRMs have three main functions: to enhance the body's immunologic function, to destroy or interfere with tumor activities, and to promote differentiation of stem cells. Further indications for BRM uses are being investigated. Two agents are used to treat chemotherapy side effects by stimulating specific bone marrow production of blood cells. The first is ery-thropoietin (Epogen, Procrit), which is used to treat patients with anemia by stimulating RBC production. The second is filgrastim (Neupogen) which binds to bone marrow cells and stimulates the growth of neutrophils—key components of the immune system.

Other BRM agents are interferons and interleukins. Interferon is a natural protein that boosts immune cells so they are better able to attack cancerous cells. It can also change the structure of cells to make them more normal in their behavior and less like cancer. Interferon is used to treat a specific type of leukemia and for use in an acquired immunodeficiency syndrome-related tumor called Kaposi's sarcoma. Interleukins are a group of proteins that are produced by the body's WBCs. They have been found to contain antitumor effects, especially in renal cell cancers and malignant melanoma.

SEARCH FOR A CURE

Epidemiology is the science that studies factors that determine and influence the frequency and distribution of disease and its cause to find a cure. The epidemiology of cancer reflects patterns based on gender, age, geographic location, and socioeconomic status. In the United States for example, lung cancers are equally likely to occur in men and women. In women, the leading sites of fatal cancers are the lung, breast, colon, and rectum. In men, leading sites are the lung, prostate, colon, and rectum.

Etiology is the cause of disease. As previously stated, the exact cause of cancer (its etiology) is not known. Evidence suggests that cellular genes (which are responsible for cellular metabolism, division, and growth) convert to malignant oncogenes (these are genes found in chromosomes of tumor cells) that cause uncontrolled cell growth and replication. We do know there are cancer-causing substances. These are known as **carcinogens**. For example, tobacco is the most important known carcinogen in the United States. It is estimated that 30% of all cancer deaths could be avoided by eliminating tobacco.

Research is ongoing regarding the uses of antineoplastic agents. Relatively few agents have been discovered in the last decade; however, new combinations of agents and higher doses have shown promise for positive results in cancer treatment. The newest class of antineoplastic agents is angiogenesis inhibitors. These medications work to block the construction of new capillaries (i.e., blood supply) to cancerous tumor cells. This prevents the cells from receiving nutrients, and the tumor stops growing or in some cases regresses, or shrinks, to a microscopic dormant lesion.

Another area of science and technology that focuses on atomic- and molecular-scale structures is nanotechnology. To measure these supersmall particles, a nanometer is used. A nanometer is one billionth of a meter, so nanoscale particles and devices can enter most cells. With the ability to manipulate particles on this level, researchers want to use nanoparticles as image contrast agents, for diagnostic purposes, and in medication delivery. One application would be to coat gold shells onto nanoparticles and use these nanoshells in the circulatory system. The nanoshells would absorb light and could be used for deep tissue imaging. Other potential applications include blood testing, optical triggered medication delivery, and targeting cancer cells in the body for destruction. By modifying nanoshells, they could seek out abnormal cells, or tumors, that could then be imaged, biopsied, and targeted with light to provoke the cell's death.

KEY CONCEPTS

- Cancer is also called carcinoma or CA.
- Cancer is the second leading cause of death in the United States.
- The exact cause, or etiology, of cancer is unknown.
- The term *malignant* describes cancer cells that have disrupted cell division and have uncontrolled growth.

- The term *benign* describes cells that resemble normal tissue and do not normally spread to surrounding areas.
- The term *metastasis* describes a tumor that has spread to other areas of the body.
- Chemotherapy is the use of pharmaceutical agents to treat cancers.
- Chemotherapeutics, or antineoplastic agents, are divided into classifications according to their mechanism of actions: alkylating agents, antimetabolites, mitotic inhibitors, antineoplastic antibiotics, hormones, and hormone antagonists.
- BRMs are agents used to enhance the body's immune system.
- Epidemiology is the science that studies factors that influence the frequency and distribution of disease.
- Carcinogens are cancer-causing substances; an example is tobacco.
- The newest class of antineoplastic agents is angiogenesis inhibitors, which target the tumor's blood supply.
- Nanotechnology is being applied to medical diagnostics, medication delivery, and treatment of neoplasms.

Unit Three

Anesthesia

As a surgical technologist, you'll observe the administration of anesthesia in the operating room nearly every day. Why is it necessary to learn about anesthesia? After all, administration of anesthetic agents is far outside the realm of the technologist's clinical practice. The fact is, understanding the terminology, methods, and agents of anesthesia will give you a more complete picture of surgical patient care. And it will make you a more effective member of the surgical team if you know the names and classification of anesthetic and supplemental agents, as well as their purposes. As team members, you'll be asked to obtain medications with whose generic and trade names you must be familiar. And to facilitate smooth flow of patient care, you'll need to understand preoperative and intraoperative anesthesia routines and medications. In both routine and emergency situations, all team members must contribute maximum effort to achieve the best possible patient outcome. For the surgical technologist, part of that effort includes learning the rudiments of pharmacology as it relates to anesthesia.

PREOPERATIVE MEDICATIONS

Medications Covered in Chapter 13

Generic Name	Brand Name	Category
diazepam	Valium	Sedative
lorazepam	Ativan	Sedative
midazolam	Versed	Sedative
morphine	Astramorph	Opioid analgesic
meperidine	Demerol	Opioid analgesic
fentanyl	Sublimaze	Opioid analgesic
atropine	Atropine	Anticholinergic
glycopyrrolate	Robinul	Anticholinergic
scopolamine	Transderm Scop	Anticholinergic
sodium citrate	Bicitra	Antacid
cimetidine	Tagamet	Antacid
famotidine	Pepcid	Antacid
ranitidine	Zantac	Antacid
ondansetron	Zofran	Antiemetic
metoclopramide	Reglan	Antiemetic

OBJECTIVES

After completing this chapter, you should be able to:

1. Define terminology related to preoperative medications.
2. Identify the purpose of preoperative patient evaluation.
3. List sources of patient information used for preoperative evaluation.
4. List the components of a preoperative evaluation.
5. Identify classification of preoperative medications.
6. Identify the purpose of each group of preoperative medications.
7. State examples of medications in each classification.

KEY TERMS

amnestic	aspiration	mg/kg
analgesia	benzodiazepine	NPO
anesthesiologist	certified registered nurse	opioid
anterograde	anesthetist (CRNA)	sedative
anticholinergic	hematocrit	vagolysis
antisialagogue	hemoglobin	
anxiolysis	mcg/kg	

Preoperative preparation is necessary to maximize the safety and comfort of every surgical patient. The surgical technologist may, on occasion, work in a preoperative care unit or assist in preoperative preparation of patients requiring elective or emergency surgery. To effectively assist the anesthesia care team, surgical technologists should understand the classifications, purposes, and common pharmacologic agents used to prepare the patient for surgery.

PREOPERATIVE EVALUATION

A preoperative evaluation, or assessment, is performed on all surgical patients and is conducted by the anesthesia provider. The anesthesia provider may be either an **anesthesiologist** (MD) or a **certified registered nurse anesthetist (CRNA)**. The purpose of a preoperative evaluation is to gather pertinent patient information to determine the optimal anesthetic plan. Information is gathered from several sources, including the patient's medical records, a preoperative patient interview, physical examination, and preoperative testing results. The preoperative evaluation is used to confirm the patient's surgical disease and to assess concurrent medical conditions. It also identifies any medications the patient may be taking and allergies and physical status. Special emphasis is placed on assessment of diseases of the cardiovascular and respiratory systems and diabetes. The evaluation usually consists of a questionnaire (Fig. 13–1) to be completed by the patient and an interview with the anesthesia provider (Fig. 13–2), who then completes a preanesthesia evaluation form (Fig. 13–3). The preanesthesia physical examination is a complete assessment of the patient's physical status. In addition, the patient's airway is evaluated. Additional preoperative testing may be ordered depending on the findings of the preoperative evaluation. Examples of preoperative tests that may be indicated include electrocardiogram (ECG), chest radiograph, pulmonary function studies, **hemoglobin** and **hematocrit** measurements, coagulation studies, and serum chemistry panels. When all the necessary information is obtained, the patient's physical status is classified according to criteria established by the American Society of Anesthesiologists (Table 13–1).

PREOPERATIVE MEDICATIONS

During the preoperative evaluation, the MD or CRNA will determine the patient's need for preoperative medications. Some preoperative medications are given to prepare the patient physically, and some prepare the patient psychologically. Preoperative medications can be classified by action, each group having a specific purpose.

Table **13–1**	American Society of Anesthesiologists' Physical Status Classification
I	A normal, healthy patient
II	A patient with mild systemic disease
III	A patient with severe systemic disease that limits activity but is not incapacitating
IV	A patient with an incapacitating systemic disease that is a constant threat to life
V	A moribund patient not expected to survive 24 hours with or without operation
E	In the event of an emergency operation, an E is placed after the Roman numeral

(From American Society of Anesthesiologists: Manual for aesthesia department organization and management, 2004, www.asahq.org/clinical/physicalstatus.htm, accessed October 4, 2005.)

Preanesthesia Questionnaire

The information you supply below assists in the development of your anesthesia care.
Please complete this questionnaire accurately and completely.

Patient Name _____

Age _____ **Weight** _____ **Height** _____ **Date** _____

Allergies _____

_____

Current Medications (Prescription and Nonprescription)_____

_____

Prior Operations _____

_____

Preanesthesia Questionnaire

Please answer the following questions. These responses will help us provide the anesthetic
that is best for you.

Yes	No	Question
[ ]	[ ]	Have you recently had a cold or the flu?
[ ]	[ ]	Are you allergic to latex (rubber) products?
[ ]	[ ]	Have you experienced chest pain?
[ ]	[ ]	Do you have a heart condition?
[ ]	[ ]	Do you have hypertension (high blood pressure)?
[ ]	[ ]	Do you experience shortness of breath?
[ ]	[ ]	Do you have asthma, bronchitis, or any other breathing problem?
[ ]	[ ]	Do you (or did you) smoke?
		Packs/day _____. Number of years _____.
		Date you quit _____.
[ ]	[ ]	Do you consume alcohol?
		Drinks/week _____.
[ ]	[ ]	Do you take or have you taken recreational drugs?
[ ]	[ ]	Have you taken cortisone (steroids) in the last six months?
[ ]	[ ]	Do you have diabetes?
[ ]	[ ]	Have you had hepatitis, liver disease, or jaundice?
[ ]	[ ]	Do you have a thyroid condition?
[ ]	[ ]	Do you have or have you had kidney disease?
[ ]	[ ]	Do you have ulcers or other stomach disorders?
[ ]	[ ]	Do you have a hiatal hernia?
[ ]	[ ]	Do you have back or neck pain?
[ ]	[ ]	Do you have numbness, weakness, or paralysis of your extremities?
[ ]	[ ]	Do you have any muscle or nerve disease?
[ ]	[ ]	Do you or any of your family have sickle cell trait?
[ ]	[ ]	Have you or any blood relatives had difficulties with anesthesia?
[ ]	[ ]	Do you have bleeding problems?
[ ]	[ ]	Do you have loose, chipped, false teeth, or bridgework?
[ ]	[ ]	Do you have any oral piercings, (such as studs or rings) in your tongue or lip?
[ ]	[ ]	Do you wear contact lenses?
[ ]	[ ]	Have you ever received a blood transfusion?
[ ]	[ ]	(Women) Are you pregnant?
		Due date _____.

Figure **13–1.** Sample preoperative patient questionnaire. (From American Association of Nurse Anesthetists: AANA's Public Information and Patient Resources Center, 2005. www.aana.com/patients/preop.asp, accessed October 4, 2005.)

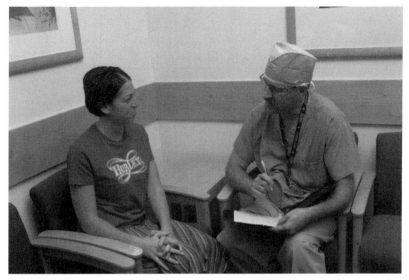

Figure **13–2.** The anesthesia provider conducts a preoperative interview with the patient.

SEDATIVES

Sedatives are given to relieve anxiety (**anxiolysis**), which is common in surgical patients. In most patients, these drugs produce a mild drowsiness, and they may have **amnestic** and antiemetic effects. The most common sedatives used preoperatively are the **benzodiazepines.** In low doses, benzodiazepines produce anxiolysis and at higher doses produce sedation and **anterograde** amnesia. The patient will remain conscious, but will not remember events while under sedation. Diazepam (Valium), lorazepam (Ativan), and midazolam (Versed) are benzodiazepines. Midazolam (Fig. 13–4) is the most common benzodiazepine administered preoperatively, and it is administered in weight-dependent doses (**mg/kg**), ranging from 0.5 to 2 mg intravenously. Effects are seen in 1 to 5 minutes, peak between 5 and 30 minutes, and last from 2 to 6 hours.

ANALGESICS

Opioids may be used preoperatively as necessary to relieve pain (**analgesia**) and reduce the amount of anesthesia needed for the surgical procedure. The term *opioid* refers to all drugs, natural, semisynthetic, or synthetic, having morphine-like actions. Opioids

PREANESTHESIA EVALUATION

Age	Sex M F	Height in/cm	Weight lb/kg

Proposed procedure	Pre-procedure vital signs
	B/P P R T

Previous anesthesia/operations	None ☐	Current medications	None ☐

Family history of anesthesia complications	None ☐	Allergies	NKDA ☐

AIRWAY/TEETH/HEAD AND NECK

History from:
☐ Patient   ☐ Significant other
☐ Parent/guardian   ☐ Chart
☐ Communication//language problems
☐ Poor historian

SYSTEM	WNL	COMMENTS	DIAGNOSTIC STUDIES
RESPIRATORY	☐	Tobacco use: ☐ Yes ☐ No _____ packs/day for _____ years	EKG
Asthma — Productive cough Bronchitis — Recent URI COPD — SOB Dyspnea — Tuberculosis Orthopnea Pneumonia			Chest X-ray
CARDIOVASCULAR	☐		
Abnormal EKG — Hypertension Angina — MI ASHD — Murmur CHF — Pacemaker Dysrhythmia — Rheumatic fever Exercise tolerance — Valvular disease			Pulmonary studies
HEPATO/GASTROINTESTINAL	☐	Ethanol use: ☐ Yes ☐ No Frequency _____ "Street drug" use: ☐ Yes ☐ No Frequency _____	Other
Bowel obstruction — Muscle weakness Cirrhosis — Neuromuscular Dis. Hepatitis/Jaundice — Paralysis Hiatal henia/reflux — Paresthesia Nausea and Vomiting — Syncope Ulcers — Seizures			
NEURO/MUSCULOSKELETAL	☐		**LABORATORY STUDIES**
Arthritis Back problems CVA/Stroke/TIAs DJD Headaches/↑ ICP Loss of consciousness			Hgb/Hct/CBC
RENAL/ENDOCRINE	☐		Electolytes
Diabetes Renal failure/dialysis Thyroid disease Urinary retention Urinary tract infection Weight loss/gain			Urinalysis
OTHER			Other
Anemia — Immunosuppressed Bleeding tendencies — Pregnancy Cancer — Sickle cell dis./trait Chemotherapy — Recent steroids Dehydration — Tranfusion history Hemophilia			

Problem list/diagnoses	PHYSICAL STATUS 1 2 3 4 5 E	POSTANESTHESIA NOTE
Planned anesthesia/special monitors		
		Signed _____ Date_____ Time_____

Pre-anesthesia medications ordered	PATIENT IDENTIFICATION

Evaluator signature	Date Time

Figure **13–3.** Sample preanesthesia evaluation. (From American Association of Nurse Anesthetists: Preanesthesia Evaluation. 1991, www.aana.org.)

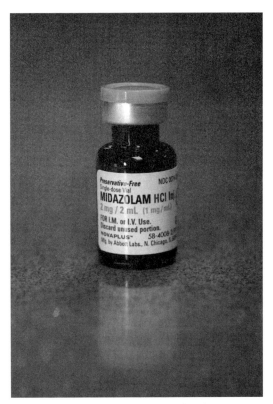

Figure **13–4.**   Vial of midazolam.

cause analgesia and mild sedation in usual doses. Slowing of respiration and reduced intestinal motility are expected. Because of slowed respiration, supplemental oxygen may be given and the patient monitored with a pulse oximeter (see Chapter 14). The patient's level of consciousness should be assessed frequently when opioids are administered. Opioids are not usually the first choice of agents when analgesia is necessary preoperatively. Contraindications to the use of opioids preoperatively include outpatient surgery due to the prohibitively intense patient monitoring required. The sedative effect of benzodiazepines often preempts the need for opioids.

Morphine (Astramorph, Duramorph) is a natural opioid that may be used preoperatively. Although rarely used, morphine may be indicated for patients experiencing significant pain preoperatively who expected to be admitted as inpatients after surgery. Morphine is given intravenously in doses of 2.5 to 15 mg, depending on the patient's ability to tolerate the drug. Onset of action is expected in 2 to 5 minutes, with peak in 10 to 15 minutes, and effects often last well over 2 to 4 hours.

The most common synthetic opioids are meperidine (Demerol) and fentanyl (Sublimaze). Meperidine is administered intravenously in doses of 75 to 100 mg to provide preoperative analgesia. Onset of effect occurs in 1 to 3 minutes, peaks at 5 to 20 minutes, and provides analgesia for 2 to 4 hours. Fentanyl is 75 to 125 times more potent than morphine; it is characterized by rapid onset (30 seconds) and short duration (30 to 60 minutes). It is administered in doses of 1 to 2 micrograms per kilogram **(mcg/kg)** for preoperative analgesia. See Table 13–2.

☞ **Note:** Opioids are covered under federal and state controlled substances acts (see Chapter 2) and must be handled according to hospital policy. The surgical technologist must be thoroughly familiar with institutional procedures regarding controlled substances.

ANTICHOLINERGICS

Anticholinergics are used for several purposes preoperatively. These medications block certain receptors on the vagus nerve (**vagolysis**), so they are used to inhibit mucous secretions of the respiratory and digestive tract (**antisialagogue** effect), and increase heart rate. The anticholinergics most frequently used preoperatively are atropine, glycopyrrolate (Robinul), and scopolamine. Atropine is given intravenously in doses of 0.4 to 1.0 mg; onset is almost immediate and duration is 15 to 30 minutes. Glycopyrrolate is administered intravenously preoperatively in doses of 0.1 to 2 mg, onset occurring within 1 minute and lasting 2 to 3 hours. Scopolamine is given intravenously in doses of 0.3 to 0.6 mg; onset is immediate and effects are seen for 30 to 60 minutes. Scopolamine may also be administered in a dermal patch to prevent postoperative nausea and vomiting. See Table 13–3.

☞ **Note:** Anticholinergics may also be used intraoperatively to block the vagal response (bradycardia) to certain stimuli such as

Table **13–2** Comparison of Analgesics Used Preoperatively					
Generic Name	Trade Name	Dosage	Onset (min)	Peak (min)	Duration (hours)
morphine	Astramorph	2.5–15 mg	2–5	10–15	2–4
meperidine	Demerol	75–100 mg	1–3	5–20	2–4
fentanyl	Sublimaze	1–2 mcg/kg	0.5	5–15	0.5–1

Table **13–3** Comparison of Anticholinergics Used Preoperatively				
Generic Name	*Trade Name*	*Dosage*	*Onset (min)*	*Duration (hours)*
atropine	Atropine	0.4–1.0 mg	Immediate	0.25–0.5
glycopyrrolate	Robinul	0.1–2 mg	1	2–3
scopolamine	Transderm Scop	0.3–0.6	Immediate	0.5–1

stretching the peritoneum during open abdominal procedures, bowel manipulation, cervical traction in gynecologic cases, or stretching eye muscles during retinal procedures.

GASTRIC AGENTS

Anxiety and fear, so often seen in surgical patients, initiates a stress response mediated by the sympathetic nervous system, which may slow down or stop the digestive process (Insight 13–1). The presence of food in the stomach and the acidic nature of gastric contents present a significant hazard to surgical patients. During induction of general anesthesia, the lower esophageal sphincter may relax to an extent that a reflux of gastric contents may occur. In addition, some agents administered at this time may cause nausea, with an increased risk for vomiting. If the patient

---

Insight 13–1   **Gastric Physiology Review**

The digestive system is responsible for intake and processing of nutrients and elimination of nutrient waste. The stomach, which is part of the digestive system, processes food by two means—mechanical and chemical. The mechanical process of digestion is due to the peristaltic motions of the muscles and folds (rugae) of the stomach, which mix food with gastric secretions. This mixture becomes a thin liquid, called chyme, which is propelled in small amounts through the pylorus into the duodenum. The chemical process of digestion is due to the action of an enzyme called pepsin. In the presence of hydrochloric acid, pepsin becomes active and breaks down protein contained in the ingested food. Hydrochloric acid is produced by the parietal (oxyntic) cells of the stomach and is the chemical responsible for the acidic nature of gastric contents. Secretion of these chemicals is controlled by both the nervous system and the endocrine system. The nervous system regulates production of gastric chemicals via stimulation of the parasympathetic fibers of the vagus nerve. The sight and smell of food also initiate stimulation of gastric glands to produce digestive chemicals. Ingestion of food causes stretching of the stomach, which is transmitted through the nerves, and a response is generated that produces more stimulation of gastric glands. For further explanation of digestion, consult a physiology textbook.

vomits or gastric reflux occurs during induction of anesthesia, gastric contents can enter the lungs, causing mild to severe damage. This complication is called **aspiration**, which may result in aspiration pneumonia. Even though elective surgical patients are **NPO**, gastric secretions are still present. Patients at increased risk for aspiration include those with gastrointestinal obstruction, history of gastroesophageal reflux disease (GERD), diabetes, or obesity. In addition, patients presenting with a need for emergency surgery may have a full or partially full stomach. When indicated in patients with risk factors for gastric reflux and possible aspiration, several different agents may be used for preoperative prophylaxis, alone or in combination with other agents.

Nonparticulate antacids may be administered preoperatively to neutralize the acidity of stomach contents (gastric acid normally has an acidity, or pH, of 2) to minimize the amount of damage that may be caused by reflux and aspiration. Sodium citrate with citric acid (Bicitra) is the most frequently used preoperative oral antacid. Sodium citrate is metabolized to sodium bicarbonate—a base that neutralizes gastric acid. Sodium citrate is given orally in a dose of 15 to 30 mL. Effects are immediate and the duration is approximately 2 hours.

Gastric acid secretion blockers interfere with the production of gastric acid by parietal cells. These agents are called histamine (H_2) receptor antagonists or blockers. The most common H_2 blockers given preoperatively are cimetidine (Tagamet), famotidine (Pepcid), and ranitidine (Zantac). Cimetidine is given intravenously as a preoperative medication in a dose of 2 to 4 mg/kg. Effects occur within 4 to 5 minutes and last approximately 4 hours. Famotidine may be given orally in a dose of 20 to 40 mg the night before or the morning of surgery or intravenously in a dose of 20 mg. Onset of effects is noted in 20 to 45 minutes, and effects last for 7 to 9 hours. Ranitidine is administered intravenously preoperatively, 50 mg, with effects occurring within 15 minutes and lasting 6 to 8 hours.

Antiemetics are administered preoperatively to reduce nausea and minimize the possibility of vomiting. Ondansetron (Zofran) is given intravenously in doses of 2 to 4 mg with effects lasting 12 to 24 hours, which is helpful in preventing postoperative nausea and vomiting as well. Ondansetron may be given in combination with dexamethasone (Decadron) 8 mg for prevention of postoperative nausea and vomiting, which increases duration of effects to 36 to 54 hours.

Droperidol (Inapsine) is an antiemetic drug with sedative properties that is less frequently used in current practice. The Food and Drug Administration requires a black-box warning on droperidol,

Table **13–4** Gastric Agents Used Preoperatively				
Generic Name	*Trade Name*	*Dosage*	*Onset (min)*	*Duration (hours)*
Antacid				
sodium citrate	Bicitra	15–30 mL	Immediate	2
cimetidine	Tagamet	2–4 mg/kg	4–5	4
famotidine	Pepcid	20–40 mg	20–45	7–9
ranitidine	Zantac	50 mg	15	6–8
Antiemetic				
ondansetron	Zofran	2–4 mg	5–10	12–24
metoclopramide	Reglan	10 mg	1–3	1–2

the most serious warning for an FDA-approved drug. Indications for use of droperidol have been limited, and its use is restricted to second-line only, because of an increased risk of fatal cardiac arrhythmias. When indicated, droperidol is administered intravenously, 15 mcg/kg, with effects in 3 to 10 minutes and duration of 2 to 4 hours.

Metoclopramide (Reglan) is a gastrointestinal motility agent given preoperatively for its antiemetic effects. It stimulates motility of the upper gastrointestinal tract without stimulating gastric acid secretion. Metoclopramide is administered intravenously, 10 mg (adult dose), with onset expected in 1 to 3 minutes and duration of 1 to 2 hours. See Table 13–4.

ADVANCED PRACTICES FOR THE SURGICAL FIRST ASSISTANT
Chapter 13—Preoperative Medications

KEY TERMS

bowel prep   convulsions   hypertension

MEDICATIONS FROM THE MEDICAL TO THE SURGICAL SETTING

In addition to the preoperative medicines described in the chapter, others must be considered before the patient undergoes a surgical procedure. Medications are prescribed either for surgical preparation or as part of a current therapy for an unrelated condition. One of the most

(continued on following page)

ADVANCED PRACTICES FOR THE SURGICAL FIRST ASSISTANT   *(continued)*

common preparations for all patients undergoing elective gastrointestinal procedures is the **bowel prep**. Healthcare workers often discount this procedure, even though it affects the patient systemically. Other medicines that patients may be taking preoperatively are antihypertensive or anticonvulsive drugs. Patients may remain on these medicines throughout the surgical procedure, usually under the advice of the anesthesia provider. The surgical first assistant should be aware of these medicines and preparations and of their effects on the surgical patient.

Bowel Prep

All patients undergoing an abdominal surgical procedure in which the small bowel, colon, or rectum may be involved are required to perform a preoperative bowel prep. Bowel preps eliminate any bowel content before surgery as well as significantly reduce the population of *Escherichia (E.coli)* and other bacteria normally found in the gastrointestinal tract. The bowel prep is in two phases that the patient performs at home, usually the day before the procedure. This consists of a mechanical phase and a antibiotic phase.

The mechanical phase requires medications to evacuate all feces from the colon. An example of one such medication is the administration of 4 liters of polyethylene glycol-electrolyte solution (PEG-ES). This preparation is taken by mouth, at home, and begins working within an hour. It is mainly performed to facilitate the procedure, not necessarily to prevent wound infections. Polyethylene glycol-electrolyte solution is available in the pharmacy under trade names such as Colyte, NuLytely, and GoLYTELY.

☞ **Note:** There are also medications given in tablet form, as enemas, or as bowel suppositories to achieve the same purpose.

Because these preparations cause diarrhea in order to evacuate fecal material, patients undergoing a bowel prep experience a significant fluid loss. This fact combined with the patient's NPO status requires administration of more fluids intra- and postoperatively. Patients with other medical problems may not tolerate this fluid shift and require hospitalization to complete the prep. The PEG-ES preparation may cause nausea in some patients. Reglan 10 milligrams orally may be prescribed to alleviate the nausea in order to retain the prep.

The antibiotic phase of the bowel prep is to eliminate the bowel of resident bacteria that may cause a wound infection if introduced by spillage. The most notable is *Escherichia (E. coli)*. Antimicrobial medications are administered to the patient preoperatively. The most effective antimicrobial medicines used for bowel preps are neomycin and erythromycin. The regimen consists of the administration of 1 gram neomycin and 1 gram of erythromycin at three selected time intervals the day before surgery as determined by the surgeon. The administration of 1 gram cefazolin and 750 milligrams of metronidazole, intravenously, may also be beneficial when given 30 minutes to one hour before surgery.

Anticonvulsants

Convulsions affect approximately 0.5% to 2% of the population and are treated with medication referred to as anticonvulsants. These medications act on the neurons in the brain by depressing their discharge and preventing seizure activity. Patients require a continuous level

ADVANCED PRACTICES FOR THE SURGICAL FIRST ASSISTANT   *(continued)*

of anticonvulsants to prevent a seizure event. Therefore, surgical patients may need to remain on this therapy throughout the procedure and postoperatively. Anticonvulsants can be placed in several categories, which include benzodiazepines, barbiturates, hydantoins, oxazolidine-diones, and succinimides. There are also several miscellaneous anticonvulsants that are available. Examples of specific medicines are listed in Table A.

HYPERTENSION MEDICINES

Hypertension is defined as a blood pressure greater than 140/90, and affects approximately 25% of the population. The vast majority of hypertensive patients require an antihypertension drug therapy to control the blood pressure. Any interruption of this therapy causes the patient's blood pressure to rise and may have an adverse affect on the outcome of the surgical procedure. Therefore, patients being treated for hypertension are instructed to take their daily medications the morning of surgery.

Physicians today have many medicines in their arsenal to control hypertension. These medicines are grouped according to their effects on the body. There are five groups: diuretics, beta-blockers, angiotensin-converting enzyme (ACE) inhibitors, calcium channel blockers, and alpha-blockers. Patients may require a combination of several in order to control the hypertension. When treating hypertension, it is best to take the staged approach. The patient is prescribed one type of medicine while the healthcare worker monitors the blood pressure. Additional medications from other groups are added until the blood pressure returns to normal level.

Table **A**   Anticonvulsants

Benzodiazepines

diazepam, clonazepam, clorazepate, lorazepam

Barbiturates

omabarbital, phenobarbital, metharbital, mephobarbyial, primidone

Hydantoins

ethotoin, fosphenytoin, mephenytoin, phenytoin

Oxazolidinediones

paramethadione, trimethadione

Succinimides

ethosuximide, methsuximide, phensuximide

Miscellaneous

valproic acid, acetazolamide, carbamazepine, gabapentin, lamotrigine

Key Concepts

- A preoperative assessment is made by the anesthesia team to determine the appropriate anesthetic method.
- A preoperative evaluation consists of a patient interview, physical examination, and medical records review.
- Several general categories of medications are used to prepare the patient both physically and psychologically for surgery. These include sedatives, analgesics, anticholinergics, and several types of gastrointestinal drugs.
- To assist the anesthesia care team, the surgical technologist should be familiar with drugs administered preoperatively and their purposes.

PATIENT MONITORING AND LOCAL AND REGIONAL ANESTHESIA

Medications Covered in Chapter 14		
Generic Name	*Brand Name*	*Category*
lidocaine	Xylocaine	Amide anesthetic
bupivacaine	Marcaine, Sensorcaine	Amide anesthetic
mepivacaine	Carbocaine, Polocaine	Amide anesthetic
cocaine	N/A	Ester anesthetic
midazolam	Versed	Sedative
fentanyl	Sublimaze	Opioid analgesic
alfentanil	Alfenta	Opioid analgesic
meperidine	Demerol	Opioid analgesic
propofol	Diprivan	Intravenous induction anesthetic

OBJECTIVES

After completing this chapter, you should be able to:

1. Define terminology related to patient monitoring and anesthesia.
2. Describe types of patient-monitoring devices.
3. Compare and contrast local anesthesia, monitored anesthesia care, and regional anesthesia.
4. List surgical procedures that may be performed under local or regional anesthesia.
5. Identify common agents used in local anesthesia and regional anesthesia.
6. Discuss the use of epinephrine in local anesthetic agents.
7. Describe types of regional blocks.

KEY TERMS

ABGs
asystole
auscultation
blood pressure
bradycardia
capnometry
central venous pressure–monitoring catheter (CVP line)
dysrhythmias
electrocardiography
electroencephalogram
epidural

exsanguination
intrathecally
laryngospasm
local anesthesia
monitored anesthesia care (MAC)
precordial
premature ventricular contraction (PVC)
pulse oximetry
regional anesthesia
tachycardia
vasoconstrictor
vasodilation

Surgical intervention and the administration of anesthetic agents is a complex and challenging process that places enormous physiologic stress on the patient. Thus, the physiologic status of each surgical patient is closely monitored throughout any surgical procedure by assessing the patient's vital signs. Monitoring the patient's physiologic status during surgery has become more comprehensive and precise, enabling continuous assessment of critical indicators. The surgical technologist must become familiar with the various means of patient monitoring, components of the devices, and purposes. Although the primary focus of the scrubbed surgical technologist is at the surgical site, it is crucial that each team member be aware of the patient's well-being at all times, to provide support to the anesthesia provider and patient when necessary.

The term *anesthesia* means "without sensation." The patient may be conscious or unconscious, but while receiving any type of anesthesia, he or she should not perceive pain. The precise chemical and physiologic means by which anesthetics work is not yet fully clear; but we do know that the mechanism depends on the type of agent being administered. Some drugs, for instance, induce amnesia, whereas others induce unconsciousness or change the perception of pain. There are three major types of anesthetic techniques: local, regional, and general. This chapter presents basic information on local and regional anesthesia. Basic concepts of general anesthesia are covered in Chapter 15.

PATIENT MONITORING

Each of the patient's vital signs is continuously monitored during surgical intervention. Physiologic vital signs monitored on all surgical patients include heart rate and rhythm, respirations, oxygen saturation, and blood pressure. During general anesthesia, additional monitors include temperature, **capnometry**, and level of awareness. Certain patient conditions and some particular surgical procedures may require advanced or invasive monitoring methods such as placement of arterial or venous pressure lines. See Table 14–1 for a summary of the most common physiologic functions monitored in the surgical patient.

ELECTROCARDIOGRAPHY

The patient's heart rate and rhythm will be continually assessed using **electrocardiography**. Electrodes that sense the electrical activity of the heart are placed on the patient's skin and attached to leads, which transmit those electrical impulses to the electro-

Table **14–1** Summary of the Most Common Physiologic Functions Monitored in Surgical Patients
Electrocardiogram (ECG, EKG)
Pulse oximetry
Blood pressure
Temperature
Capnometry
Consciousness
Neuromuscular function
Arterial pressure
Central venous pressure
Pulmonary artery pressure

cardiogram (ECG) device. The electrical activity of the heart is recorded and displayed on a screen. The ECG device may be set to record a tracing of the electrical activity on a strip of paper or emit an audible signal to indicate heart rate.

The ECG may be recorded using 3-lead or 5-lead systems. The surgical technologist in the circulating role may assist the anesthesia provider in placing the electrodes, which should be securely adhered to areas of clean, dry skin. The electrodes should be protected from prep solutions and placed so that a change in the patient's position (e.g., supine to lateral) will not disrupt electrode contact. In a 5-lead system, electrodes are placed on each shoulder, each hip, and in the fifth intercostal space near the left anterior axillary line. A baseline reading is obtained, and the ECG is used to monitor changes in the heart rate and rhythm during surgery.

The ECG is supplemented by **auscultation** (listening to the sounds of the chest, i.e., the heart rate, rhythm, and pulmonary sounds) with a **precordial** stethoscope. A modified version of a standard stethoscope, the precordial stethoscope is taped onto the patient's chest at the level of the diaphragm or at the suprasternal notch. A long piece of tubing extends from the stethoscope to a specialized earpiece placed in the anesthesia provider's ear.

A review of basic physiology of the electrical conduction system of the heart is highly recommended. The surgical technologist should be able to interpret a normal ECG cycle, including the meaning of the P wave, QRS complex, and T wave. By listening to the audible ECG in the background noise of the operating room, the surgical technologist should be able to appreciate various types of **dysrhythmias**, including **bradycardia, tachycardia,** and **asystole.** In addition, the surgical technologist should be able to identify a **premature ventricular contraction (PVC)** and the presence of an active pacemaker by its characteristic spike. Each of these abilities contributes to the surgical technologist's value as a surgical team member. The ability to recognize and appreciate the importance of changes in heart rate and rhythm enables the surgical technologist to provide assistance to the anesthesia provider and patient when necessary.

PULSE OXIMETRY

Pulse oximetry is a noninvasive measure of the oxygen saturation of blood. A two-sided sensor probe is attached to a finger, toe, or earlobe (Fig. 14–1). The probe emits red and infrared light, which is absorbed while passing through tissue. Remaining light is detected by the opposite side of the sensor probe and used to

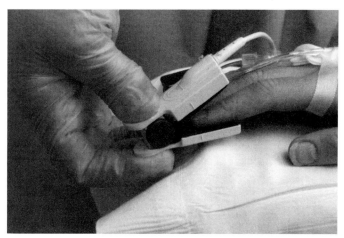

Figure **14–1.**   A sensor probe clip for the pulse oximeter is attached to the patient's finger.

calculate the saturation of peripheral oxygen (SpO_2 or SaO_2). Ideally, the saturation should be above 95%. An audible signal reflects pulse rate and the signal tone indicates saturation. The deeper the tone, the lower the saturation. Readings may be affected by intense room lighting, administration of intravenous dyes such as methylene blue, patient movement, or hypothermia.

> Even while cleaning up the back table after a procedure, the surgical technologist should be alert to the rate and tone of the pulse oximeter. A slow pulse or dropping oxygen saturation during emergence from anesthesia may signal an emergency situation such as **laryngospasm** (see Chapter 16). The surgical technologist must be able to identify such a situation, stop cleanup duties, and turn full attention to the patient and the needs of the anesthesia provider until the crisis has been resolved.

BLOOD PRESSURE

Blood pressure (BP) is a measure of the force of blood against the vessel walls. Normal blood pressure in an adult is considered to be less than 130 mm Hg systolic and less than 85 mm Hg diastolic. Recent discussion, however, indicates that opinions may be changing regarding what is considered a normal blood pressure measurement. In adults over age 50, a measurement that was once accepted as normal blood pressure may be considered prehypertensive. Multiple variables affect blood pressure, including ventricular contraction strength, capillary resistance, vessel wall elasticity, and blood volume. An inflatable cuff of appropriate size is placed on the patient's upper arm, preferably not the arm that has the intravenous cannula in place. The cuff is connected to a device that automatically measures blood pressure at specified intervals. The machine can be set to emit an audible alarm if blood pressure is not within preset parameters.

TEMPERATURE

All patients under general anesthesia are at risk for mild to significant hypothermia and the rare event of malignant hyperthermia. Pediatric and geriatric patients are particularly vulnerable to a drop in temperature. Several precautions are taken to minimize heat loss, and the patient's body temperature is continually monitored to verify the effectiveness of those precautions. Temperature may be taken from any number of locations, including skin, axilla, bladder, esophagus, and ear. Normal core temperature varies within a limited range near 98° F (37° C), so a baseline measurement is obtained and changes are monitored and assessed.

CAPNOMETRY

Capnometry is a measurement of carbon dioxide (CO_2) exhaled by the patient during general anesthesia, called end-tidal CO_2. An adapter is connected to the breathing circuit and a small tubing extends from the adapter to the analyzer (Fig. 14–2). The concentration of expired CO_2 is measured and displayed as a continuous graph and in numerical value. Capnometry is an extremely valuable tool in the assessment of respiratory function and can serve a critical role in early detection of problems such as compromised ventilation or malignant hyperthermia (see Chapter 16).

MONITORING CONSCIOUSNESS

Traditionally, the depth of various components of general anesthesia has been monitored in several ways, including basic vital signs and nerve stimulation. However, traditional monitoring methods were not sufficient to adequately assess the level of patient awareness under anesthesia. Patient awareness while under anesthesia is a rare but significant concern (see Chapter 15) estimated to occur in approximately 1 to 2 of 1000 patients under-

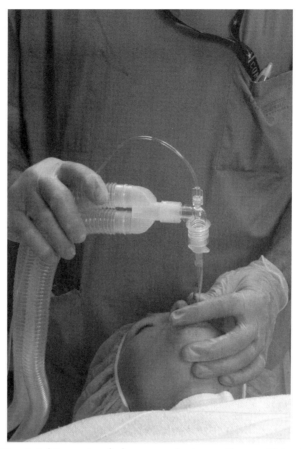

Figure **14–2.**   A tubing extends from an adapter on the ventilator tubing to the respiratory analyzer to measure expired CO_2.

going general anesthesia. In an effort to assist the anesthesia provider in assessing the depth of consciousness (hypnosis) under anesthesia, another monitoring tool, the Bispectral Index Monitor (BIS), has been developed. The BIS monitor is a modified **electroencephalogram** (EEG) used to determine the level of consciousness. EEG information is obtained from a sensor placed on the patient's forehead. The BIS monitor interprets the information and displays a reading between 0 and 100, indicating the level of consciousness. A number near 100 indicates that the patient is fully awake and responsive and a number less than 60 indicates an appropriate depth of general anesthesia with a low probability of explicit recall (see Chapter 15).

NEUROMUSCULAR FUNCTION

During general anesthesia, muscle relaxants are administered to allow endotracheal intubation (see Chapter 15). A nerve stimulator is used to assess neuromuscular function and the extent of blockade. A stimulus is delivered to the nerve from a surface electrode or probe, often placed at the ulnar nerve or a branch of the facial nerve. Four stimuli (train of four, or TOF) are administered, and the extent of the block is estimated based on the twitch response. The presence of four of the four twitches indicates no muscle relaxation, whereas zero of the four twitches indicates full muscle relaxation. Nerve stimulation is used to determine if the vocal cords are adequately relaxed for intubation and to determine when additional muscle relaxants should be administered during a surgical procedure. Nerve stimulation is also used to assess the extent to which muscle relaxants are wearing off and the patient is becoming ready to breathe on his or her own after surgery.

ADVANCED MONITORING

Certain patient conditions and surgical procedures may require additional monitoring. These invasive monitoring techniques include arterial catheterization and pressure monitoring, central venous catheterization and pressure monitoring, and pulmonary artery catheterization (Swan-Ganz catheter). An arterial pressure–monitoring catheter (often referred to as an arterial line or art-line) is usually placed in the radial artery and allows continuous, immediate, and highly accurate measurement of blood pressure. Placement of an arterial line is indicated for a number of reasons, including potential for rapid changes in blood pressure, frequent sampling of arterial blood for blood gas analysis (**ABGs**), or when routine blood pressure measurement is inaccurate. A **central venous pressure–monitoring catheter (CVP line)** is positioned in the vena cava and is used to assess the volume of blood returning to the heart. A CVP line is also used to assess the need for fluid replacement and to prevent fluid overload. A pulmonary artery (PA) catheter (such as a Swan-Ganz catheter) is guided through the heart into a branch of the pulmonary artery to obtain measurements of central venous pressure, pulmonary artery pressure, pulmonary capillary wedge pressure, and cardiac output. PA catheters are most frequently used in adult patients during cardiac surgery, lung transplantation, and liver transplantation.

When the patient has been admitted to the operating room and all the appropriate basic monitoring devices are in place, baseline measurements are recorded and the patient is ready for administration of anesthesia. Invasive monitoring devices may be placed after the patient is anesthetized.

LOCAL AND REGIONAL ANESTHESIA

To accomplish anesthesia, transmission of the sensation of pain through nerve impulses may be interrupted at several locations, including nerve endings, groups of nerves, or at the brain. **Local anesthesia** is the administration of an anesthetic agent to nerve endings in the surgical site. **Regional anesthesia** is accomplished by the administration of the same type of agents, but at a group of nerves called a plexus. Regional anesthesia provides both sensory and motor block to an entire area of the body, because a group of nerves is anesthetized. General anesthesia (see Chapter 15) interferes with the brain's ability to interpret pain impulses coming from anywhere in the body.

LOCAL ANESTHESIA

A local anesthetic is administered to the immediate surgical site. Whether injected into tissue or applied topically to mucosal membranes, it affects a small, circumscribed area. Local anesthetics, such as lidocaine, interfere with sensory nerve endings in the operative area; thus, they block transmission of pain impulses to the brain. When local anesthesia is used without an anesthesia provider present, it is imperative that a registered nurse be assigned to monitor the patient's vital signs during the surgical procedure. The registered nurse assesses the patient's physical condition and psychological status so that appropriate measures can be taken to maintain patient safety and comfort. Heart rate and electrical activity are measured by ECG, whereas blood pressure, respirations, and oxygen saturation are monitored continuously. The registered nurse may also administer sedatives as ordered by the surgeon. Only physically healthy and psychologically stable patients undergoing brief, uncomplicated surgical procedures are appropriate candidates for local anesthesia without monitoring by an anesthesia provider.

Applications for Local Anesthesia

Local anesthesia without anesthesia provider standby has several applications. In general surgery, local injections are appropriate for excision or biopsy of small soft tissue masses such as lipomas, nevi, or lesions. In orthopedic surgery, local anesthesia is used for limited work on digits, such as repair of finger lacerations or toenail excisions. Local injection is used in otorhinolaryngology and plastic surgery for minor facial procedures, such as excision of lesions, and for nasal procedures such as septoplasty. In urology, cystoscopy may be performed with a topical anesthetic agent. Because local anesthesia blocks sensory nerve impulses only at the site of injection or application, the patient cannot feel pain in that area but is still able to move muscles and feel pressure.

Agents Used for Local Anesthesia

The three most common local anesthetic agents used in surgery are lidocaine, bupivicaine, and mepivicaine (Fig. 14–3). Each of these agents may be combined with dilute epinephrine (see Chapter 8) to increase the duration of effect. Recall that epinephrine is a potent **vasoconstrictor.** When combined with a local anesthetic agent, epinephrine causes local vasoconstriction slowing the absorption of the agent into the circulatory system. This action keeps the local anesthetic in the surgical site longer, thus increasing the duration of effect.

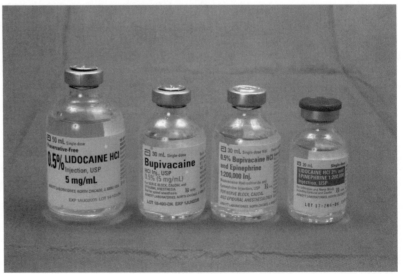

Figure **14–3.** Lidocaine and bupivacaine are available with and without epinephrine.

⚠ **CAUTION**

Epinephrine premixed in a local anesthetic agent is present in very tiny amounts (most commonly one part of epinephrine to 100,000 or 200,000 parts of the anesthetic). The surgical technologist must be aware that epinephrine is also available separately in the very high concentration of 1:1000, 100 times or 200 times stronger than the dose intended for injection (see Chapter 8). It is vital to administer epinephrine in the correct concentration for the correct purpose and by the correct route. If the high 1:1000 concentration of epinephrine is inadvertently injected, severe tachycardia (rapid heart rate) and hypertension will result, increasing the potential for cardiac arrest. All medications present on the sterile field must be correctly labeled (name and dose) and identified when passing to the surgeon to avoid medication administration errors.

The most common local anesthetic agent in use today is lidocaine (Xylocaine), which is classified chemically as an aminoamide compound. Lidocaine is fast acting and rapidly metabolized. The duration of anesthesia with infiltrated lidocaine is 30 to 60 minutes. If epinephrine is added to a lidocaine solution, the duration of effect is increased by approximately 50%. In addition, epinephrine will slow systemic absorption of lidocaine resulting in prolonged effect. Lidocaine is available in solutions of 0.5%, 1%, 1.5%, and 2%, with and without epinephrine 1:100,000 and 1:200,000. See Table 14–2 for a comparison of common local anesthetic agents.

☞ **Note:** Many people mistakenly refer to lidocaine as Novocain, which is a completely different agent. Novocain is the trade name for procaine, which was used by dentists for many years, but is seldom used currently. Procaine is classified chemically as an aminoester–type anesthetic. Aminoester–type anesthetics cause more allergic reactions than aminoamide–type anesthetics. Patients

Table **14–2** Comparison of Common Local Anesthetic Agents

Generic Name	Trade Name	Solutions Available	Duration (hours)
lidocaine	Xylocaine	0.5%, 1%, 1.5%, 2%	0.5–1.5
with epinephrine			1–2
bupivacaine	Marcaine, Sensorcaine	0.25%, 0.5%, 0.75%	4
with epinephrine			8–12
mepivacaine	Carbocaine, Polocaine	1%, 1.5%, 2%, 3%	0.75–1.5
cocaine	N/A	4%, 10%	0.5–2

who are allergic to Novocain do not usually have allergies to lidocaine, because these agents have different chemical structures.

Bupivacaine (Marcaine, Sensorcaine) is an aminoamide anesthetic, which is about four times more potent than lidocaine and has a longer duration, up to 4 hours. Bupivicaine is available in solutions of 0.25%, 0.5%, and 0.75%, with and without epinephrine 1:200,000. When combined with epinephrine, the action of bupivicaine may last for 8 to 12 hours.

Mepivacaine (Carbocaine, Polocaine) is another aminoamide anesthetic that has a similar potency to lidocaine, with slightly longer duration (45 to 90 minutes). Mepivacaine is available in solutions of 1%, 1.5%, 2%, and 3% solution and may be combined with epinephrine.

The only aminoester–type anesthetic agent used in surgery is cocaine. Cocaine is a naturally occurring alkaloid derived from coca leaves. It has long been known to have a numbing effect when used topically on mucous membranes. Today, it is used frequently in nasal surgery.

 CAUTION

Cocaine is for topical use only; it is never injected.

Cocaine comes in 4% and 10% solutions; thus it may be administered on cotton applicators or nasal packing, or it may be sprayed directly on the mucosal surface. In addition to its anesthetic properties, cocaine is the only local anesthetic agent that is also a powerful vasoconstrictor. This means it reduces bleeding and helps shrink mucous membranes. Thus it's particularly useful in nasal surgery because it allows better visualization in the nasal cavity. It also means that dosage is critical. Dosages must be carefully calculated, both to the patient's age and physical condition, using the lowest dose necessary to achieve the required anesthetic effect. Concentrations greater than 4% increase potential for systemic toxic reactions. The maximum safe dose is 1.5 mg/kg. Adverse effects are seen primarily in the central nervous system. These include excitement and depression, and may lead to respiratory arrest.

 CAUTION

Cocaine is a controlled substance. It should never be left unattended in the operating room, and any cocaine solution dispensed but unused should be returned to the pharmacy or destroyed. At least two people should witness the destruction of unused cocaine to verify that it has not been used for illicit purposes (see Chapter 2).

Table **14–3** Comparison of Approximate Maximum Dosages of Local Anesthetics for Infiltration			
Agent	*Concentration*	*Volume (mL)*	*Dose (mg/kg)*
lidocaine without epinephrine	0.5%	up to 60	up to 4.5
with epinephrine		up to 100	up to 7
bupivacaine	0.25%	up to 70	up to 2
mepivacaine	1%	up to 40	up to 7

Note: This table is intended for comparison only and not for use as clinical dosage recommendations.

Adverse reactions to amide local anesthetics are primarily dose-related and affect both the central nervous system and the cardiovascular system. See Table 14–3 for a comparison of maximum dosages of local anesthetics. Adverse central nervous system effects are variable, from drowsiness at low doses to excitement or agitation at higher doses. Excitement may or may not occur, and the patient may go from a drowsy state to unconsciousness and into respiratory arrest. Nausea and vomiting may also occur. Cardiovascular adverse effects are also dose-related and include hypotension, bradycardia, and ventricular arrhythmias leading to possible cardiac arrest.

Monitored Anesthesia Care

Monitored anesthesia care (MAC) is a term used to indicate the presence of an anesthesia provider during a surgical procedure performed under local anesthesia. The anesthetic method is the same as regular local anesthesia; that is, the use of a topical or injected local anesthetic agent at the surgical site is the same. The anesthesia provider is present for a number of reasons, including more complicated surgical procedures, potential need for conscious sedation, and patients with conditions necessitating a higher level of care. Common applications for MAC include transvenous pacemaker insertion, venous access port or catheter insertion, or placement of a dialysis access graft. The anesthesia provider monitors the patient's heart rate and ECG, blood pressure, respirations, and oxygen saturation continuously. In some cases, the anesthesia provider must also administer supplemental sedation or pain control to ensure that the patient is relaxed and comfortable. Common sedatives and analgesics that may be administered include midazolam (Versed), fentanyl (Sublimaze), alfentanil (Alfenta), meperidine (Demerol), and propofol (Diprivan).

REGIONAL ANESTHESIA

Regional anesthesia blocks nerves (not just nerve endings) at specific locations; thus, it provides a larger anesthetized area. Whereas local anesthesia involves injection of a local anesthetic at the operative site, regional anesthesia involves injecting a local anesthetic into the nerves that supply the operative region. Regional blocks affect sympathetic, sensory, and motor nerve supply, so an anesthetized limb becomes immobile as well as numb. Regional blocks are effective for many types of surgical procedures. Various types of regional anesthetic techniques are named for the areas of the body to be blocked. Although nearly any group of nerves can be blocked, we discuss only the most frequently used regional anesthetic techniques in this text.

Spinal Anesthesia

In spinal anesthesia, agents are injected **intrathecally,** that is, through the dura mater, into the subarachnoid space, usually in the lumbar area of the spine (Fig. 14–4). This technique anesthetizes the entire lower body. The circulator commonly assists the anesthesia provider during injection of a spinal anesthetic by helping the patient to get into optimum position (Fig. 14–5). The patient may be positioned laterally to facilitate correct needle placement. That is, patients may lie on the side, with knees bent and chin on chest. Thus, the patient is usually instructed to curl up as much as possible, pushing his or her lower back out toward the anesthesia provider. This position spreads the vertebral bodies apart so the spinal needle may be more easily inserted. It is, however, difficult for some patients, especially the elderly, to curl their backs. These patients may be assisted gently into position, using caution to avoid injury. Alternatively, patients may be in a sitting position for administration of a spinal anesthetic (Fig. 14–6). The patient may sit on the operating bed with his or her back to the anesthesia provider.

Spinal anesthesia is often used for transurethral resection of the prostate gland or bladder tumors, for lower leg vascular procedures such as embolectomy, orthopedic procedures, and for cesarean sections. Most local anesthetics can be used for spinal injection.

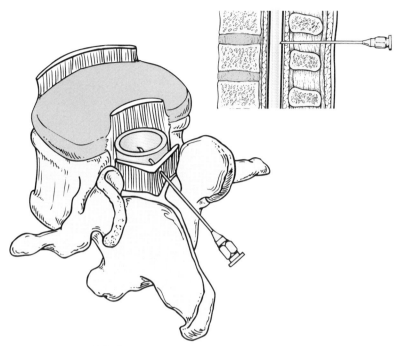

Figure **14–4.**   Location of spinal anesthesia injection.

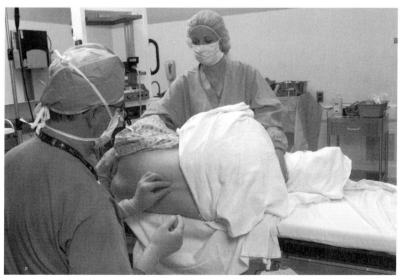

Figure **14–5.**   Patient positioned laterally for spinal administration.

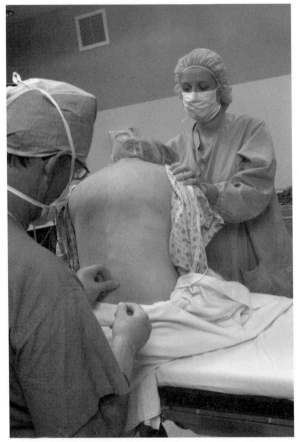

Figure **14–6.**   Patient in a sitting position for spinal administration.

A drop in blood pressure may occur with administration of a spinal or epidural anesthetic because of **vasodilation** (sympathectomy).

Epidural Anesthesia

In **epidural** anesthesia, an anesthetic agent is injected into the space surrounding the dura mater (Fig. 14–7). A single injection may be administered, or a catheter may be placed for continuous injection. Positioning for administration of an epidural anesthetic is identical to that described for a spinal anesthetic. Epidural anesthesia is used to relieve the pain of labor and vaginal delivery, as well as to provide anesthesia for cesarean section. Epidural blocks

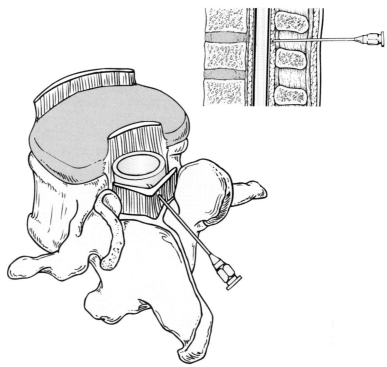

Figure **14–7.** Location of epidural anesthesia injection.

may also be used as an adjunct to general anesthesia to minimize the amount of agents needed; they may also be used for postoperative pain control after such procedures as thoracotomy.

Caudal Block

Caudal anesthesia is a type of epidural block injected into the epidural space via the sacral canal (Fig. 14–8). Caudal blocks used for vaginal childbirth are administered in the obstetrical unit rather than in the surgical suite. Caudal blocks may also be used in conjunction with general anesthesia for lower-extremity procedures in children and for postoperative pain management.

Retrobulbar Block

Retrobulbar blocks are injected behind the eye into the muscle cone (Fig. 14–9). These blocks may be used for procedures requiring a motionless, anesthetized eye. Retrobulbar blocks may be

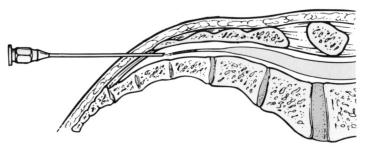

Figure **14–8.** Location of caudal block.

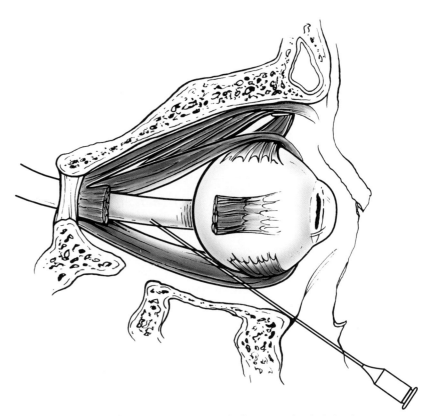

Figure **14–9.** Location of retrobulbar anesthesia injection.

administered by an ophthalmologist or an anesthesia provider. To minimize patient discomfort, a sedative may be given intravenously prior to retrobulbar injection. Once the most common anesthesia technique for cataract extraction, retrobulbar blocks are less frequently used today.

Extremity Block

There are several techniques for extremity (distal arms and legs; particularly, the hand and fingers, foot and toes) block. These techniques vary depending on the anesthesia provider's expertise and preference, but in practice the upper extremities (arm, hand, fingers) are more frequently blocked than the lower extremities. The arm may be blocked at several locations—including the median, radial, and ulnar nerve—whereas the leg may be blocked at the femoral, obturator, or sciatic nerves. Depending on the surgical site, portions of the hand, foot, and digits may also be blocked.

In some cases, the arm is blocked via the axillary approach (at the armpit) at the brachial plexus (a network of nerves that serve the arm). In this case, the entire arm is numbed and immobilized when an anesthetic is injected into the tissue surrounding the brachial plexus, as shown in Figure 14–10. Because it is important not to penetrate the nerve sheath or damage nearby blood vessels when performing this technique, a needle attached to a nerve stimulator is inserted first. This allows the anesthesia provider to precisely locate the nerves of the brachial plexus. This technique is used for manipulation and casting of fractures in patients who present a high risk for complications of general anesthesia; thus, it's a favored technique for use in alcohol-intoxicated patients whose central nervous system is already depressed.

One of the most common extremity blocks is the Bier block. Bier block, or intravenous block, is a technique that involves pre-

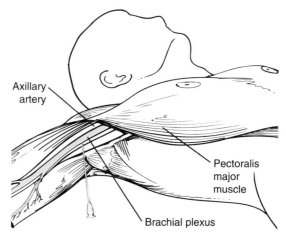

Figure **14–10.**   Location of axillary block injection.

liminary **exsanguination**—that is, the extremity is first rendered bloodless by constriction and elevation. This technique can be employed for procedures on upper and lower distal extremities, although it is most frequently used for procedures on hands (such as release of carpal tunnel, trigger finger, or Dupuytren's contracture). It is seldom used for fracture reduction because of the discomfort occasioned by exsanguination. For a procedure on the hand, for example, a pneumatic or electric double-cuffed tourniquet is placed around the proximal (upper) arm. An intravenous catheter is inserted in a vein of the hand and blood is forced from the distal limb by wrapping the arm with a rubber bandage (Fig. 14–11). One cuff of the tourniquet is inflated, the bandage is removed, and a local anesthetic is injected into the catheter. The

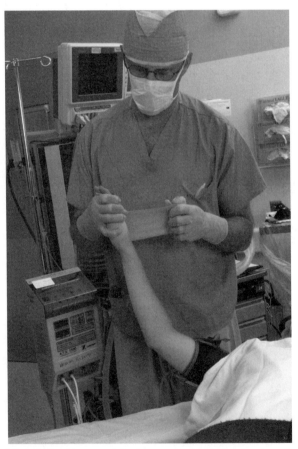

Figure **14–11.**   Patient's extremity is exsanguinated prior to administration of a Bier block.

tourniquet remains inflated throughout the procedure to keep the anesthetic agent in the area. If the cuff pressure becomes too uncomfortable for the patient, the second cuff is inflated and the first cuff is deflated, which provides a measure of relief. Once the surgical procedure is completed, the tourniquet cuff is released slowly to avoid rapid infusion of the anesthetic into the systemic circulation. Bier block is both rapid and effective; but there may be some discomfort caused by exsanguination and tourniquet use. Often the patient requires mild sedation.

Most regional extremity blocks have one primary disadvantage—it takes time for them to take effect. This means they may delay surgery. Extremity blocks may therefore be administered in the preoperative holding area. However, it is difficult to time the block so that the patient is ready when the operating room becomes available. Any type of regional anesthesia requires continuous monitoring of the patient's vital functions, including heart rate and ECG, blood pressure, respirations, and oxygen saturation.

ADVANCED PRACTICES FOR THE SURGICAL FIRST ASSISTANT
Chapter 14—Patient Monitoring and Local and Regional Anesthesia

KEY TERMS

circumoral   para-aminobenzoic acid (PABA)
erythema   urticaria

CLASSIFICATIONS OF LOCAL ANESTHETIC

Local anesthetics are classified into two groups: aminoesters (esters) and aminoamides (amides). The structural difference of these two agents is the pathway in which they are metabolized and their allergic potential. Esters are relatively unstable in solution and are rapidly hydrolyzed in the body by acetylcholinesterase at the neuromuscular junction. One of the metabolic products of hydrolysis is **para-aminobenzoic acid (PABA),** which is associated with hypersensitivity and allergic reactions. Ester agents include cocaine, procaine, tetracaine, and chloroprocaine. Amides are relatively stable in solution, and are slowly metabolized by the enzymes in the liver. Allergic reactions are extremely rare and so amides are more commonly used in current clinical practice. Amides include lidocaine, prilocaine, bupivacaine, and mepivacaine.

(continued on following page)

ADVANCED PRACTICES FOR THE SURGICAL FIRST ASSISTANT   *(continued)*

CAUTION

Because amides are metabolized in the liver, care should be used in patients with severe liver disease or patients taking medication that interferes with the metabolism. Monitoring for signs of toxicity is critical.

ADVERSE EFFECTS OF LOCAL ANESTHETIC

In the surgical first assistant role, it is imperative to understand that the principal adverse effects of local anesthetics are allergic reactions and systemic toxicity. Keep in mind that aminoamides are less allergenic than aminoesters (because of the metabolic product PABA) and that although rare, allergic reactions can be life-threatening.

Allergic reactions are classified into two categories: local and systemic. A local allergic reaction (hypersensitivity) is similar to allergic contact dermatitis. Clinical signs may include **erythema, urticaria,** and edema. Systemic allergic reactions (anaphylactic signs) may include generalized erythema, urticaria, facial edema, wheezing, bronchoconstriction, cyanosis, nausea, vomiting, hypotension, and cardiovascular collapse. Treatment is symptomatic and supportive (see Chapter 16).

Systemic toxicity of local anesthesia is due to excess concentration of the medication in the blood. This effect is most often encountered after an accidental intravascular injection or administration of an excessive dose of the anesthetic (Table A).

Systemic toxicity of local anesthetics involves the central nervous system (CNS) and the cardiovascular system. Signs and symptoms of CNS toxicity may include tinnitus, **circumoral** numbness, metallic taste in mouth, lightheaded, visual disturbances, nausea and vomiting, slurred speech, muscular twitching, seizures, and coma.

Table **A**   Maximum Dosages of Local Anesthetic Agents

Anesthetic	Duration (min)	Duration with Epinephrine (min)	Maximum Dose (mg/kg)	Maximum Dose with Epinephrine (mg/kg)
Esters				
cocaine	45	—	2.8	—
procaine	15–30	30–90	7.1	8.5
tetracaine	120–240	240–480	1.4	—
Amides				
lidocaine	30–120	60–400	4.5	7.0
mepivacaine	30–120	03–120	4.5	7.0
bupivacaine	120–240	240–480	2.5	3.2

ADVANCED PRACTICES FOR THE SURGICAL FIRST ASSISTANT *(continued)*

Cardiovascular toxicity can produce reduced cardiac contractility, vasodilation, and dysrhythmias. Severe systemic toxicity is treated by maintaining the patient's airway, and administering oxygen and fluids. Seizures are controlled with diazepam, thiopental, or succinylcholine. Cardiac instability may be managed with vasodilators, antiarrhythmics, and inotropes. Systemic absorption of the anesthetic can be reduced by one third with the addition of vasoconstrictor such as epinephrine.

CONCENTRATION OR DOSAGE

Local anesthetics are presented in percent of concentration or percent of strength. They are calculated as the number of grams of medication in 100 mL of solution. Therefore, a 2% lidocaine solution is 2 grams of medication in 100 mL of solution. A further breakdown of this concept would be 2 grams equals 2000 mg; therefore, each 100 mL of solution contains 2000 mg of lidocaine. Breaking it down further, 1 mL contains 20 mg of lidocaine. A quick calculation is to move the decimal point one place to the left, because this will determine mg/mL of local anesthetic. Examples are:

2.0% = 20 mg/mL
1.0% = 10 mg/mL

EPINEPHRINE ADDITIVE TO LOCAL ANESTHETICS

Epinephrine acts as a vasoconstrictor that not only decreases bleeding but also slows the rate of systemic absorption of the aesthetic. This allows the body more time to metabolize the anesthetic and prolongs the anesthetic effects. Given the slower absorption rate, a larger volume of anesthetic with epinephrine can be injected without causing toxicity. Epinephrine can be used in a variety of surgical procedures. An example of this is septoplasty with inferior turbinectomies. A local anesthetic with epinephrine is beneficial because of the vascularity of the nasal mucosa and the confined space within the nasal cavity.

ASSISTANT ADVICE

Local anesthetics containing epinephrine will have red labels or red printing noting the concentration of epinephrine.

(continued on following page)

ADVANCED PRACTICES FOR THE SURGICAL FIRST ASSISTANT   *(continued)*

Concentrations of epinephrine are described as a ratio (for example, 1:100,000 or 1:200,000) and are calculated as the number of grams of the agent in a given volume of solution. The previous examples show 1 gram of epinephrine in 100,000 mL of solution and 1 gram of epinephrine in 200,000 mL of solution respectively. If the number of grams is always one, then the greater the number on the other side of the ratio, the less concentrated the solution becomes. A 1:100,000 solution of epinephrine is stronger than a 1:200,000 solution.

 CAUTION

Local anesthetics containing epinephrine should never be used in an area in which vascular supply is minimal, such as fingers, tip of nose, penis, and toes.

POSTOPERATIVE PAIN MANAGEMENT WITH LOCAL AND REGIONAL ANESTHETICS

Traditionally oral or intramuscular anesthetics or opioids have been used for postoperative pain management. Despite the belief that opioids provide optimal pain relief, studies have shown that more than half of the surgical patients receiving opioids remain in moderate to severe pain. The recognition that unrelieved pain contributes to perioperative morbidity and mortality has inspired new pre-emptive analgesic techniques to control postoperative pain. The surgical first assistant may be involved with implementing various techniques for pain control during the procedure.

Local anesthetics can be administered into the incision sites or intra-articularly. An example is bupivacaine, which can provide approximately six hours of pain control. The maximum dose of bupivacaine for infiltration is 175 mg (70 mL of 0.25% solution). Another alternative is continuous local infusion therapy (site-specific infusion) when a catheter is placed in the incision site or intra-articularly, and a continuous infusion or boluses of local anesthetic can be administered with patient controlled pumps. The pump dispenses 2 mL or 4 mL of local anesthetic to the surgical site per hour. Depending on the type of pump, a 4-mL-bolus chamber can be squeezed, providing additional medication to the site. These pumps are disposable and have 2- or 4-day duration.

KEY CONCEPTS

- The vital signs of all patients undergoing surgical intervention must be closely monitored.
- Vital signs monitored on all patients include heart rate and rhythm, oxygen saturation, blood pressure, and respirations.
- Additional parameters measured under general anesthesia include temperature, expired CO_2, consciousness level, and neuromuscular function.

- Certain patient conditions and surgical procedures may require additional invasive monitoring such as arterial pressure, central venous pressure, and pulmonary artery pressure.
- When basic monitoring parameters are established, the appropriate anesthetic method is administered. More invasive monitors are placed after the patient is under anesthesia.
- Three main types of anesthesia methods are used: local (with or without MAC), regional blockade, and general.
- Several agents are used to produce local and regional anesthesia, and there are many applications for these techniques.

15

GENERAL ANESTHESIA

Medications Covered in Chapter 15

Generic Name	Brand Name	Category
midazolam	Versed	Sedative
diazepam	Valium	Sedative
lorazepam	Ativan	Sedative
thiopental	Pentothal	Hypnotic agent (barbiturate)
methohexital	Brevital	Hypnotic agent (barbiturate)
propofol	Diprivan	Hypnotic agent
ketamine	Ketalar	Hypnotic agent
etomidate	Amidate	Hypnotic agent
fentanyl	Sublimaze	Opioid analgesic
alfentanil	Alfenta	Opioid analgesic
sufentanil	Sufenta	Opioid analgesic
remifentanyl	Ultiva	Opioid analgesic
nitrous oxide (N_2O)	N/A	Inhalation anesthetic
isoflurane	Forane	Inhalation anesthetic
desflurane	Suprane	Inhalation anesthetic
sevoflurane	Ultane	Inhalation anesthetic

(continued on following page)

Medications Covered in Chapter 15   *(continued)*

Generic Name	Brand Name	Category
succinylcholine	Anectine	Depolarizing muscle relaxant
atracurium besylate	Tracrium	Nondepolarizing muscle relaxant
mivacurium chloride	Mivacron	Nondepolarizing muscle relaxant
pancuronium bromide	Pavulon	Nondepolarizing muscle relaxant
rocuronium bromide	Zemuron	Nondepolarizing muscle relaxant
tubocurarine chloride	Curare	Nondepolarizing muscle relaxant
vecuronium bromide	Norcuron	Nondepolarizing muscle relaxant
naloxone	Narcan	Reversal agent for opioid analgesics
nalmefene	Revex	Reversal agent for opioid analgesics
naltrexone	ReVia, Trexan	Reversal agent for opioid analgesics
flumazenil	Mazicon	Reversal agent for benzodiazepines
neostigmine	Prostigmin	Reversal agent for nondepolarizing muscle relaxants
edrophonium	Tensilon	Reversal agent for nondepolarizing muscle relaxants

OBJECTIVES

After completing this chapter, you should be able to:

1. Define terminology related to anesthesia.
2. Discuss indications for general anesthesia.
3. Identify anesthesia equipment.
4. Explain the basic components of a general anesthetic.
5. List methods of inducing general anesthesia.
6. Define the phases of general anesthesia.
7. Discuss options for airway management.
8. Describe the process of endotracheal intubation.
9. Discuss the concept of awareness under anesthesia.
10. List agents used to accomplish general anesthesia.
11. Identify the purposes and categories of agents used in general anesthesia.
12. Identify generic and trade names of common agents used in anesthesia.
13. State the phase of anesthesia in which various agents are administered.
14. Compare and contrast depolarizing and nondepolarizing muscle relaxants.

KEY TERMS

amnestic
anesthesia
depolarization
emergence phase
emulsion
endotracheal (ET) tube
extubation
fasciculation
induction phase
intubation

lacrimation
laryngeal masked airway (LMA)
maintenance phase
minimum alveolar concentration (MAC)
nebulizer
opioid
postanesthesia care unit (PACU)
preinduction phase
rapid sequence induction (RSI)
repolarization

Geneeral **anesthesia** is a systemic state of anesthesia, rather than anesthesia in a large area (regional) or a specific site (local). The decision to use a general anesthetic is based both on the surgical procedure to be performed and on the individual patient. For instance, a general anesthetic is used when there are multiple operative sites or for a procedure on an area that is difficult to block regionally, such as the thoracic or abdominal cavities. Examples of surgical procedures on multiple locations include skin grafts, breast reconstruction, and autologous bone grafts. Surgical procedures that require an absolutely motionless field, such as retinal surgery, are also performed under general anesthesia. In addition, the expected duration of the surgical procedure may influence the choice of general anesthesia because of patient discomfort when the patient is required to lie flat on the operating room bed for a long period of time.

Patient factors that influence the selection of general anesthesia include patient age, cognitive ability, mental or emotional state, and (when possible) patient preference. Patient age is a primary consideration in that children are almost never candidates for regional or local anesthesia, regardless of the surgical procedure being performed. General anesthesia is usually indicated when the patient's cognitive ability is impaired, causing an inability to understand, communicate, or cooperate with directions required in regional or local anesthesia. For example, mentally disabled patients or those with Alzheimer's disease may not be capable of understanding what is happening to them, so general anesthesia is the method of choice. Patient preference is taken into account when possible; for example, if a patient is very frightened at the idea of a spinal needle being inserted into the back and is in otherwise good health, general anesthesia may be a more appropriate choice than a regional.

Historically, early agents used to produce general anesthesia had unwanted side effects—they were extremely toxic to the patient or they were explosive (Insight 15–1). However, modern advances in the pharmacology of anesthesia have produced many agents that accomplish general anesthesia with a high degree of safety. Several classes of drugs are used to achieve general anesthesia, often in combination. The desired effect is a patient who (1) remains unconscious, (2) is pain free, (3) retains no memory of the event, (4) is immobile, and (5) maintains normal cardiovascular function. Although several theories have been suggested, the exact mechanism of agents used to induce and maintain general anesthesia is still not clearly understood. Different categories of agents affect different parts of the body at the cellular level; for example:

- Drugs used to produce an unconscious state affect the reticular activating system in the brain stem.

Insight 15–1   **Yesterday and Today: Anesthesia**

In today's world, surgery and anesthesia are inseparable concepts. However, this was not always true. Surgery can actually be divided into two eras: preanesthesia and postanesthesia. In the preanesthesia era, surgery was based on speed, because the patient would often die from hemorrhage, shock, or the trauma of the operation. Ironically, shock may have helped to relieve some of the pain before death occurred. The postanesthesia era began in the 19th century when discoveries were finally published, accepted, and used.

Attempts to alleviate pain probably date back as far as humankind has experienced suffering. These first attempts treated pain as an evil spirit or demon, and the idea was to frighten it away. Thus, early anesthesia involved tattoos, jewelry, talismans, amulets, and charms. Pain relievers existed and were used in ancient times, but they were impure, unsafe, and unreliable. Ancient pain remedies documented include a Babylonian clay tablet from approximately 2250 BCE that gives the remedy for a toothache. Early Egyptian surgeons applied pressure to nerves or blood vessels, which caused insensibility to a specific part of the body for an operation.

Many early methods of pain control used drugs. Alcohol was often used in the form of spirits or wines. Along with opium and marijuana, ancient literature contains many references to the mandragora (mandrake, or mandragon) plant as a pain reliever that produced a confused mental state. Dioscorides, a first-century Greek physician, administered the mandragora root boiled in wine to his patients before they went under his knife. Mandragora was also

---

Insight 15–1   **Yesterday and Today: Anesthesia**   *(continued)*

known as the "potion of the condemned," because it was given to criminals to decrease the agonies of crucifixion.

Besides drugs, other pain-control methods were used in the preanesthesia era. One method was to produce unconsciousness by compressing the carotid arteries to decrease heart rate; another was to place a wooden bowl over the patient's head and strike the bowl to cause a concussion. Another method came from China in the form of acupuncture, which decreased pain sensations. A third method was cryothermia. This was documented in England in 1050 in an Anglo-Saxon manuscript that instructed the surgeon to wait a while before making the incision as the patient sat in cold water "until it can become deadened."

The word *anesthesia* comes from the Greek word *anaisthesis,* which means "no sensation." *Anesthesia* appeared in *Bailey's English Dictionary* in 1721. However, the term itself was reportedly coined by Oliver Wendell Holmes in a letter in 1846.

Unfortunately, many agents with anesthetic properties were known for generations but were not applied in surgery. The great alchemist Paracelsus (1493?–1541) mixed sulfuric acid with alcohol and distilled his concoction. He believed this mixture, called sweet vitriol, could quiet suffering and relieve pain. We know this mixture today as ether. Nitrous oxide was discovered by Joseph Priestly in 1772. However, both nitrous oxide and ether were popularized by traveling "professors" as entertainment tools. Volunteers would inhale the gases and become intoxicated. This fad produced "laughing gas parties" and "ether frolics." Little known to the public at the time was the fact that in 1800 a man named Humphrey Davy had described the use of nitrous oxide to relieve pain produced by a wisdom tooth.

It was after one of these public demonstrations of ether that a young physician named Crawford W. Long contemplated its use as an anesthetic during surgery. He was inspired when he saw friends receive injuries without pain while under the vapor's influence. So, on March 30, 1842, Dr. Long administered ether to James M. Venable and successfully removed a tumor from the patient's neck. A dentist named Horace Wells observed a similar demonstration of nitrous oxide in 1844 and used it in his dental practice for many years to relieve pain from tooth extractions. Unfortunately, Wells's demonstration to Harvard Medical School was not a success, possibly because of incomplete administration of the gas, and nitrous oxide was not accepted. Wells's partner, Dr. William T.G. Morton, realized that although nitrous oxide was unreliable, an alternative could be found in ether vapor. After numerous experiments, Morton contacted Dr. John Warren, a senior surgeon of the Massachusetts General Hospital. A demonstration was arranged for October 16, 1846. This demonstration was a success as a tumor was removed from the jaw of a 20-year-old male, who remained insensible throughout the procedure. Thus the postanesthesia era was officially accepted with Dr. Warren's famous remark, "Gentlemen, this is no humbug."

The widespread use of anesthesia began in England on April 7, 1853, when Queen Victoria accepted the use of chloroform during childbirth. Her physician was Dr. Sir James Young Simpson. Chloroform had been discovered in 1831; however, its use by the queen now led to its acceptance by the medical community. From these beginnings, anesthesia has developed into the vital branch of medicine we know today.

- Agents used to produce analgesia (opioids) bind with receptors on cell membranes in the brain and spinal cord, suppressing the perception of pain.
- Muscle relaxants work at the neuromuscular junction of skeletal muscles.

The ability to accomplish general anesthesia is an art as well as a science. The anesthesia provider manages a delicate balance of agents to achieve the necessary components of general anesthesia while maintaining the patient in a stable physiologic state. In addition, the anesthesia provider manages the timing of these agents so that the anesthetic effect is wearing off as the surgical procedure is concluding. In most situations, the goal is to have patients awake, alert, and breathing on their own before transport to the **postanesthesia care unit (PACU)**.

In addition to pharmacologic agents, the anesthesia provider uses various pieces of equipment to assist in the process of accomplishing general anesthesia. Much of this equipment is contained on the anesthesia machine, such as manual and automatic ventilation systems, oxygen and nitrous oxide (N_2O) central pipeline hoses and backup tanks, vaporizers (for volatile gases), flowmeters, breathing circuits, and gas-scavenging systems. A number of physiologic monitors are used, including electrocardiogram, pulse oximeter, blood pressure monitor, and capnograph (see Chapter 14). Each component is checked for proper function prior to admitting the patient to the operating room. Additional equipment used to assist the delivery of anesthesia and provide physiologic support to the patient includes infusion control devices (see Chapter 11, Fig. 11–3), thermoregulatory devices, fluid warmers (see Chapter 11, Fig. 11–7), and fluid pumps.

COMPONENTS OF GENERAL ANESTHESIA

General anesthesia is accomplished by administering agents to achieve four major goals. These goals, or components, of general anesthesia are unconsciousness (a state of being unaware), analgesia (painlessness), amnesia (memory impairment), and muscle relaxation (Table 15–1). That is, the patient must remain uncon-

Table **15–1**   Components of General Anesthesia
Amnesia
Analgesia
Muscle relaxation
Unconsciousness

scious, pain free, and immobile while retaining no explicit memory of the event. Different agents are used to accomplish each of these required components. The anesthesia provider monitors the effects of the agents administered and works to maintain the patient's cardiovascular stability throughout the course of anesthesia.

ADMINISTRATION METHODS

Two methods, or routes, are used to administer general anesthetic agents: inhalation and intravenous injection. An inhalation anesthetic is administered as a gas the patient breathes, whereas intravenous agents are administered directly into the bloodstream through a small catheter placed in a vein (see Chapter 1, Fig. 1–11 and Chapter 11, Fig. 11–1). The term *balanced anesthesia* refers to the technique that uses a combination of inhalation and intravenous agents. Another (but much less common) anesthesia technique uses a combination of a regional block, such as an epidural, and a light general anesthetic. This technique is useful for select patients undergoing major vascular procedures because it decreases the amount of general anesthetic agents required, helping to maintain cardiovascular stability, and provides an effective means of postoperative pain control.

PHASES OF GENERAL ANESTHESIA

There are five phases of general anesthesia: preinduction, induction, maintenance, emergence, and recovery (Table 15–2). Preinduction includes preoperative assessment and preparation of the patient, both physically and psychologically (see Chapter 13). The intraoperative phases of general anesthesia are induction, maintenance, and emergence. Recovery is the postoperative phase. Phases of general anesthesia are not to be confused with the concept of stages of anesthesia (Insight 15–2), which was based on the effects of ether.

Table **15–2**   Phases of General Anesthesia

Preinduction
Induction
Maintenance
Emergence
Recovery

Insight 15–2   **Stages of Anesthesia**

Classic texts describe four stages of anesthesia. These stages are based on the physiologic effects of ether, one of the first anesthetic agents. Each stage was based on observations of body movement, respiratory rhythm, oculomotor reflexes, and muscle tone.

Stage 1. *Amnesia:* Induction to loss of consciousness.

Stage 2. *Delirium* (or excitement): Patient is unconscious but still responding reflexively and unpredictably to certain stimuli.

Stage 3. *Surgical anesthesia:* Adequate depth of anesthesia is reached so that an incision can be made and procedure performed without negative patient response (such as hypertension or tachycardia).

Stage 4. *Overdose* (or medullary depression): Level of anesthesia is so deep that cardiovascular and respiratory function is compromised to the point of collapse due to depression of those centers in the brain.

It is important to note that the stages as traditionally described are no longer as useful in anesthesia practice. Current anesthetic agents are able to bring the patient more quickly through stages 1 and 2, and so may exhibit different signs during induction and make the early stages more difficult to identify. These signs, based on muscular responses, are also invalidated with the current frequent practice of administration of muscle relaxants. In addition, modern anesthetic agents are much more predictable than ether, so stage 4 is less likely to occur.

PREINDUCTION PHASE

The **preinduction phase** begins as the patient is admitted to the preoperative holding area and continues up to the point of administration of anesthetic agents. In this phase, the patient is assessed and prepared for anesthesia and surgery. Appropriate medications are administered during this phase as ordered by the anesthesia provider (see Chapter 13). One goal of the preinduction phase is to have the patient arrive in the operating room calm, physiologically stable, and fully prepared for anesthesia.

The preinduction phase continues as the patient is transported to the operating room and transferred to the operating room bed. The circulator secures the safety belt over the patient's thighs and obtains warm blankets for patient comfort. The anesthesia provider begins by attaching monitoring devices to the patient and obtaining baseline vital signs. The vital functions of all patients receiving a general anesthetic are continuously monitored (see Chapter 14). Heart rate and electrocardiogram, blood pressure, respirations, oxygen saturation, expired gases (end-tidal CO_2), and temperature are closely observed to constantly assess the physiologic status of the patient. A breathing mask is usually placed over the patient's nose and mouth, and 100% oxygen is administered, a process known as preoxygenation. This practice is performed to bring the oxygen saturation of the patient's blood to the highest possible level prior to induction.

INDUCTION PHASE

The **induction phase** begins when medications are administered to initiate general anesthesia and concludes when an adequate depth of anesthesia is reached and the patient's airway is secured.

 CAUTION

The patient may experience a period of agitation or excitement during induction. The effect of loud noises and sudden movement may be intensified during this time, inducing a stress reaction in the patient. The stress response may be characterized by unstable cardiovascular functions, which is potentially harmful to the patient. In addition, moving the patient suddenly at this time can trigger laryngospasm. Thus, the surgical technologist and all members of the surgical team must make every effort to minimize unnecessary operating room noise and movement of the patient during induction.

Induction agents are usually administered by intravenous injection. The option of masked induction with an inhalation anesthetic may be chosen for children to avoid the emotional impact of starting an intravenous drip. Various induction agents are used to produce an unconscious state, amnesia, and analgesia. A variation of standard induction technique called neuroleptanesthesia (Insight 15–3) was used in specific situations but is rarely used in current practice. When the patient becomes unconscious, the anesthesia provider ensures that an adequate airway is maintained.

Airway Management

The exchange of oxygen and carbon dioxide (respiration) is a vital function that must be sustained throughout any surgical procedure. An unconscious patient requires additional support to ensure optimal respiratory function and various methods of airway management are used to provide that support. The patient's airway may be managed with a mask for surgical procedures of short duration when muscle relaxation is not required, such as myringotomy with placement of pressure equalization

---

Insight 15–3   **Neuroleptanesthesia**

Occasionally, you may hear the term *neuroleptanesthesia* used in surgery. This strange-sounding term is used to indicate an anesthetic state that produces sedation and analgesia while allowing the patient to breathe on his or her own and move on command. Also called a dissociative anesthetic state, its effects are similar to those of ketamine. Fentanyl and droperidol are the agents used to produce neuroleptanesthesia. When indicated, this technique was used for induction of anesthesia in high-risk patients undergoing vascular procedures because of the minimal negative impact on cardiovascular and hemodynamic stability. Recently, however, the FDA has required a black-box warning on droperidol due to an associated increased risk of fatal cardiac arrhythmias. Thus, the use of droperidol is significantly limited, and as a result the technique of neuroleptanesthesia is used rarely if at all in current practice.

(PE) tubes. When the patient becomes unconscious, a pharyngeal (oral) airway may be placed in the mouth as needed to hold the tongue in position and facilitate air exchange through the mask. The mask is held in position with straps and the anesthesia provider supports the airway by maintaining the patient's head in a chin-lift position.

In select patients undergoing procedures of fairly short duration, the airway may be managed with a **laryngeal masked airway (LMA)** (Fig. 15–1). After induction of anesthesia, an LMA is inserted and positioned in the laryngopharynx to cover the epiglottis and larynx. The LMA cuff is inflated to provide a seal, and the tube is connected to the breathing circuit. The patient may continue to breathe on his or her own (if no muscle relaxant is needed for the surgical procedure), or respirations may be controlled with the use of a ventilator (if muscle relaxants are administered). The LMA, which does not require laryngoscopy or muscle relaxation, is particularly useful for ambulatory surgical procedures. Contraindications to LMA include procedures on the oral cavity, obesity, hiatal hernia, gastroesophageal reflux disease (GERD), and low pulmonary compliance. Several variations of the LMA are available, allowing for expanded applications in select patients.

Many patients are not appropriate candidates for masked or laryngeal masked airway and require more precise control of the airway. In addition, many surgical procedures are of longer duration, require deep muscle relaxation, or are performed in a lateral or prone position, all of which require a more highly controlled airway. Deep muscle relaxation is achieved by the administration of neuromuscular blockers, which cause temporary relaxation of

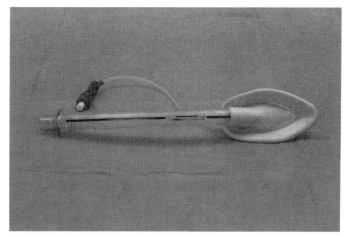

Figure **15–1.**   Laryngeal masked airway.

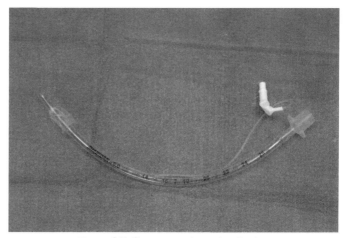

Figure **15–2.**   An endotracheal tube.

skeletal muscles including the muscles of respiration. During a surgical procedure requiring deep muscle relaxation, the patient will not be breathing on his or her own, so respirations are controlled by mechanical ventilation through an **endotracheal (ET) tube** (Fig. 15–2). The ET tube is placed through the patient's mouth into the trachea to establish the most direct and precisely controlled airway.

The process of **intubation** begins after induction agents are administered to render the patient unconscious.

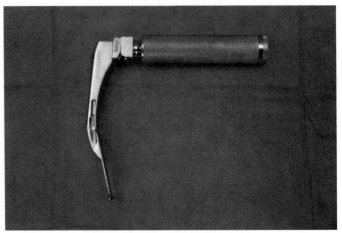

Figure **15–3.** A laryngoscope.

TECH TIP

The circulator assists the anesthesia provider during intubation and should be present at the patient's head as soon as induction begins.

When the patient's airway is adequately managed with masked ventilation, a short-acting muscle relaxant (neuromuscular blocker) is administered to relax the vocal cords and facilitate placement of the ET tube. When the patient is adequately relaxed to suppress the laryngeal reflex, an ET tube is inserted past the epiglottis, through the larynx, and into the trachea under direct visualization with a laryngoscope (Fig. 15–3). An intubating laryngoscope is somewhat similar to an operating laryngoscope and is used to retract the tongue and lift the jaw to visualize the larynx and vocal cords. A flexible stylet may be placed inside the ET tube to guide the tube along the correct path, and the circulator may be asked to remove the stylet when the tube is in position.

A variation on standard induction technique called **rapid sequence induction (RSI)** may be used for patients who are at an increased risk for gastric reflux and pulmonary aspiration. RSI is used for patients who have not been NPO (especially trauma patients), and those with a history of hiatal hernia, GERD, previous gastrointestinal surgery, diabetes, or obesity. Rapid sequence induction is used to secure and control the airway quickly. Key elements of RSI include preoxygenation and application of cricoid

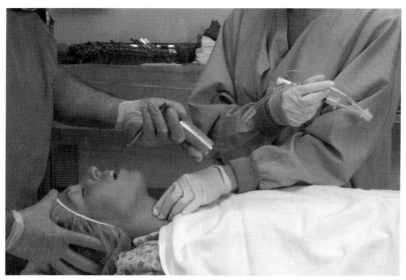

Figure **15–4.**   Application of cricoid pressure prior to endotracheal intubation.

pressure (Fig. 15–4). Cricoid pressure (also known as the Sellick maneuver) is applied to the cricoid cartilage, gently compressing the esophagus, in an effort to prevent gastric contents from entering the trachea and lungs. Cricoid pressure is maintained until the ET tube is in correct position.

In certain circumstances, other intubation techniques may be indicated. Nasal intubation may be used for particular surgical procedures performed in the oral cavity, such as repair of mandibular fractures, when the presence of the ET tube in the mouth may not be desirable. The ET tube is inserted through the nose to the oropharynx, a laryngoscope is used to visualize the vocal cords, and a McGill forceps may be used to guide the ET tube into place.

If the preoperative evaluation indicates a potential significant problem for ventilation and intubation, the patient may be intubated while awake. This technique is reserved for patients with specific conditions such as morbid obesity, a history of difficult intubation, facial deformities, laryngeal cancer, or other conditions that may compromise the airway. Preparation for an awake intubation begins with administration of an antisialagogue (an agent to dry salivary secretions) such as glycopyrrolate (Robinul) approximately 30 minutes before intubation. Lidocaine may be administered through a **nebulizer** to anesthetize the entire airway. Sedation is administered so that the patient can tolerate the intubation and yet continue to breathe and protect his or her own airway. An awake intubation may be accomplished by nasal or oral route, depending on the situation. If a nasal intubation is selected, vasoconstrictors such as cocaine or phenylephrine may be used intranasally to prevent bleeding (epistaxis). Regardless of the intubation route, various topical anesthetic agents such as lidocaine or benzocaine (Cetacaine) are used to gradually anesthetize the airway. The ET tube is loaded over a flexible fiber-optic bronchoscope, and the scope is gently guided into the trachea. The ET tube is placed in position and the bronchoscope removed.

Regardless of the method, once intubation is accomplished the ET tube is connected to a breathing circuit leading to the ventilator (Fig. 15–5). The ET tube position is verified by auscultation

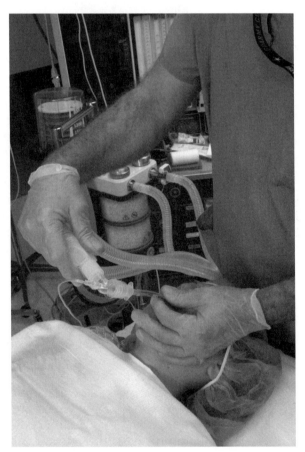

Figure **15–5.**   The endotracheal tube is connected to the ventilator.

during the delivery of manual ventilations. When proper ET tube position is confirmed, respirations are controlled with mechanical ventilation set to the appropriate volume and rate. The ET tube is secured in position, and an adequate depth of anesthesia is achieved to begin the surgical procedure, concluding the induction phase of anesthesia.

MAINTENANCE PHASE

The **maintenance phase** begins as the patient's airway is established and secured and continues until the surgical procedure has been completed. Additional anesthetic agents are administered during the maintenance phase as needed to maintain a depth of anesthesia appropriate to the surgical procedure. Abdominal and thoracic procedures require a much deeper level of anesthesia than superficial procedures, for example. The patient is maintained in an unconscious state by using a combination of intravenous and inhalation agents, some of which also produce amnesia and analgesia. Muscle relaxants are administered as needed to keep the patient immobile and facilitate retraction and visualization of the surgical site. The anesthesia provider maintains the delicate balance of administering the appropriate agents in the appropriate amounts at the appropriate times to achieve a level of anesthesia neither too deep nor too light for the surgical procedure while maintaining a stable cardiovascular state in the patient.

The anesthesia provider uses direct measurements of vital signs and clinical observation to continually assess the patient's status and need for additional anesthetic agents. For example, if the analgesic agents are wearing off most surgical patients demonstrate a measurable physiologic response to pain such as an increase in blood pressure or heart rate. Indirect measures (clinical observations) such as sweating and **lacrimation** are also considered reliable indicators of pain response. However, these signs may also indicate an insufficient depth of consciousness. In addition, specific conditions may cause some of these responses as well. For example, an increased heart rate may be caused by hypovolemia rather than a painful stimulus. Some medications the patient may be taking preoperatively, such as beta-blockers and calcium channel blockers (agents administered for specific heart conditions), can prevent the normal heart rate increase in response to pain. Each patient and each surgical situation present unique challenges in assessing and responding to patient needs under anesthesia.

Awareness Under Anesthesia

A disturbing phenomenon known as awareness under anesthesia is emerging as one of the most challenging problems in current anesthesia practice. For reasons that remain unclear, some patients do not demonstrate characteristic (measurable or observable) physiologic responses to pain or have inadequate depth of consciousness during surgery. The result is that the patient may have direct recall, or explicit memory (Insight 15–4), of intraoperative

---

Insight 15–4   **Explicit and Implicit Memory Under Anesthesia**

The term *explicit memory* refers to the ability to recall events—that is, conscious recollection. When a patient has explicit memory of events during surgery, it may be quite traumatic. Although explicit memory may be somewhat vague, some patients have been able to recall specific comments and conversations that took place during their surgical procedure. Much effort is being directed at preventing such occurrences.

But what is *implicit* memory? *Implicit memory* is the term used to describe subconscious processing of information by the brain, demonstrated by changes in the performance of tasks. For example, you know how to tie your shoelaces, but you may not remember exactly how or when you learned to do so. Another example of implicit memory is posthypnotic suggestion. Popular nightclub acts offer hypnosis to audience volunteers. The volunteer is hypnotized and asked to perform some particular behavior when a cue is given. The volunteer is awakened from the hypnotic state and the cue is given, causing the volunteer to display the suggested behavior. The experience occurred, and the behavior was displayed, but the volunteer has no conscious recollection (explicit memory) of why he or she is doing so.

A few experiments have shown that some learning (similar to hypnotic suggestion) is possible while under anesthesia, indicating that implicit memory during anesthesia exists in some form. Surgical patients who agreed to participate in these studies were routinely anesthetized for surgery. During the surgical procedure, verbal instructions were given asking the patient to perform a simple task (such as scratching the nose) on cue during the postoperative interview. On the prearranged cue, a surprising number of patients displayed the suggested behavior, yet without remembering why they were doing so. These studies seem to indicate that a significant number of surgical patients hear and remember what is said (implicit memory), but without conscious recall (explicit memory). The potential impact of implicit memory and the surgical patient is enormous and much remains unknown. Could pessimistic comments made by the surgeon and other surgical team members during surgery have a negative effect on the patient's recovery? Could positive suggestions given under anesthesia actually speed recovery? Until the impact of implicit memory is clearly identified, all surgical team members should consider making only positive, affirming comments and keeping conversations on an encouraging and professional level during surgery. After all, it appears that our patients may be hearing and implicitly remembering everything we say throughout their operations.

events. When muscle relaxants are used, the patient is unable to move or speak and therefore is unable to communicate this awareness to the anesthesia provider. Various studies report that an average of 0.1% to 0.2% of all patients undergoing general anesthesia experience some sort of awareness. Because about 20 million patients in the United States receive general anesthesia each year, an estimated 20,000 to 40,000 cases of awareness under anesthesia may be occurring yearly. The risk of awareness appears to be greater when it is necessary to use the lowest possible dose of anesthesia medications to avoid undesirable side effects. Patients who are hemodynamically unstable (such as trauma patients) are also at greater risk for awareness under anesthesia, as well as those undergoing cardiac and obstetric procedures. Although the extent of awareness is highly variable, about half of these patients report auditory recall, half report a sensation of being unable to breathe, and one third recall pain. A number of these patients reportedly go on to develop post-traumatic stress disorder as a result.

Previously, the surgical team was periodically reminded that the patient's hearing is the last sense to go and the first to return. Inherent in that statement is a belief that what was said during a patient's surgical procedure did not affect the patient. What we now understand about explicit and implicit memory and the number of patients who experience auditory recall (explicit memory) should motivate us to try to effect significant change in surgical team behaviors. We can no longer assume that the patient is unaffected by our conversations and comments during surgery. As surgical technologists, we can support the anesthesia providers in their efforts to bring this new understanding to the attention of all surgical team members.

Additional methods of patient monitoring have been developed in an effort to predict and prevent awareness under anesthesia. Rather than measure physiologic responses, these devices monitor brain activity and are modified types of electroencephalography. These devices may be known as level-of-consciousness or anesthesia-depth monitors. The most common is the bispectral index (BIS) monitor (see Chapter 14). It is important to note, however, that although these monitors may provide additional information on patient consciousness, there is not yet a perfect system for preventing awareness under anesthesia.

Muscle Relaxation

Whereas a short-acting muscle relaxant is administered to allow intubation, a long-acting muscle relaxant is given during the maintenance phase to facilitate exposure of the surgical site. The amount of muscle relaxation required depends on the surgical procedure, abdominal procedures requiring the deepest relaxation. In addition to depth, timing of relaxation is a crucial factor. The duration of a long-acting muscle relaxant and the anticipated length of the surgical procedure are taken into consideration when selecting and administering the appropriate agent.

The level of muscle relaxation is monitored with the use of a peripheral nerve stimulator. The peripheral nerve stimulator administers an electrical stimulus to a nerve–muscle group and the motor response is measured, indicating the extent of muscle blockade. An electrode is placed at the desired location, usually the wrist, and connected to the unit. Alternately, the unit may have two probes attached that are placed directly on the desired location, often at a branch of the facial nerve. Different stimuli patterns may be used as indicated, but one of the most common is the train-of-four (TOF) pattern, a series of four electrical stimuli delivered approximately 10 seconds apart. Recall from Chapter 14 that the presence of four of the four twitches indicates no muscle relaxation, and zero of the four twitches indicates full muscle relaxation. The patient's motor response is measured and used to determine when and how much additional muscle relaxant is necessary to maintain optimal surgical exposure. Ideally, muscle relaxation is present through closure of the deep wound layers and wears off as superficial layers are closed.

EMERGENCE PHASE

As the procedure is completed, the **emergence phase** begins, during which anesthetic agents are discontinued and allowed to wear off. If indicated, the duration of certain anesthetic agents may be shortened by the administration of reversal agents to permit the patient to gradually awaken. The emergence phase ends when the patient is transported to the PACU.

 CAUTION

The emergence phase of anesthesia is another time when the patient is hypersensitive to loud noises and movement. Because the surgical procedure has concluded and pressure exists to minimize the operating room turnover time, surgical technologists in the scrub role are busy with various tasks to break down the sterile back table. These tasks involve manipulation of instruments and metal pans and basins, which can produce loud noises. In addition, the surgical technologist in the circulating role may be performing various duties around the patient, such as dressing application, replacement of blankets, and preparation for patient transfer. Each of these activities may cause a sudden movement of the patient, which in turn may cause laryngospasm. The surgical technologist must always maintain an awareness of the surgical patient's status and make every effort to minimize movement of the patient and noise during the emergence phase of anesthesia.

As the patient awakens and becomes able to maintain his or her own airway, the items used to provide airway support are removed. In masked airway, the pharyngeal airway is removed (if present), but the mask may be left in place to administer oxygen. If an LMA was used, it is removed and replaced with a regular mask for oxygen administration as needed. If the patient has been intubated, particular care is used to assess the appropriate timing for removal of the endotracheal tube, a process called **extubation.** The patient must be breathing on his or her own, with airway reflexes present, and must demonstrate sufficient muscle strength to be able to maintain the airway independently. A mask may be used to administer oxygen if necessary. When vital signs are stable, the patient is carefully moved to a transport stretcher and taken to PACU for the recovery phase. The anesthesia provider gives a detailed report to the PACU staff nurses, who closely monitor the patient during the recovery phase. When it is deemed safe, the patient is discharged from PACU to the appropriate care location.

AGENTS USED FOR GENERAL ANESTHESIA

Several different classes of drugs have been used to achieve general anesthesia. Multiple agents are used to provide an unconscious state, analgesia, amnesia, and muscle relaxation. These medications are presented by category, and the phases of general anesthesia in which they are administered are indicated. The broad categories covered are sedatives and hypnotic agents, analgesics, inhalation agents, neuromuscular blocking agents, and reversal agents (Table 15–3).

INTRAVENOUS INDUCTION AGENTS

Intravenous induction agents are administered to produce a rapid loss of consciousness. Agents used to induce unconsciousness are

Table **15-3** Major Categories of Anesthesia Medications
Intravenous induction agents Analgesics Inhalation agents Neuromuscular blocking agents Reversal agents

classified as either sedatives or hypnotics. Benzodiazepines are sedatives (see Chapter 13) used for induction. Hypnotic agents used for induction include barbiturates (thiopental and methohexital), ketamine, etomidate, and propofol.

Benzodiazepines, which have both sedative and **amnestic** effects, are used preoperatively and occasionally as induction agents. Benzodiazepines are not commonly used for induction because of the high doses required to induce an unconscious state. Recall that the benzodiazepines include midazolam (Versed), diazepam (Valium), and lorazepam (Ativan). Benzodiazepines rapidly penetrate the blood–brain barrier, producing a loss of consciousness in 45 to 90 seconds. Benzodiazepines do not provide analgesia.

Barbiturates are ultra–short-acting hypnotic agents derived from barbituric acid. The most frequently used barbiturates are thiopental (Pentothal) and methohexital (Brevital). Thiopental, for instance, takes just 15 seconds to travel from the injection site to the brain; thus, it is rapidly taken up by the brain, but it is also rapidly eliminated. Barbiturates induce anesthesia, but they have no analgesic effect; patients may therefore be agitated and disoriented during the emergence phase because of the pain they may begin to feel.

Ketamine (Ketalar) is a dissociative hypnotic agent used for induction and maintenance of general anesthesia. Chemically related to the drug PCP (phencyclidine or "angel dust"), ketamine is a powerful analgesic—the only hypnotic agent with this property. The onset of action is 30 to 60 seconds after intravenous injection. When ketamine is used, patients appear to be awake and their eyes may be open; however, they are dissociated from their environment and they do not consciously recall surgical events. Ketamine can cause hallucinations and involuntary movements, making patients difficult to handle. It also exaggerates the effect of sudden loud noises. Ketamine is most often used for superficial procedures of short duration, such as painful dressing changes, debridements, or skin grafts. Ketamine does not produce any skeletal muscle relaxation.

Etomidate (Amidate) is a hypnotic agent that produces an unconscious state in less than a minute but provides no analgesia and no muscle relaxation. This agent is often used for patients with compromised heart function who cannot tolerate the drop in blood pressure often seen with other induction agents. Etomidate is ideal for brief procedures such as cardioversion. It is also useful for induction in trauma patients, who may be hypovolemic and hence unable to tolerate any additional hypotension.

Propofol (Diprivan) is a hypnotic agent chemically unrelated to any other anesthetic agent. It is an **emulsion** (a mixture of two liquids not mutually soluble) that is injected intravenously in doses of 2 to 2.5 mg/kg. Propofol produces an unconscious state within a minute. Because of its brief duration (4 to 6 minutes), patients recover alert and free of the usual side effects of an anesthetic agent. Propofol provides poor analgesia and no muscle relaxation. Among the inactive components of the propofol emulsion are soybean oil, glycerol, and egg lecithin; thus, propofol is contraindicated in patients with a known allergy to eggs. Propofol has a characteristic milky white appearance (Fig. 15–6). Strict aseptic technique must be maintained when handling propofol because it contains no antimicrobial preservatives and can support rapid growth of microorganisms. Potential adverse effects include bradycardia, hypotension, and apnea. Many patients (40% to 90%) report a stinging sensation at the injection site.

See Table 15–4 for a summary of intravenous induction agents used in general anesthesia.

ANALGESICS

Analgesic agents are given during maintenance of general anesthesia to prevent pain during surgery. If adequate pain control is achieved, the amount of other anesthetic agents required may be reduced.

Apply what you already know to assist you in learning pharmacology. The term *analgesia* literally means "without pain." An analgesic, then, is an agent given to prevent or treat pain. You are already familiar with many examples of analgesics available over the counter, such as aspirin (Bayer, Excedrin, etc.) and acetaminophen (Tylenol). Remember, just as you take aspirin or acetaminophen (analgesics) to relieve the pain of a headache (e.g., those caused by studying so hard to learn all this pharmacology information), we give analgesics (different ones, however) to our patients to relieve the pain of surgery.

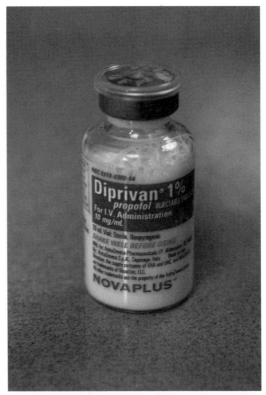

Figure **15–6.** Propofol (Diprivan) is an intravenous induction agent.

Table 15–4   Intravenous Induction Agents Used in General Anesthesia

Sedatives (benzodiazepines)

midazolam (Versed)
diazepam (Valium)
lorazepam (Ativan)

Hypnotics (barbiturates)

thiopental (Pentothal)
methohexital (Brevital)

Hypnotics (various chemical categories)

propofol (Diprivan)
ketamine (Ketalar)
etomidate (Amidate)

> *Insight* 15–5   **Papaverine**
>
> Papaverine is a chemical derived from the opium poppy *(Papaver somniferum)* that is used as a smooth-muscle relaxant during surgery. Papaverine may be administered from the sterile field during procedures on small blood vessels (such as coronary artery bypass grafts). It is injected at the vessel wall to prevent vasoconstriction from vascular muscle spasms caused by surgical manipulation.

The most common analgesic agents administered for anesthesia are classified as opioids. The term **opioid** refers to drugs that have morphine-like actions. The brain has its own natural pain suppression system, in part consisting of neurochemicals called endorphins (or endogenous opioids) and specific receptors sites for these chemicals. Opioids used in anesthesia are able to bind with the brain's natural receptor sites, initiating pain suppression.

☞ **Note:** Previously, the term *narcotic* was used to describe analgesics used for anesthesia and was associated with the production of a state of stupor. In current use, however, the word *narcotic* is used to indicate any drug that can cause dependence. Thus the term *narcotic analgesic* is no longer used in reference to anesthesia.

Opioids are available from several drug sources:

- Plants (also known as a natural source; from the opium poppy, *Papaver somniferum*)
- Semisynthetic (modified from the natural alkaloids found in the poppy)
- Synthetic (manufactured from chemicals)

Natural opioids are morphine and codeine (Tylenol 3). Although not an analgesic, another natural derivative of the poppy is papaverine (Insight 15–5), a smooth muscle relaxant.

Synthetic opioids used for anesthesia are fentanyl (Sublimaze), alfentanil (Alfenta), sufentanil (Sufenta), and remifentanil (Ultiva). These drugs are useful in anesthesia because of their relatively short action and intense analgesic effect. Synthetic opioids are more potent analgesics than morphine, but at equivalent analgesic doses, they cause the same degree of respiratory depression.

Fentanyl is 100 times more potent than morphine. This drug has a rapid onset, about 30 seconds, with a duration of 45 to 60 minutes. Fentanyl provides analgesia plus some sedation. When used as the sole anesthetic agent, the dose for induction is 30 to 100 mcg/kg of body weight. When used in addition to other agents, the dose is 1 to 10 mcg/kg. Alfentanil has one fourth the potency of fentanyl; it has a slower onset, about 1 to 2 minutes,

Table **15–5**	Comparison of Opioids Used for Analgesia During General Anesthesia			
Generic Name	Trade Name	Dosage (mcg/kg)	Onset	Duration (min)
fentanyl	Sublimaze	1–10	30 sec	45–60
alfentanil	Alfenta	10–25	1–2 min	10–15
sufentanil	Sufenta	0.2–0.6	Immediate	20–45
remifentanyl	Ultiva	0.5–1.0 per min	1–3	5–10

and lasts just 10 to 15 minutes. Alfentanil is classified as an ultra–short-acting opioid. When used as a sole anesthetic agent, the induction dosage is 50 to 150 mcg/kg. When used in combination with other agents, the dose is 10 to 25 mcg/kg. Sufentanil is 5 to 10 times more potent than fentanyl, but it is more rapidly cleared from the body, providing a very rapid recovery. Onset is immediate, with effects lasting 20 to 45 minutes. When used as a sole anesthetic agent, the induction dose is 2 to 10 mcg/kg. If used with other agents, the dose is 0.2 to 0.6 mcg/kg. Remifentanil (Ultiva) is the newest ultra–short-acting opioid and is 20 to 40 times more potent than alfentanil. Onset of effects occurs in 1 to 3 minutes, but duration is only 5 to 10 minutes. If used for general anesthesia, remifentanil is given as a continuous infusion of 0.5 to 1.0 mcg/kg/minute.

See Table 15–5 for a comparison of opioids used for analgesia during general anesthesia.

INHALATION AGENTS

The first inhalation anesthetics used were ether, chloroform, nitrous oxide, and cyclopropane. Of these, only nitrous oxide is in use currently. Ether and cyclopropane are explosive and chloroform is toxic to the liver, so use of these agents was discontinued as new agents were developed. Halothane (Fluothane), introduced in 1956, was the first nonexplosive inhalation agent. Additional inhalation agents have been developed, each generation of new agents improving on previous agents.

Inhalation anesthetics (also called volatile anesthetics) are distributed in liquid form packaged in bottles. The liquid agent is poured into the appropriate vaporizer on an anesthesia machine, and the administration rate is adjusted as needed (Fig. 15–7). The vaporizer turns the liquid agent into a gas that is relatively easy

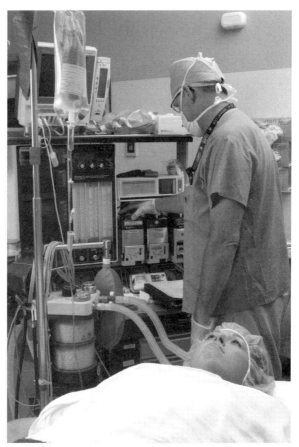

Figure **15–7.** Concentration of inhalation anesthetics is controlled in an anesthesia machine.

to administer via breathing mask, LMA, or endotracheal tube. Inhalation agents, which are measured by the percentage of vapor present in the mixture the patient inhales, diffuse into the blood from the air in the alveoli, then rapidly diffuse out of the blood and into the brain—the site of action. Inhalation anesthetics are eliminated from the body quickly, most via the pulmonary, hepatic, and renal systems. The potency of inhalation agents is compared using a measurement called **minimum alveolar concentration (MAC).** The minimum alveolar concentration is the concentration, at one atmosphere of pressure, that stops the motor response to a painful stimulus in 50% of patients.

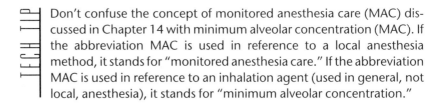

Don't confuse the concept of monitored anesthesia care (MAC) discussed in Chapter 14 with minimum alveolar concentration (MAC). If the abbreviation MAC is used in reference to a local anesthesia method, it stands for "monitored anesthesia care." If the abbreviation MAC is used in reference to an inhalation agent (used in general, not local, anesthesia), it stands for "minimum alveolar concentration."

The disadvantages of inhalation agents include an increased potential for cardiovascular depression and lack of postoperative analgesia. The selection of an inhalation agent is influenced by factors such as solubility of the gas and the patient's cardiac output. The most common inhalation agents in use today include the gas nitrous oxide and three volatile liquid anesthetics, isoflurane (Forane), desflurane (Suprane), and sevoflurane (Ultane).

Nitrous oxide (N_2O)—a colorless, odorless, tasteless gas—is the most widely used inhalation anesthetic in clinical practice. Nitrous oxide provides rapid onset and emergence and is completely eliminated by the lungs. Its mild analgesic and amnestic characteristics make it an excellent adjunct to volatile liquid inhalation anesthetic agents. Nitrous oxide is often used in conjunction with volatile anesthetics to reduce the amount of the latter needed. A muscle relaxant must also be given if needed.

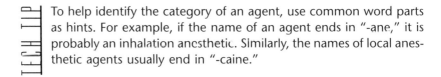

To help identify the category of an agent, use common word parts as hints. For example, if the name of an agent ends in "-ane," it is probably an inhalation anesthetic. Similarly, the names of local anesthetic agents usually end in "-caine."

The three most common volatile liquid anesthetics are isoflurane (Forane), desflurane (Suprane), and sevoflurane (Ultane). These agents are quite similar to previous volatile liquid anesthetic agents, except that they provide more precise control of maintenance and more rapid induction and emergence. See Table 15–6 for a list of inhalation anesthetic agents.

 CAUTION

Inhalation anesthetic agents (except for nitrous oxide), either alone or in combination with succinylcholine, have been identified as triggering agents of a rare but life-threatening condition called malignant hyperthermia (see Chapter 16).

Table **15–6** Inhalation Anesthetics	
Generic Name	*Trade Name*
Gas	
nitrous oxide (N$_2$O)	N/A
Volatile liquid (vapor)	
isoflurane	Forane
desflurane	Suprane
sevoflurane	Ultane

Insight 15–6   **The First Muscle Relaxant**

The earliest known muscle relaxant was curare. It is a toxin that is extracted from plants found in the rain forest. Indigenous peoples on three separate continents—South America, Africa, and Southeast Asia—used curare on the tips of darts to immobilize monkeys and other tree-dwelling animals. Once discovered by Western culture, curare was used in the experimental laboratory for various purposes. A German report in 1912 described the use of curare on humans as an adjunct to anesthesia; however, the report was generally ignored. Not until 1942 was curare first used in surgery to relax abdominal muscles of a patient undergoing an appendectomy. Discovery of the benefits of curare radically changed anesthesia practice. Patients could now be routinely intubated, a sporadic practice prior to the use of curare. Since the introduction of curare, many agents have been developed to provide muscle relaxation.

NEUROMUSCULAR BLOCKING AGENTS

Patients under general anesthesia may be unconscious, pain free, and memory free, but their skeletal muscles continue to respond to stimuli. To receive an endotracheal tube, the patient must be adequately relaxed; that is, the muscles must be relaxed. And during the surgical procedure, the patient's muscles must be relaxed to facilitate exposure of the surgical site, especially in the abdomen (Insight 15–6). Agents categorized as neuromuscular blockers are administered to relax skeletal muscles for intubation and surgery.

Muscle Physiology Review

There are three types of muscle tissue: cardiac, smooth, and skeletal. Muscles function in circulation, labor and delivery, and intestinal movements, as well as in body movement. For a muscle to contract, it must be stimulated by a motor nerve. The neuromuscular junction is an area where the motor nerve axon is very near the muscle fiber. The space between an axon and a muscle fiber is called a synapse. When a neurotransmitter called acetylcholine (ACh) is released from the axon, it diffuses across the synapse and binds to receptor sites on the surface of the muscle fiber (the sarcolemma). Acetylcholine causes an impulse to spread across the muscle fiber to the sarcoplasmic reticulum, releasing calcium ions from storage. Calcium ions alter muscle filaments, exposing myosin-binding sites; this results in muscle contraction, known as **depolarization. Repolarization** is the process of muscle fiber relaxation, that is, returning to a resting state. For muscle fibers to return to a resting state, ACh must diffuse away from the receptor sites and be broken down, or recycled, by an enzyme called acetylcholinesterase. This enzyme, which is present on the sarcolemma, breaks down ACh and terminates the contraction. Calcium ions are then transported back into the sarcoplasmic reticulum for storage and later release. Depolarizing muscle relaxants act like ACh; they bind with receptor sites and initiate a contraction (depolarization). Such contractions are observed as **fasciculations.** Subsequent contractions are prevented as long as the depolarizing muscle relaxant stays on the binding sites. Nondepolarizing muscle relaxants are ACh antagonists; they block receptor sites and prevent ACh binding, thus preventing a contraction (see Fig. 1–15 from Chapter 1).

☞ **Note:** Students should consult an anatomy and physiology text to review the physiology of muscle contraction in more depth.

There are two basic types of muscle relaxants classified according to their action on the motor end-plate: depolarizing and nondepolarizing. Examples of each type are listed with a brief description.

Succinylcholine (Anectine) is the only depolarizing muscle relaxant in use. Succinylcholine acts similarly to the neurotransmitter acetylcholine (ACh), but its duration is longer. It causes persistent depolarization (sustained contraction) and produces fasciculations followed by flaccidity. Succinylcholine acts rapidly, and its effects are seen in 30 to 60 seconds. Duration of effects is also short, usually only 4 to 6 minutes; but because no antagonist or reversal agent is currently available, succinylcholine must be allowed to wear off. Some adverse effects associated with administration of succinylcholine include increased intracranial pressure, increased intraocular pressure, increased intragastric pressure (which increases the potential for regurgitation), and muscle soreness postoperatively. Elevated serum potassium levels have been noted in burn patients receiving succinylcholine. Patients with pseudocholinesterase deficiency may experience prolonged respiratory paralysis because succinylcholine is not eliminated effectively without that enzyme.

 CAUTION

Succinylcholine has been identified as a triggering agent for malignant hyperthermia. See Chapter 16 for additional information.

There are several nondepolarizing muscle relaxants. These include atracurium besylate (Tracrium), mivacurium chloride (Mivacron), pancuronium bromide (Pavulon), rocuronium bromide (Zemuron), tubocurarine chloride (Curare), and vecuronium bromide (Norcuron). Nondepolarizing muscle relaxants prevent muscle contractions by binding to cholinergic receptors, preventing acetylcholine from binding to the receptor sites. Nondepolarizing muscle relaxants do not cause fasciculations and may be used prior to administration of succinylcholine to prevent fasciculations. The selection of a particular nondepolarizing muscle relaxant depends on its pharmacologic properties, such as onset and duration of effects, and side effects, such as those seen in the cardiovascular system. See Table 15–7 for a comparison of the duration of effects of neuromuscular blocking agents. Adverse effects of nondepolarizing muscle relaxants on the cardiovascular system include hypotension or hypertension, tachycardia, bradycardia, and arrhythmias. Dosage is variable, depending on onset time and depth of block required. Nondepolarizing muscle relaxants may be reversed if necessary with an antagonist such as neostigmine (Prostigmine). Neostigmine works by competing

Category	Generic Name	Trade Name	Duration (min)
Depolarizing	succinylcholine	Anectine	4–6
Nondepolarizing	atracurium besylate	Tracrium	20–35
	mivacurium chloride	Mivacron	6–10
	pancuronium bromide	Pavulon	40–65
	rocuronium bromide	Zemuron	15–85
	vecuronium bromide	Norcuron	25–30

Table **15–7**   Comparison of Duration of Neuromuscular Blocking Agents

Table 15–8 Reversal Agents for Anesthetics	
Reversal Agent	*Used to Reverse*
naloxone (Narcan)	Opioid analgesics
nalmefene (Revex)	Opioid analgesics
naltrexone (ReVia, Trexan)	Opioid analgesics
flumazenil (Mazicon)	Benzodiazepines
neostigmine (Prostigmin)	Nondepolarizing muscle relaxants
edrophonium (Tensilon)	Nondepolarizing muscle relaxants

with acetylcholine for attachment to acetylcholinesterase. This competition causes a buildup of acetylcholine, which facilitates transmission of impulses across the neuromuscular junction.

REVERSAL AGENTS

Occasionally, the surgical procedure may be completed sooner than expected. An example of this situation is a radical hysterectomy. This procedure is expected to take several hours, and so several different long-acting anesthetic agents are administered. If unexpected metastases are discovered in the liver or scattered over the intestines, the procedure may be terminated without resection. This situation may require the administration of reversal agents to counteract specific anesthetic agents. Naloxone (Narcan), nalmefene (Revex), and naltrexone (ReVia, Trexan) are used to reverse opioid analgesics if necessary. Benzodiazepines may be reversed with flumazenil (Mazicon). When indicated, nondepolarizing muscle relaxants may be reversed with neostigmine (Prostigmin) or edrophonium (Tensilon). See Table 15–8 for a list of reversal agents for various anesthetics.

ADVANCED PRACTICES FOR THE SURGICAL FIRST ASSISTANT
Chapter 15—General Anesthesia

According to its definition, the term *anesthesia* means "lack of sensation." How this effect is achieved may employ many methods. In addition to the ones mentioned in this chapter, the surgical first assistant should be familiar with some of these alternate anesthesia methodologies. Cryoanesthesia, also known as frost or refrigeration anesthesia, is defined as a local anesthesia produced by chilling a part of the body or peripheral nerves to near-freezing

ADVANCED PRACTICES FOR THE SURGICAL FIRST ASSISTANT   *(continued)*

temperature to numb the area against pain. This technique uses an applicator (cryoprobe) or sprays such as Frigiderm (dichlorotetrafluoroethane), Fluro-Ethyl (ethyl chloride), and Cryoesthesia. It is used in surgical specialties as dermatology for dermabrasion and gynecology for endometrial cryoablation. Hypnosis has long been associated with entertainment; however, there is a therapeutic hypnosis used in medical applications as well. It was approved by the American Medical Association in 1958 as an alternative form of medicine and has been used by dentists, obstetricians, and midwives in place of local anesthesia for many years. In a hypnotized state, a part of the central nervous system shows greater activity and influence on the patient's senses (as feeling and thoughts) and on the sensation of pain. Acupuncture originated in China more than 2000 years ago and is one of the oldest and most commonly used medical procedures worldwide. This group of procedures involves the stimulation of anatomical points of the body by varying methods. The most studied scientifically is the penetration of the skin with thin, metallic needles that are manipulated by hand or by an electrical stimulation. The U.S. Food and Drug Administration approved acupuncture needles for use by licensed practitioners in 1996. According to acupuncture theory, pain signals travel from the area of the injury to the spinal cord and brain. Acupuncture generates a stimulus that travels faster and crowds out the pain signals to effectively block and prevent them from reaching the brain. The result is that the patient never experiences the pain.

Key Concepts

- Accomplishing anesthesia is an art as well as a science. Various drugs and techniques have been used to achieve a state of anesthesia. Although several theories have been proposed, the exact mechanism of action of anesthetic drugs remains unclear.
- In some cases, it is important that the patient be under general anesthesia, that is, unconscious, pain free, and immobile. General anesthesia may be necessary because of patient factors or the nature of the surgical procedure.
- Four major components must be accomplished in general anesthesia: hypnosis, analgesia, amnesia, and muscle relaxation.
- There are five phases of administration of a general anesthetic: preinduction, induction, maintenance, emergence, and recovery.
- The two methods or routes used to deliver general anesthetics are intravenous and inhalation.
- Intravenous induction agents include barbiturates, benzodiazepines, ketamine, etomidate, and propofol.
- Analgesics administered as an adjunct to general anesthesia are fentanyl, alfentanil, sufentanil, and remifentanil.

- Common inhalation agents include the gas nitrous oxide and many volatile liquid anesthetics such as isoflurane, desflurane, and sevoflurane.
- Muscle relaxants, given as an adjunct to general anesthesia, are categorized as depolarizing and nondepolarizing neuromuscular blockers.
- Agents that may be administered during emergence include naloxone, nalmefene, naltrexone, flumazenil, neostigmine, and edrophonium.
- Anesthesia is a complex physiologic state, often taken for granted by operating room personnel. To function effectively on the surgical team, the surgical technologist must understand the basic concepts of anesthesia and the names of common agents used.

16

EMERGENCY SITUATIONS

Medications Covered in Chapter 16

Generic Name	Brand Name	Category
albuterol	Proventil, Ventolin	Beta-adrenergic agonist
terbutaline	Breathaire, Bicanyl	Beta-adrenergic agonist
epinephrine	Adrenalin	Hormone
atropine	Atropine	Anticholinergic
ipratropium	Atrovent	Anticholinergic
dopamine	Intropin	Adrenergic agonist
dobutamine	Dobutrex	Beta-adrenergic agonist
phenylephrine	Neo-Synephrine	Alpha-adrenergic agonist
diphenhydramine	Benadryl, Allergan 50	Antihistamine
succinylcholine	Anectine	Depolarizing muscle relaxant
amiodarone	Cordarone	Antiarrhythmic agent
procainamide	Pronestyl	Antiarrhythmic agent
lidocaine	Xylocaine	Antiarrhythmic agent
isoproterenol	Isuprel	Beta-adrenergic agonist
methoxamine	Vasoxyl	Alpha-adrenergic agonist
norepinephrine bitartrate	Levophed	Beta-1 agonist
labetalol	Normodyne	Beta-adrenergic antagonist
atenolol	Tenormin	Beta-adrenergic antagonist
nicardipine	Cardene	Calcium channel blocker
nifedipine	Procardia	Calcium channel blocker
verapamil	Isoptin	Calcium channel blocker
nitroglycerine	Transderm-Nitro, Nitrodisc	Nitrovasodilator
nitroprusside	Nipride	Nitrovasodilator
digoxin	Lanoxin	Inotropic agent
dantrolene	Dantrium	Skeletal muscle relaxant
mannitol	Osmitrol	Diuretic
furosemide	Lasix	Diuretic

OBJECTIVES

After completing this chapter, you should be able to:

1. Define terminology related to emergency situations.
2. Identify emergency situations associated with anesthesia.
3. Identify medications used in emergency situations.
4. State the purpose of drugs used in emergency situations.
5. Identify the category of specified emergency medications.
6. Discuss the role of the surgical technologist during a cardiac emergency in surgery.
7. List clinical signs of malignant hyperthermia.
8. Outline basic course of treatment for malignant hyperthermia.
9. Discuss the role of the surgical technologist in a malignant hyperthermia crisis.

KEY TERMS

anaphylaxis	capnography	hypermetabolic
asystole	cyanosis	pyrexia
bolus	desaturation	tachycardia
bradycardia	diaphoresis	tachypnea
bronchospasm	hemoglobinuria	urticaria

One goal of anesthesia is to maintain the patient in a stable physiologic state throughout the course of anesthesia and surgery. However, surgery and anesthesia are complex processes that place a significant impact on the human physiologic state. In addition, many patients requiring surgery are critically ill and have multiple organ system failure. The most common anesthesia emergency situations, which vary from mild to life-threatening, merit careful study by the surgical technologist. Emergency situations in the operating room may be due to existing disease, trauma, the surgical procedure, anesthesia, or may be of unknown origin and may occur at any point during the patient's care. This chapter is specifically focused on anesthesia-associated emergencies that require pharmacologic treatment. Two of the most pertinent to the surgical technologist—cardiac arrest and malignant hyperthermia (MH)—are discussed at length. The surgical technologist should be able to respond appropriately as a surgical team member to any patient emergency. To function in a competent manner, the surgical technologist must have a thorough knowledge of the medications frequently used in emergency situations.

RESPIRATORY EMERGENCIES

Intraoperative respiratory impairment or obstruction may be caused by a number of factors including swelling from trauma or inflammation, bronchospasm, or laryngospasm.

BRONCHOSPASM

Bronchospasm (impaired breathing from contraction and inflammation of the bronchi) may occur as a result of an acute asthma attack, as a complication of obstructive pulmonary disease (COPD), or secondary to an allergic reaction. When intraoperative bronchospasm is diagnosed, 100% oxygen is administered and the patient is ventilated manually. The underlying condition, such as foreign body or secretions in airway, incorrect endotracheal (ET) tube placement, pulmonary edema, or pneumothorax is identified and corrected. Several different categories of medications may be used to treat bronchospasm. A group of drugs called beta-adrenergic agonists (classified by physiologic action, see Chapter 1) are particularly effective. Examples of beta agonists include albuterol (Proventil, Ventolin), which is aerosolized and administered via the ET tube, and terbutaline (Breathaire, Bicanyl), which may be aerosolized or administered subcutaneously or intravenously. Epinephrine (Adrenalin) is a hormone (see Chapter 8) that may be aerosolized through the ET tube or given subcutaneously for bronchospasm. Anticholinergics (see Chapter 13) such as atropine and ipratropium (Atrovent) may also be administered aerosolized through the ET tube to treat bronchospasm. Corticosteroids such as methylprednisolone do not have an immediate effect, but may be administered as needed. Corticosteroids may be delivered aerosolized, but are usually given intravenously.

ANAPHYLAXIS

Anaphylactic shock (**anaphylaxis**) may result from a severe allergic reaction to medications, anesthetics, latex, or blood administered in surgery. Anaphylactic shock occurs rapidly and is potentially lethal. Early signs include hives and **urticaria** (wheals), followed by bronchospasm, dyspnea (labored breathing), respiratory obstruction, and circulatory collapse. Under general anesthesia, however, the first sign usually noted is hypotension. Hypotension is treated with intravenous fluids, and medications used to raise blood pressure (vasopressor or inotropic agents) are administered as needed. Vasopressor agents include dopamine

(Intropin) and dobutamine (Dobutrex). Agents such as ephedrine or phenylephrine (Neo-Synephrine) may also be used to treat hypotension associated with allergic reaction.

Treatment for anaphylaxis differs from treatment for a mild allergic reaction. If early signs of a mild allergic reaction appear, potentially triggering medications being administered may be discontinued and a dose of diphenhydramine (Benadryl) may be given intravenously. Diphenhydramine (Benadryl, Allergan 50) is an antihistamine; it is used to treat allergic reactions or as an adjunct in treatment of anaphylaxis. Normal dosage is 25 to 50 mg intravenously. If this treatment is effective, surgery may continue, but without the use of the suspected agent. If conservative treatment is not effective, the allergic reaction may quickly progress to anaphylaxis and possible cardiac arrest.

☞ **Note:** Medications that cause the most frequent allergic reactions include penicillin, codeine, contrast media, morphine, meperidine, atracurium, and thiopental.

Transfusion (Hemolytic) Reaction

Blood transfusion reaction is an infrequent, but important, type of intraoperative allergic reaction. Any adverse reaction to the administration of blood or blood products in surgery is a condition treated and managed by the anesthesia provider. Transfusion reactions may be one of three types: febrile nonhemolytic, allergic, or hemolytic. Febrile nonhemolytic reaction is rarely seen during surgery and is usually treated with antipyretic agents, such as acetaminophen. Allergic transfusion reaction is treated as previously discussed. Hemolytic transfusion reaction occurs when ABO type–incompatible blood or blood products are administered (see Chapter 11). Numerous safety precautions are taken during all phases of blood replacement to ensure that the patient receives only compatible blood, but errors can occur. Hemolytic transfusion reaction may be characterized by hypotension, **hemoglobinuria** (hemoglobin in urine), anuria or oliguria, fever, and disseminated intravascular coagulopathy (DIC). Hemolytic transfusion reactions are first treated by discontinuation of blood products, followed by control of hypotension as described previously. Diuretics such as mannitol may be administered to maintain kidney function.

LARYNGOSPASM

Laryngospasm is an involuntary constriction of the vocal cords. It may occur during intubation or shortly after extubation as a reaction to the endotracheal tube. Laryngospasm is seen more frequently in children and infants, and is characterized by a high-pitched crowing sound on inspiration. Positive airway pressure is administered by masked ventilation in an effort to break the spasm. If the spasm does not respond to positive pressure ventilation, and pulse oximetry shows oxygen **desaturation,** a dose of the depolarizing muscle relaxant succinylcholine (Anectine) will be administered intravenously or intramuscularly. (For further discussion of succinylcholine, see Chapter 15.) Succinylcholine is used to relax muscles to allow reintubation, which may be necessary to achieve adequate ventilation and oxygenation.

CARDIAC ARREST

Cardiac arrest may occur at any time before, during, or after an anesthetic. Cardiac arrest may be attributed to several causes. For example, some anesthetic agents can cause cardiac irritability or arrhythmias; in other cases, the patient may have an existing condition, such as cardiac disease, low serum potassium, or hypovolemia that might precipitate a cardiac arrest. Cardiac or respiratory arrest in surgery is usually called a code blue or code 99. When cardiac arrest occurs in other departments of the hospital, an announcement is usually made throughout the hospital over the public address system to notify members of the code blue team (including an emergency physician and designated members of the anesthesia and respiratory care departments) to report to the location of the arrest. Most surgery departments do not announce the code blue to the entire hospital, however, because the surgical team is its own code blue team.

All surgical technologists should be certified in basic cardiac life support at the healthcare provider level by the American Heart Association. Surgical technologists should know exactly what must be done to treat cardiac arrest in the operating room. Cardiac arrest in surgery could occur in any number of possible scenarios, so it is helpful to use critical thinking techniques to analyze each situation. The surgical technologist must be familiar with the roles of various team members and understand the functions performed by each team member during cardiac resuscitation.

Usually, it is the anesthesia provider who makes the diagnosis, officially calls the code blue, and initiates treatment. The ABCDs of cardiopulmonary resuscitation techniques (airway, breathing, circulation, and defibrillation) are followed. The anesthesia provider manages the airway and breathing. If the ET tube has not been placed when the cardiac arrest occurs, an immediate laryngoscopy is performed, the ET tube is placed, and mechanical ventilation is initiated. If the patient has been intubated prior to the arrest, mechanical ventilation continues. Cardiac compressions may be administered by any member of the surgical team trained in cardiopulmonary resuscitation, depending on the situation. For example, if the operation has not yet begun, any member of the team may begin compressions. If the operation is in progress, the surgeon may administer cardiac compressions from the sterile field. Alternately, the circulator may perform cardiac compressions under the sterile drapes. A designated team member calls for, or goes to get, the crash cart, which contains emergency medications and a cardiac defibrillator (Fig. 16–1). The defibrillator is brought into the operating room and prepared for use. Defibrillator paddles are placed on the patient's chest by a physician or registered nurse and used to deliver electric shocks to the patient's heart in an effort to reinstate normal cardiac rhythm. If the thoracic cavity is open, sterile internal defibrillator paddles are opened and placed by the surgeon into direct contact with the heart muscle.

Several factors influence the tasks the surgical technologist performs in resuscitation efforts, including the time of day (how much help is available) and whether or not an incision has been made (need to protect sterility of the surgical site). In addition, the tasks may vary depending on the role the surgical technologist is performing on the surgical team: first scrub, second assistant, first or surgical assistant, or circulator. In the first scrub role, the surgical technologist may remain sterile to cover the wound if necessary, prepare the internal defibrillator paddles for use, or

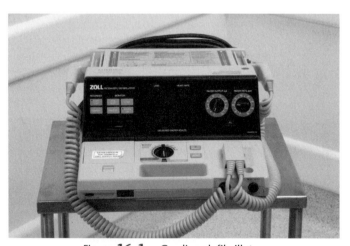

Figure **16–1.** Cardiac defibrillator.

(rarely) prepare to open the chest cavity for open-heart massage. If an additional surgical technologist is scrubbed in as a second assistant, he or she may be asked to break scrub to obtain the crash cart. If necessary, the second assistant may be designated as the official record keeper, documenting all medications given, dosages, and times of events on a special cardiac resuscitation form provided on the crash cart. A surgical technologist in the first or surgical assistant role may perform cardiac compressions, close the surgical incision if needed, or serve as recordkeeper. In the circulating role, the surgical technologist may notify appropriate personnel of the situation, bring in or call for the crash cart, assist the anesthesia provider, perform cardiac compressions, or serve as recordkeeper.

Regardless of the role, it is vital that the surgical technologist be familiar with medications given during a cardiac emergency, their usual dosages, and their purposes. The following is a brief synopsis of drugs frequently used in treatment of a cardiac arrest (Table 16–1).

Epinephrine (Adrenalin) is a hormone (see Chapter 8) that acts as a cardiac stimulant. During cardiac arrest, epinephrine may be administered intravenously in an effort to restore both force and rate of myocardial contractions. Intravenous dosage of epinephrine for cardiac arrest is usually 1 mg **bolus** (depending on patient's weight), which may be repeated every 3 to 5 minutes as needed. Rarely, epinephrine may be administered directly into the cardiac muscle (intra-cardiac injection). An alternate choice instead of epinephrine is vasopressin (Pitressin), which is given in a one-time dose of 40 units intravenously.

☞ **Note:** Epinephrine is also used in nonemergency situations to prolong the duration of local anesthetics (see Chapter 14) or provide limited topical hemostasis.

Table **16–1** Summary of Cardiac Resuscitation Drugs	
Generic Name	*Purpose*
epinephrine	Cardiac stimulant
vasopressin	Cardiac stimulant
lidocaine	Ventricular arrhythmias
procainamide	Ventricular arrhythmias
amiodarone	Ventricular or atrial arrhythmias
magnesium sulfate	Hypomagnesemia
sodium bicarbonate	Metabolic acidosis

Additional medications that may be administered during cardiac arrest include amiodarone (Cordarone), procainamide (Pronestyl), and lidocaine (Xylocaine), anti-arrhythmic agents used in an effort to restore normal cardiac rhythm. Magnesium sulfate (1 to 2 mg bolus intravenously) may be administered to correct hypomagnesemia if present. Sodium bicarbonate is used to treat metabolic acidosis, which is frequently seen in cardiac arrest. Hyperventilation and effective cardiac compressions usually correct acidosis, so sodium bicarbonate is indicated only when blood gas analysis demonstrates significant acidosis. Sodium bicarbonate neutralizes excess hydrogen ion concentration in the blood, thus raising blood pH. When administered during cardiac arrest, the dose of sodium bicarbonate is 1 mEq/kg intravenously, repeated 0.5 mEq/kg every 10 minutes.

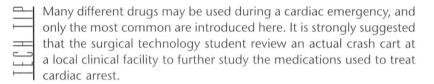

Many different drugs may be used during a cardiac emergency, and only the most common are introduced here. It is strongly suggested that the surgical technology student review an actual crash cart at a local clinical facility to further study the medications used to treat cardiac arrest.

MISCELLANEOUS CARDIOVASCULAR DRUGS

There are a huge number of cardiovascular drugs, only a few of which are of concern to the practice of surgical technology. The surgical patient may be taking various cardiovascular medications to manage chronic heart problems such as angina or congestive heart failure. In addition, some cardiovascular medications may be administered during the course of anesthesia and surgery. These agents are classified in several categories (Insight 16–1), and only the most common agents are discussed in this chapter.

Adrenergic Agonists

Dobutamine (Dobutrex) is a beta-adrenergic agonist and inotropic agent used to treat cardiac failure (medically, for chronic conditions) and hypotension (intraoperatively, for acute situations).

Dopamine (Intropin) is an adrenergic agonist used to increase blood pressure and cardiac output.

Isoproterenol hydrochloride (Isuprel) is a beta-adrenergic agonist administered to increase the rate and force of myocardial contractions. It is also used to treat bradyarrhythmias and serves as a bronchodilator.

Insight 16–1   **Cardiovascular Medications and the Autonomic Nervous System**

The majority of cardiovascular drugs are agonists or antagonists (see Chapter 1). Recall that agonists are drugs that bind to or have an affinity (attraction) for a receptor, causing a particular response. Antagonists, then, are drugs that bind to a receptor and prevent a response, also called receptor blockers. Cardiovascular drugs affect the autonomic nervous system; adrenergic agents affect the sympathetic system and cholinergic agents affect the parasympathetic system. Recall from physiology class that neurotransmitters are the natural chemicals that cause responses in the autonomic nervous system. The sympathetic neurotransmitters are epinephrine and norepinephrine, and the major cholinergic neurotransmitter is acetylcholine. Adrenergic agonists, therefore, are agents that mimic the effect of epinephrine and norepinephrine (sympathomimetics) and cholinergic agonists mimic the effects of acetylcholine (parasympathomimetics). Adrenergic antagonists block the effects of epinephrine and norepinephrine (sympatholytics) and cholinergic antagonists (called anticholinergics) block the effects of acetylcholine (parasympatholytics).

Adrenergic receptors are further divided into alpha-receptors and beta-receptors, and each subtype is divided into two further subtypes: alpha-1 and alpha-2, and beta-1 and beta-2. Alpha-adrenergic receptors respond to norepinephrine and beta-adrenergic receptors respond to epinephrine. An additional type of adrenergic receptor responds to the neurotransmitter dopamine (called dopaminergic receptors).

Adrenergic agonists include the catecholamines epinephrine (alpha-1, beta-1, beta-2), norepinephrine, dopamine, dobutamine, and isoproterenol (beta-1 and beta-2). Other adrenergic agonists are ephedrine, phenylephrine, and methoxamine. Selective beta-2 adrenergic agonists are albuterol and terbutaline, used as bronchodilators.

Adrenergic antagonists (blockers) include the alpha-blocker prazosin (Minipress) used to treat hypertension, the beta-blockers metoprolol (Lopressor) used to treat hypertension, angina, and heart failure and propranolol (Inderal) used to treat hypertension, angina, and arrhythmias, and a nonselective adrenergic antagonist labetalol (Normodyne) used to manage hypertension.

Cholinergic agonists include pilocarpine (used in ophthalmology for miosis and treatment of open-angle glaucoma) and neostigmine (used to reverse nondepolarizing muscle relaxants).

Cholinergic antagonists (anticholinergics) include atropine glycopyrrolate, and scopolamine (preoperative medications; see Chapter 13). Atropine in low doses slows the heart rate, in high doses increases the heart rate by blocking vagus nerve's ability to inhibit the SA and AV nodes of the intrinsic rate mechanism of the heart. Ipratropium (Atrovent) is an anticholinergic used to reverse bronchoconstriction associated with chronic obstructive pulmonary disease (COPD).

In addition to the classification as agonists or antagonists, several other medical terms are used to classify cardiac drugs by their action on the heart. Inotropic agents increase the force of cardiac muscle contractions. Dromotropic agents increase the conductivity of nerve or muscle fibers. Chronotropic agents influence the rate of cardiac contractions.

Phenylephrine (Neo-Synephrine) and methoxamine (Vasoxyl) are alpha-adrenergic agonists used to treat cardiac arrhythmias and to treat hypotension by causing peripheral vasoconstriction.

Norepinephrine bitartrate (Levophed) is a beta-1 agonist and potent peripheral vasoconstrictor used to raise blood pressure, subsequently increasing coronary artery blood flow.

Albuterol (Proventil, Ventolin) and terbutaline (Breathaire, Bicanyl) are beta-adrenergic agonists used to treat bronchospasm.

Adrenergic Antagonists

Labetalol (Normodyne) and atenolol (Tenormin) are beta-adrenergic antagonists, or beta-blockers, that slow the heart rate and are used to treat cardiac arrhythmias and hypertension.

Cholinergic Agents

Cholinergic agonists are not used in the treatment of cardiac conditions, but cholinergic antagonists (anticholinergics) may be used in certain instances. Atropine sulfate is a cholinergic antagonist used to block the effects of the vagus nerve on the sinoatrial (SA) node of the heart. Recall that atropine or a similar drug, glycopyrrolate (Robinul), may be given preoperatively (see Chapter 13) to dry oral secretions (antisialagogue). Blocking the effects of the vagus nerve also prevents **bradycardia** resulting from a stimulus such as stretching the peritoneum or placing traction on eye muscles. If **asystole** (absence of heartbeat) occurs as a response to such actions, cardiac resuscitation is initiated. Additional amounts of atropine may be injected during the resuscitation process.

Antiarrhythmics

Lidocaine (Xylocaine) is a local anesthetic that also has antiarrhythmic effects. As a cardiac antiarrhythmic agent, lidocaine is administered intravenously to treat ventricular arrhythmias such as premature ventricular contractions (PVCs). Lidocaine in a 1% or 2% solution is administered slowly intravenously in doses of 1 mg/kg. This may be repeated 0.5 mg/kg every 2 to 5 minutes as needed. Additional antiarrhythmic agents include amiodarone (Cordarone) and procainamide (Pronestyl) to treat atrial fibrillation, lidocaine-resistant ventricular arrhythmias, and paroxysmal atrial tachycardia (PAT).

Calcium Channel Blockers

Nicardipine (Cardene) and nifedipine (Procardia) are arterial vasodilators used to treat hypertension and stable angina. Verapamil hydrochloride (Isoptin) is a calcium channel blocker also used to treat hypertension and angina, and is helpful in treating tachyarrhythmias.

Vasodilators

Nitroglycerine (Transderm-Nitro, Nitrodisc) and nitroprusside (Nipride) are nitrovasodilators used to treat hypertension, angina, and cardiogenic shock.

Inotropic Agents

Digoxin (Lanoxin) is an inotropic agent used to treat congestive heart failure (CHF), atrial fibrillation and flutter, and paroxysmal atrial tachycardia (PAT). Digoxin is administered intravenously, 0.5 to 1.0 mg in divided doses.

MALIGNANT HYPERTHERMIA

Malignant hyperthermia is a rare but life-threatening reaction triggered in susceptible individuals by administration of certain anesthetic agents. MH is an inherited muscle condition that causes a **hypermetabolic** state in patients exposed to those specific trigger agents. When trigger agents are administered, massive amounts of calcium accumulate in muscle cells causing sustained contractions, glycolysis, and heat production. If untreated, mortality is nearly 80%. Agents known to trigger this disease are succinylcholine (Anectine) and all inhalation anesthetics except nitrous oxide. Although the condition is rare, it is crucial that the surgical technologist understand the signs, treatment, and pharmacology involved in such a crisis in order to provide competent assistance to the anesthesia team.

 CAUTION

Once MH has been triggered, the patient can die in as little as 15 minutes, so prompt diagnosis and treatment are vital.

CLINICAL SIGNS OF MALIGNANT HYPERTHERMIA

Contrary to popular belief, **pyrexia** is *not* an early indicator of MH (Table 16–2). A rise in patient temperature indicates that a full crisis is in effect. The earliest sign presented is an increase in end-tidal carbon dioxide. An increase of even 5 mm Hg could be significant. End-tidal CO_2 can increase for several reasons other than MH; but when other possibilities have been ruled out, the anesthesia provider may begin to alert the operating room staff that potential exists for an MH crisis.

Additional early signs include **tachycardia** and **tachypnea**. These conditions may have other causes, but in combination with the signs described here, tachycardia and tachypnea are classic symptoms of MH. Both tachycardia and tachypnea are means the body uses to eliminate the excess carbon dioxide that is accumulating because of the hypermetabolic crisis. Tachypnea may even override the ventilator setting.

Muscle rigidity, especially masseter muscle rigidity (MMR), can be an early warning of MH; but there are other, benign causes of MMR. Opinions vary on the correlation here; but if MMR is present, the patient should be closely monitored for MH. In combination with signs described previously, MMR is considered a classic sign of MH. In addition, the patient may exhibit an unstable blood pressure, arrhythmias, **cyanosis, diaphoresis**, and a rapid increase in body temperature. Temperatures of higher than 42° C have been reported.

MALIGNANT HYPERTHERMIA TREATMENT PROTOCOL

Once MH has been identified, the surgical procedure is stopped if possible and all triggering agents are discontinued. The patient is

Table **16–2**   Clinical Signs of Malignant Hyperthermia
Increase in end-tidal CO_2
Tachycardia
Tachypnea
Masseter muscle rigidity (MMR)
Unstable blood pressure
Arrhythmias
Cyanosis
Diaphoresis
Pyrexia

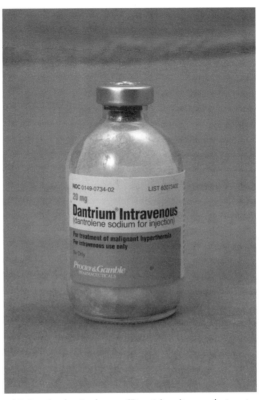

Figure **16–2.** Vial of dantrolene (Dantrium) used to treat malignant hyperthermia.

hyperventilated with 100% oxygen to help eliminate the excess CO_2 that accumulates in the blood. Ventilator circuit tubing is changed to prevent exposure to residual inhalation agents. Dantrolene sodium (Dantrium), a skeletal muscle relaxant developed specifically to treat MH, is administered intravenously (Fig. 16–2). Initial dosage is a bolus of 2.5 mg/kg. Dantrolene is packaged, freeze-dried, in vials of 20 mg with 3 g of mannitol, and must be reconstituted with 60 mL of sterile water. In an adult patient weighing 80 kg (176 lb), 200 mg of dantrolene (10 vials) is required to begin treatment. Dosages may reach 10 mg/kg, so in this case 800 mg (40 vials) of dantrolene may need to be reconstituted. If appropriate, the scrubbed surgical technologist may break scrub to help reconstitute the dantrolene. Once sterile water has been injected into the vial, the mixture must be shaken vigorously until the solution becomes clear yellow, indicating complete reconstitution. Dantrolene may be repeated in a dose of

2 mg/kg every 5 minutes, then 1 to 2 mg/kg/hr, and is administered until symptoms disappear. MH may also be seen in children, so the number of vials reconstituted is adjusted accordingly by patient weight. Sodium bicarbonate is given intravenously in doses of 1 to 2 mEq/kg to treat the metabolic acidosis resulting from high concentrations of lactate in the blood. Blood gasses are monitored frequently. The patient must be rapidly cooled to prevent brain damage. Ice packs are applied to groin, neck, and axilla in an effort to lower the temperature. Iced lavage of stomach, rectum, or bladder may be performed to cool the patient's core temperature. Diuretics such as 20% mannitol (Osmitrol) or furosemide (Lasix) are given intravenously to keep the kidneys functioning properly. Muscle cells are destroyed during an MH crisis, and the myoglobin that is released in this process tends to accumulate in the kidneys, obstructing flow. Procainamide or lidocaine is given intravenously to treat arrhythmias secondary to electrolyte imbalances. Procainamide (Procan SR, Pronestyl) and lidocaine (Xylocaine) are antiarrhythmic agents used to control cardiac arrhythmias seen in MH. Glucose and insulin are administered to treat hyperkalemia, frequently seen because potassium (K^+) is released as muscle cells are destroyed. All these treatment steps are taken virtually simultaneously and are arranged to help remember key points. All patient vital functions are monitored closely to determine response to treatment. **Capnography** is crucial, as are arterial lines, frequent blood gas assessment, and accurate temperature measurement. A Foley catheter should be in place to measure urine output. Basic treatment steps for an MH crisis are summarized in Table 16 3. For additional information, visit the Malignant Hyperthermia Association of the United States website: http://www.mhaus.org.

A 24-hour hotline staffed by volunteer physicians has been established to assist with information to treat an MH crisis:
1-800-MH HYPER (1-800-644-9737)

Table **16–3** Malignant Hyperthermia Treatment Steps

Hyperventilate—with 100% oxygen
Dantrolene—administer 2.5 to 10 mg/kg intravenously
Sodium bicarbonate—administer intravenously to treat metabolic acidosis
Temperature management—ice packs and lavage
Diuretics—administer mannitol or furosemide intravenously
Insulin—treat hyperkalemia

Treatment can be considered successful when vital signs and blood gases return to within normal limits. Elective surgery is discontinued. Life-threatening surgery is resumed, but with different anesthetic agents and a different anesthesia machine to prevent residual inhalation agent from triggering a second crisis. On cancellation or completion of the surgical procedure, the patient is transported to the intensive care unit (ICU) or PACU accompanied with the replenished MH cart, because another episode could yet occur. Always consult and follow individual institution policies covering an MH crisis. The surgical technologist should become familiar with all institutional policies covering any emergency situation, including MH. In addition, the surgical technologist should be familiar with signs, treatment, and pharmacology of MH.

KEY CONCEPTS

- A number of emergency situations arise associated with anesthesia, including respiratory conditions, cardiac arrest, and MH.
- Although not common in surgery, these situations merit careful study and continuing education. As an allied health professional, the surgical technologist must attain and maintain the proficiency required to function effectively in these emergency situations.
- Drugs used to treat cardiac arrest include epinephrine, vasopressin, amiodarone, lidocaine, procainamide, magnesium sulfate, and sodium bicarbonate.
- Numerous miscellaneous cardiovascular drugs are also administered in surgery to treat various conditions.
- MH is a hypermetabolic crisis triggered by some anesthetic agents. Signs of an MH crisis include tachycardia, tachypnea, masseter muscle rigidity, unstable blood pressure, arrhythmias, cyanosis, diaphoresis, and pyrexia. Basic treatment steps for MH include hyperventilation with 100% oxygen, intravenous injection of dantrolene and sodium bicarbonate, temperature management, and administration of diuretics.

Index

Note: Page numbers in *italics* refer to illustrations; page numbers followed by t refer to tables.